AF879442

Implementing Hemodialysis in the Home:

A Practical Manual

Edited by

Mark R. Marshall, MD

Faculty of Medical and Health Sciences, University of Auckland, Auckland, New Zealand;
Department of Renal Medicine, Counties Manukau District Health Board, Auckland, New Zealand.

Christopher T. Chan, MD

Division of Nephrology, University Health Network, Toronto, Ontario, Canada

on behalf of the Global Forum for Home Hemodialysis

iSHD
International Society for Hemodialysis

International Society for Hemodialysis
Indianapolis, IN

First Edition

Copyright © 2016 International Society for Hemodialysis

All rights reserved. This book is protected by copyright. No part of this book may be reproduced or transmitted in any form or by any means, including as photocopies or scanned-in or other electronic copies, or utilized by any information storage and retrieval system without written permission from the copyright owner, except for brief quotations embodied in critical articles and reviews. Materials appearing in this book prepared by individuals as part of their official duties as U.S. government employees are not covered by the above- mentioned copyright.
To request permission, please contact International Society for Hemodialysis at 911 East 86th Street, Suite 202, Indianapolis, IN, 46240, via email at info@ishd.org, or via our website at ishd.org.

9 8 7 6 5 4 3 2 1

Supported by an unrestricted educational grant from Baxter Healthcare. This content is also available as a 2015 supplement in ***Hemodialysis International***, at this weblink: http://onlinelibrary.wiley.com/doi/10.1111/hdi.2015.19.issue-s1/issuetoc

The editorial and management support as well as graphic design contributions, of JB Ashtin are gratefully acknowledged.

Cover art: Shutterstock, Denphumi

Cover design and interior page design adaptation for printing: Aleksandra Godlevska and Oleksiy Serdyuk

DISCLAIMER: Care has been taken to confirm the accuracy of the information presented and to describe generally accepted practices. However, the author(s), editors, and publisher are not responsible for errors or omissions or for any consequences from application of the information in this book and make no warranty, expressed or implied, with respect to the currency, completeness, or accuracy of the contents of the publication. Application of this information in a particular situation remains the professional responsibility of the practitioner; the clinical treatments described and recommended may not be considered absolute and universal recommendations.

The author(s), editors, and publisher have exerted every effort to ensure that drug selection and dosage set forth in this text are in accordance with the current recommendations and practice at the time of publication. However, in view of ongoing research, changes in government regulations, and the constant flow of information relating to drug therapy and drug reactions, the reader is urged to check the package insert for each drug for any change in indications and dosage and for added warnings and precautions. This is particularly important when the recommended agent is a new or infrequently employed drug.

Some drugs and medical devices presented in this publication have Food and Drug Administration (FDA) clearance for limited use in restricted research settings. It is the responsibility of the health care provider to ascertain the FDA status of each drug or device planned for use in his or her clinical practice.

ISHD.org

Acknowledgements

The Global Forum for Home Hemodialysis is endorsed by the International Society for Hemodialysis, and sponsored by an unrestricted grant from Baxter Healthcare Corporation. We would like to acknowledge the following people for their contributions to the website, which range from project initiation and vision to content feedback and peer review.

Markku Asola, MD

Medical Director, EMEA, Home Hemodialysis Baxter Healthcare Corporation

Dervla Connaughton, LRCP&SI, MB, MCh, BAR (Hons)

Nephrology Beaumont Hospital, Dublin

Cormac Breen, FRCP

Consultant Nephrologist Guy's and St Thomas' NHS Foundation Trust

Michelle Carver, BSN, RN, CNN

Senior Director Clinical Services Home Dialysis Plus

Bruce Culleton, MD, FRCPC, MBA

Vice President, Renal Therapeutic Area Baxter Healthcare Corporation

Richard Fluck, MBBS, FRCP, MA (Cantab)

Consultant Renal Physician Royal Derby Hospital

National Clinical Director (Renal) National Health Service, England

Michelle Hladunewich, MD, MSc, FRCP(C)

Associate Professor of Medicine University of Toronto Director, Nephrology and Obstetrics Sunnybrook Health Sciences Center

Eero Honkanen, MD, PhD

Associate Professor, Chief Physician Helsinki University Central Hospital, Division of Nephrology

Daljit Hothi, MD, MBBS, MRCPCH

Consultant Pediatric Nephrologist Clinical lead for home hemodialysis Great Ormond Street and Portland Hospitals London, UK

Anu Jayanti, MBBS, MRCP, MSc, CCT

Renal Research Fellow Manchester Royal Infirmary Manchester, UK

Peter G. Kerr, MBBS, PhD, FRACP

Director of Nephrology Monash Medical Centre

Victoria A. Kumar, MD

Internal Medicine, Nephrology Kaiser Permanente, Los Angeles Medical Center

Hoyee Leong, PhD

Associate Director, Global Medical Affairs, Home Hemodialysis Baxter Healthcare Corporation

John Moran, MBBS, FRACP, FACP

Chief Medical Officer ProMetic Life Sciences, Inc.

Ercan Ok, MD

Ege University School of Medicine Department of Internal Medicine Division of Nephrology

Virpi Rauta, MD, PhD, EMBA

Nephrologist in charge of Home Hemodialysis and Dialysis Training Department Helsinki University Central Hospital Richard Ward, PhD (retired) Professor of Medicine, University of Louisville, KY.

Contributing Authors

John Agar, MBBS, FRACP, FRCP

Conjoint Professor of Medicine, Deakin University School of Medicine and the University Hospital, Barwon Health, Geelong, Victoria, Australia.

Paul Bennett, BN, MHSM, PhD

Foundation Chair and Professor in Translational Nursing at Western Health-Deakin University Partnership in Melbourne, Australia.

Christopher Blagg, MD, FRCP

Executive Director Emeritus of the Northwest Kidney Centers (Seattle) and Professor Emeritus of Medicine in the Division of Nephrology at the University of Washington, Seattle, WA.

Christopher T. Chan, MD FRCPC

Professor of Medicine, University of Toronto
Director - Division of Nephrology - University Health Network, Toronto, Ontario, Canada.

Calli Cleland, RN, BHS

Associate clinical charge nurse in the Home Haemodialysis & Satellite Dialysis Unit, Counties Manukau District Health Board, working through Middlemore Hospital in Auckland, New Zealand.

Tom Cornelis, MD

Staff nephrologist in the Division of Nephrology of the Maastricht University Medical Centre, Maastricht, Netherlands .

Cheryl Cress, RN, CNN

Clinical Nurse Coordinator, Home Modalities, at Barnes-Jewish Dialysis Center, St. Louis, Missouri.

Deborah Eastwood, MSc

General Manager, Medicine and Health of Older People, North Shore and Waitakere Hospitals, Auckland, New Zealand.

Rose Faratro, RN, BHScN, CNephr(C)

Home hemodialysis nurse at University Health Network, Toronto General Hospital, Toronto, Canada.

Sally Fox, RGoNComp, PGCert

Renal Nurse Manager (Home Therapies and Community) for the Counties Manukau District Health Board (CMDHB), Middlemore Hospital, in Manukau City, New Zealand.

Tony Goovaerts, RN

Nurse manager, Brussels Saint-Luc University Hospital Home Hemodialysis Program, Peritoneal Dialysis Program, Self-care Satellite Unit, and the Pretreatment Counseling Program, Brussels, Belgium.

Raymond Hakim, MD

Attending physician at Vanderbilt University Medical Center, Division of Nephrology.

James Heaf, MD, DMSc

Director, Limited Care Dialysis Department at Herlev Hospital, University of Copenhagen, Copenhagen, Denmark.

Aaron Herold, MSW, LICSW

Director of Transition Care Services and Operations Support for Northwest Kidney Centers, Seattle, WA.

Kirsten Howard, MPH, MHlthEc, PhD

Professor of health economics in the Sydney School of Public Health at the University of Sydney, Australia.

Jane Jeffries, RN, MNS

Nurse unit manager of the Home Training Haemodialysis Unit, Princess Alexandria Hospital, Brisbane, Australia.

Robert S. Lockridge, Jr., MD

Now retired. Previously, clinical nephrologist in private practice with Lynchburg Nephrology and medical director of the University of Virginia's Home Dialysis program.

Jennifer MacRae, MD, MSc, FRCP

Associate Professor of Medicine, Division of Nephrology, University of Calgary, Calgary, Canada.

Mark Marshall, MBChB, MPH

Faculty of Medical and Health Sciences, University of Auckland, Auckland, New Zealand, and Department of Renal Medicine, Counties Manukau District Health Board, Auckland, New Zealand; Baxter Healthcare, Asia.

Ikuto Masakane, MD, PhD

Deputy Director of Yabuki Hospital in Yamagata, Japan.

Phil McFarlane, MD, PhD, FRCP(C)

Assistant Professor, Department of Medicine, University of Toronto; Medical director, Toronto Hospital's Home Dialysis Program, and medical codirector of the Multidisciplinary Diabetes Complications Clinic.

David Mendelssohn, MD, FRCP(C)

Professor of Medicine, University of Toronto, Toronto, Canada.

Sandip Mitra, MBBS, MD, FRCP

Consultant nephrologist at Central Manchester University Hospitals Foundation Trust; Clinical and governance lead for hemodialysis in the renal network; Senior Lecturer at the University of Manchester (Cardiovascular Sciences), Manchester, UK.

Rachel L. Morton, MSc, PhD

Senior research fellow in the Sydney Medical School, University of Sydney, Australia; and Academic Visitor at the Health Economics Research Centre, University of Oxford, UK.

Gihad Nesrallah, MD, MSc, FRCP(C)

Medical Director of Hemodialysis and the Chief of the Nephrology Program at Humber River Hospital in Toronto, Canada.

Robert P. Pauly, MD, MSc, FRCP(C)

Associate Professor of Medicine in the Division of Nephrology at the University of Alberta and Medical Director of the Northern Alberta Home Hemodialysis Program.

Anthony Perkins, RN

Clinical Nurse Specialist working in the Home Dialysis Unit at Barwon Health in Geelong, Victoria, Australia.

Jean-Philippe Rioux, MD

Director, nocturnal home hemodialysis program, Montr é al, Québec, Canada; Assistant Professor of Medicine at the University of Montréal.

Dorian R. Schatell, MS

Executive Director, Medical Education Institute, Madison, WI.

Kamal D. Shah

Director, Patient Services, at NephroPlus Dialysis Centers, Hyderabad, India.

Rosie Simmonds, RN, MN

Clinical Coordinator of the Home & Satellite Haemodialysis Training Unit at Barwon Health, University Hospital, Geelong, Australia.

Carolyn van Eps, MBBS, PhD, FRACP

Staff nephrologist at Princess Alexandra Hospital, Brisbane, Queensland, Australia. Director of the Home Training Haemodialysis Unit and the Ipswich Renal Dialysis Unit.

Rachel Walker, BN, RN, MN

Renal Nurse Practitioner, New Zealand; PhD student at the University of Sydney, Australia.

Robert J. Walker, MD, FRACP, FAHA. Professor and Chair of Medicine, University of Otago, New Zealand; Clinical Leader for the Southern District Health Board Nephrology Services; Director of "The Kidney in Health and Disease Research Group" based at the University of Otago.

Bessie Young, MD, MPH, FACP

Associate professor of nephrology at the University of Washington and staff nephrologist at the Veterans' Administration Puget Sound Health Care System in Seattle, WA.

PREFACE

There is renewed interest in home hemodialysis (HD), which has been fueled by encouraging clinical outcomes from observational and randomized controlled data in the forms of frequent HD. However, given its benefits, home HD is relatively underutilized throughout the world. With all the positive data and the great strides made in the treatment modality, why wouldn't a patient select home HD as his or her preferred method of dialysis treatment? Most data reflect that among patients, physicians, and care providers, there is a considerable lack of knowledge about home HD and its proven attributes. To encourage international uptake of home HD, it is obvious that a pragmatic solution is needed.

The Global Forum for Home Hemodialysis, an independent panel comprised of internationally recognized nephrologists, home HD nurses, administrators, patient advocates, and a long-time home HD patient, has convened with the intention of creating an open-source, comprehensive, practical manual that provides useful information to clinicians who are interested in implementing home HD.

The content of this manual was written by noted experts in the field, has undergone peer-review to ensure the highest scholarship, and presents an in-depth overview of the latest practice patterns available. These best practices, which are focused on patient- and provider-related pathways, are denoted in 10 modules that are available through an open-source web resource (www.ishd.org) and are also published in a 2015 supplement of the ISHD's journal, *Hemodialysis International*. In the future, the unique web-based manual will include additional modules and will be updated as new information about home HD becomes available. We are indebted to all contributors for their expertise.

Great advances have been made since the first home HD machine, which was made in only 3 months by the team of Drs. Scribner and Babb. As the evolution of renal replacement technology and practice pattern continues, the niche for home HD will likely become more dominant. Today, patients are more informed about their health and are taking a more active role in their treatment, and clinicians want to provide their patients with therapies that are the most effective and offer improved quality of life. It is our hope that more nephrologists and allied health professionals will continue to see the value of home HD and that a more sizable proportion of patients with end-stage renal disease will benefit from the appropriate utilization of home HD as a treatment of choice.

Disclosure: The Global Forum for Home Hemodialysis is endorsed by the International Society for Hemodialysis, and sponsored by an unrestricted grant from Baxter International, Inc.

Mark Marshall and Christopher Chan,
on behalf of The Global Forum for Home Hemodialysis

CONTENTS

Home Hemodialysis Needs You!

Authors and Affiliations:

John W M Agar, MBBS, FRACP, FRCP[1]

Dori R Schatell, MS[2]

Rachael Walker, BN, RN, MN[3]

[1]Renal Unit, University Hospital, Barwon Health, Geelong, Victoria, Australia; [2]Medical Education Institute, Inc., Madison, WI, USA; [3]Renal Department, Hawke's Bay District Health Board, Hastings, New Zealand

Introduction

Three words, "Yes, we can," were used with great effect by Barack Obama in his 2008 campaign for the American presidency. These words came to epitomize the hopes of a new generation yearning for a better way. While some may question whether those political goals have been achieved, what cannot be argued is the optimism and enthusiasm that this short phrase embodied.

The same three words "Yes, we can" also aptly apply to the provision of hemodialysis (HD) in the home; however, in this case, "yes we can" has truly become "yes, we are." For those unfamiliar with home HD or those who are unsure how to begin, this website will show you that "you can, too."

Home Hemodialysis Uptake

Despite demonstrated benefits to patients, many dialysis professionals still seem reluctant to tread a home dialysis path. In the United States, the growth of home modalities has been hindered by a system that until recently has not promoted home options to patients.[1]

Despite the early success and implementation of home HD, use of this modality in that country declined rapidly in the years that followed the passage of the Social Security Act of 1972, legislation that favored facility HD rather than home-based care.[2] Meanwhile, in other countries, such as Australia and New Zealand, legislation and funding structures developed in a way to favor home-based care instead.

The days of home HD underutilization may be coming to an end in the United States, as evidenced by the growing concerted effort of clinicians to encourage home modalities and, in particular, by working HD patients who want to maintain their employment status.

Unfortunately, the 30-year hiatus in expertise and familiarity with home modalities created by the predominance of the for-profit model has left a deep chasm in physician knowledge about and acceptance of home HD.

While governments are now realizing the dual outcome advantages of home dialysis—better clinical outcomes at lower cost to the overall health system—physician inertia now seems to be the most important remaining challenge to overcome.[1,3]

Such inertia is largely bred from unfamiliarity, as many physicians receive training that does not require experience with home HD. The unfortunate result is a lack of knowledge among physicians on how to establish home HD programs and how to adequately manage home HD training and care.

In Australia and New Zealand, all nephrology trainees have long been required to fully train in both home peritoneal dialysis and home HD.[4] Perhaps as a result, home modalities comprise more than one-third of all dialysis patients in these 2 countries, while home HD sustains 11% (Australia) and 18% (New Zealand) of all dialysis patients.[5]

Conversely, in the United States, many trainees have not been exposed to any home dialysis training. In a national survey of US nephrologists, 38% reported that they did not even feel well enough prepared to care for in-center HD patients despite success in their certification examinations, let alone care for home HD patients. Of note, however, only 6% said they would choose standard in-center HD for themselves if their kidneys failed, assuming they had to wait 5 years for a transplant.[6]

It stands to reason that if we do not train, and trainees are not exposed to home-based treatment, then it is unlikely that many clinicians will later prescribe these modalities or establish a home dialysis program. This fact, coupled with the inevitable distortions created by complex reimbursement and financial disincentives, may contribute to the extremely low uptake of home HD in the United States, which at most recent estimate was just 1.3%.[7]

Fortunately, the American Society of Nephrology recently moved to mandate a home dialysis curriculum for all trainees, with similar requirements proposed for dialysis nurses. Times are truly changing.

Educating Patients On Modality Options

What is certain is that we, the professionals who lead and inform, must accept responsibility for informing our patients of home dialysis alternatives, rather than hiding behind the easy option of center-only treatment. Growing home HD first needs YOU—the clinician—to engage with home care, and to then engage your patients.

Your patients won't "go home" unless you lead them there, and it is not primarily their fear, but their lack of awareness, that holds them back from choosing home HD.

Although the authors acknowledge that not all patients are clinically appropriate for home dialysis, dialysis providers in Australia and New Zealand have achieved a prevalence of home HD that is several-fold higher than that of the United States and many other countries.

Indeed, some clinicians in Australia and New Zealand manage more than 50% of their dialysis population on HD and peritoneal dialysis at home. Others consistently sustain >25% to 30% of all HD as home treatment.[8]

In Australia and New Zealand, dialysis decisions are commonly led, influenced, and encouraged by home–savvy clinicians who understand the benefits for patient outcomes and provider cost containment—both are part of the home equation. Further, binational survival data underpin and encourage this approach.[9]

It is not unethical to "lead" patients to choose a dialysis modality. It is essential that nephrology professionals provide expert guidance. If clinically and socially suited and provided the opportunity, many patients prefer self-care at home—as did more than 90% of both Scottish[10] and American[6] nephrologists when asked where they would prefer to dialyze. Yet, most physicians currently send the great majority of their patients to facility care that they would not accept for themselves.

While we must be careful not to send patients home who are unsuitable, this website will help you determine between those who can and cannot manage at home. Consider this: at your next regular predialysis group or one-on-one education session—you do run one, don't you?—ask your patients one simple question, "Do you drive?" Driving requires a number of key cognitive attributes: conceptualization; problem-solving; multitasking; decisions at speed; rapid responses; adequate vision and manual dexterity; and, above all, confidence, self-belief, and bravery.

These same attributes indicate that a patient is also a potential candidate for home dialysis, until proven otherwise. In addition, "driving" a home dialysis system is arguably both easier and safer than driving a car.

Creating and Expanding Home HD Programs

Many good, reliable websites have described successful programs. Among these are a basic but informative Australian website (http://www.nocturnaldialysis.org) that provides useful patient-oriented material,[11] and the US-based Home Dialysis Central (www.homedialysis.org), a not-for-profit website brimming with useful information for both patients and professionals.[12]

But among the best home advocates of all are the home HD patients themselves. They are uniquely passionate about their home care—harness their passion. Think about it: Can you name a single facility patient of yours who shows a passion for in-center care? Resignation, perhaps, but rarely passion.

The website describes, in detail, the prerequisites for successful home HD, and we hope you will read it in its entirety. Meanwhile, the following simplistic guide for patient recruitment encapsulates 6 key essentials that combine to deliver a successful program:

1. Find, educate, or become a "champion".

2. Consider forming a partnership with an experienced home HD program to assist with planning, funding, building, and staffing issues and to provide advice if or where problems might arise.

3. Invite a ready-made expert—a home dialysis professional, or better still, an experienced home HD patient—to speak at your program's education days.

4. Identify your potential home HD patients using the module in this website titled "Patient Selection and Training for Home Hemodialysis", or use the MATCH-D tool,[13] or the Renal Association's NICE Guidelines on selection of patients for home dialysis.[14]

5. Educate patients about the data supporting home HD: reduced dietary and fluid restrictions; reengagement with society, friends, and the community; return to work; and associated improved survival.

6. Provide copies of Help, I need Dialysis!,[15] and encourage the use of the My Life, My Dialysis Choice,[16] or the My Kidneys, My Choice[17] decision aids that are designed to help each patient match his or her desired lifestyle to a dialysis option

For any who still doubt the effectiveness of home HD; for any who may be uncertain about how to choose suitable patients, or to know who might benefit; for any who fear potential clinical, ethical, or legal traps and pitfalls; for any who are unfamiliar with the infrastructure, water, and machine requirements for successful support in the home; for those uncertain about funding or costs; for any concerned about misadventure or mishaps at home and, if or when they do uncommonly occur, how these should be handled—this website addresses these questions and details how others have overcome the challenges that home HD can present.

As the future affordability of all dialysis and an improved trajectory toward more optimal dialysis is now increasingly linked to home-based care, this website will show you where to start. We challenge you to start to believe that "Yes, you can," too.

References

1. Mehrotra R, Marsh D, Vonesh E, Peters V, Nissenson A. Patient education and access of ESRD patients to renal replacement therapies beyond in-center hemodialysis. Kidney Int. 2005;68:378-390.

2. Rettig RA. Origins of the Medicare Kidney Disease Entitlement: The Social Security Amendments of 1972. In: Hanna KE, ed. Biomedical Politics. Washington, DC: Division of Health Sciences Policy: Committee to Study Biomedical Decision Making, Institute of Medicine. 1991;176-214. Available from: http://www.nap.edu (accessed date: January 27, 2016).

3. Agar JWM. Home hemodialysis: A glass half-full. Nephrol News Issues. 2013;27:22.

4. Royal Australasian College of Physicians. Advanced Training in Nephrology. Available from: http://www.racp.edu.au/... (accessed date: January 27, 2016).

5. Polkinghorne K, Briggs N, Khanal N, Hurst K, Clayton P. The Australia and New Zealand Dialysis and Transplant Registry. Chapter 5: Haemodialysis (including home haemodialysis). 36th Annual Report. Adelaide: Australia, 2013. Available from: http://www.anzdata.org.au/... (accessed date: January 27, 2016).

6. Merighi JR, Schatell DR, Bragg-Gresham JL, Witten B, Mehrotra R. Insights into nephrologists, clinical practice, and dialysis choice. Hemodial Int. 2012; 16:242-251.

7. USRDS Annual Data Report. International Comparisons. Am J Kidney Dis. 2014;63(Suppl 1):e333-e334.

8. Fortnum D, Ludlow M, Morton RL. Renal unit characteristics and patient education practices that predict a high prevalence of home-based dialysis in Australia. Nephrology (Carlton). 2014; 19:587-593.

9. Marshall MR, Hawley CM, Kerr PG, et al. The effect of home haemodialysis on mortality risk in Australian and New Zealand populations. Am J Kidney Dis. 2011;58:782-793.

10. McManus SK, Mactier RA. Scottish nephrologists' dialysis preferences: exposing the gap between what we offer and what we would choose [abstract]. The Scottish Renal Association, 2009 Autumn. Abstract.

11. Agar JWM. Nocturnal Home Haemodialysis. 2012. Available from: http://www.nocturnaldialysis.org .

12. Medical Education Institute, Inc. Home Dialysis Central. 2014. Available from: http://www.homedialysiscentral.org.

13. Schatell DR, Witten B, et al. Method to assess treatment choices for home dialysis (MATCH-D). Madison, WI: Medical Education Institute, Inc. 2013. Available from: http://homedialysis.org/match-d.

14. Mactier R, Hoenich N, Breen C. The Renal Association Home Haemodialysis Guidelines (9.1-9.3). 2009. Available from: http://www.renal.org.

15. Schatell DR, Agar JWM. Help, I Need Dialysis. 2012. Available from: http://lifeoptions.org/help_book.

16. Schatell DR, Witten B, Agar JWM. My Life, My Dialysis Choice. 2014. Available from: http://mydialysischoice.org.

17. Fortnum D (for Kidney Health Australia). My Kidneys, My Choice. 2013. Available from: http://homedialysis.org.au/.

1 The Home Hemodialysis Hub: Physical Infrastructure and Integrated Governance Structure

Mark R Marshall, MBCHB, MPH, FRACP[1,2]
Bessie A Young, MD, MPH, FACP, FASN[3]
Sally J Fox, RGoNComp, PGCert[2]
Calli J Cleland, RN, BHS[2]
Robert J Walker, MBChB, MD, FRACP, FASN, FAHA[4]
Ikuto Masakane, MD, PhD[5]
Aaron M Herold, MSW, LICSW[6]

[1]Faculty of Medical and Health Sciences, University of Auckland, Auckland, New Zealand; [2]Department of Renal Medicine, Counties Manukau District Health Board, Auckland, New Zealand; [3]Veterans Affairs Puget Sound Health Care System, Kidney Research Institute, Division of Nephrology, University of Washington, Seattle, Washington, USA; [4]Department of Medicine, Dunedin School of Medicine, University of Otago, Dunedin, New Zealand; [5]Kidney and Dialysis Center, Yabuki Hospital, Yamagata City, Japan; [6]Operations Support, Administration, Northwest Kidney Centers, Seattle, Washington, USA

Implementing Hemodialysis in the Home
A Global Perspective

iSHD
International Society for Hemodialysis

CONTENTS

Abstract

An effective home hemodialysis program critically depends on adequate hub facilities and support functions and on transparent and accountable organizational processes. The likelihood of optimal service delivery and patient care will be enhanced by fit-for-purpose facilities and implementation of a well-considered governance structure. In this module, we describe the required accommodation and infrastructure for a home hemodialysis program and a generic organizational structure that will support both patient-facing clinical activities and business processes.

Introduction

A well-functioning home hemodialysis (HD) training facility is critical for the success of a program. These facilities often have wider functions than just those of home HD training, however, and need to be resourced appropriately. Most support the entire patient journey from inception into the program to eventual exit, as illustrated in Figure 1.[1] It is important to realize that this journey extends to prospective patients who are not yet receiving home HD, who should be presented with the opportunity to tour training facilities, meet home HD patients, and get to know the staff and program. For this reason, the term "home HD hub" is preferable to "home HD training facility," and better reflects its broader functionality. The hub should, therefore, have appropriate physical infrastructure and organizational structure to support optimal clinical governance and effective operations management. Inadequate facilities and support functions will inevitably lead to patients experiencing problems and delays, and having poorer outcomes and overall experiences.

In this module, we describe the required accommodation and infrastructure for a home HD program, and provide a generic organizational structure that will support both patient-facing clinical activities and business processes. However, a defining feature of successful home HD programs is the adaptability and cross-functional skill sets of staff. It is not unusual or inappropriate for 1 person to have several roles that cross the clinical-business divide; for instance, home HD clinical staff often have business functions (eg, organizing equipment, managing supply inventory, and performing troubleshooting activities), and managers are often heavily involved with clinical governance implementation (eg, patient safety programs). This is not a shortcoming, so long as everyone has clear roles and responsibilities within the program—roles should have defined accountability and performance measures (the "what"), accepting that people may fill several different roles, especially in smaller programs (the "who"). When all parties understand and accept "who" does "what," the program and the care it delivers should not be compromised.

The size and complexity of the home HD hub will depend on the number of patients in the program and whether it aims to grow. In Japan, most home HD programs are small and located within

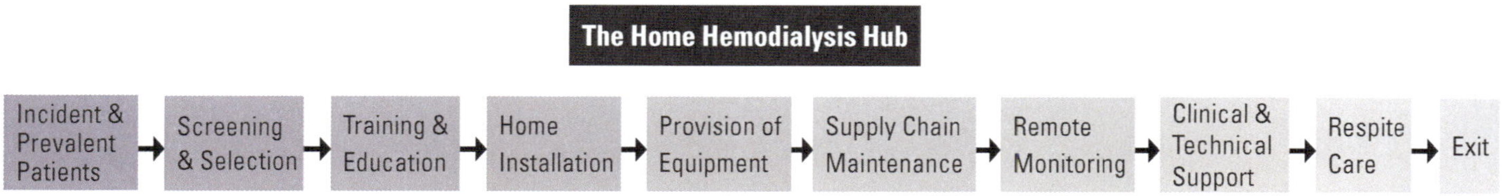

Figure 1. The home hemodialysis resource map. Adapted from Alhomayeed B, Lindsay RM. Saudi J Kidney Dis Transpl. 2009; 20:185–191.[1]

hospital HD facilities,[2] while in Australia and New Zealand, home HD programs are larger and, in most cases, enabled by specialized facilities and personnel (Figure 2).[3] In general, a program can be started and managed with modest infrastructure and simple operating mechanisms (ie, existing hospital infrastructure and personnel). When the program expands beyond 10 to 20 patients, more substantial, specialized physical and human resources are required.

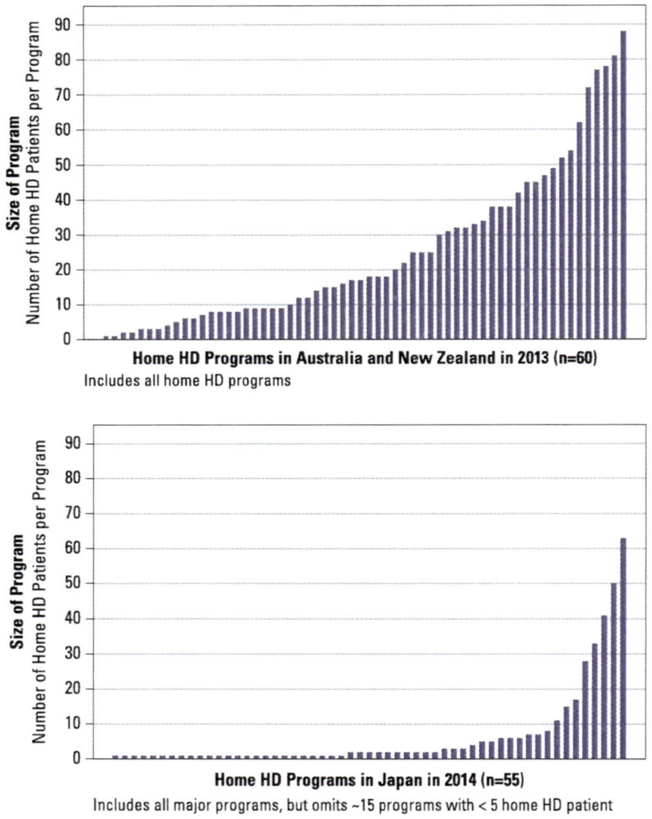

Figure 2. Size of Home HD Programs in Australia and New Zealand and Japan.[2,3]

Infrastructure

There a several key characteristics to consider for a home HD hub: its location, the number and type of training stations, and its physical and functional configuration.

Facility Location

The location of the home HD hub should be carefully considered to optimize accessibility for patients. Accessibility is defined not only by traveling distances but also by available options for patient parking and proximity to local transport. Ideally, the location for the home HD hub should have the potential for infrastructure expansion, should there be future growth of the program.

Home HD training is a core function of the hub—it can occur in a variety of settings, and there are no clear data that support the superiority of 1 setting over another. There are 4 main options for the location of home HD training, some of which are designed to allow functional integration of the hub with other dialysis services: (i) adjacent to or within hospital dialysis facilities, (ii) adjacent to or within community-based satellite dialysis facilities, (iii) a stand-alone facility, and (iv) the patient's home.[4–6] In our opinion, most locations are acceptable, although the advantages and disadvantages of each setting should be noted. A comparison of the various options for the location of the home HD hub is provided in Table 1.[6] Although less common than in-center training, the option of performing home HD training in the patient's home is an interesting one and should not be discounted. Training in the home removes options for cross-cover between trainers during training sessions and increases inefficiencies and duplication for shared tasks (eg, data management and stock management). Home training may be a financially feasible option for smaller or new programs—overall program costs are reduced by avoiding

Table 1. Comparison of Locations for Home HD Hub or Training

Considerations		Hospital	Satellite Site	Stand-Alone Site	Home
Clinical Considerations	Nephrologist on site	✓✓✓	✓✓	✓✓	–
	Allied health on site	✓✓✓	✓✓	✓✓	✓
	Laboratory on site	✓✓✓	–	–	–
	Access to specialist nurses (eg, vascular access, transplant nurses)	✓✓✓	✓✓	✓✓	✓
	Access to electronic medical records	✓✓✓	✓✓✓	✓✓	✓
	Visibility and promotion of home HD training to facility HD patients	✓✓✓	✓✓	–	–
	Staff access to facility HD patients for cultivation or assessment for home HD	✓✓✓	✓✓✓	–	–
	Options to commence preemptive home HD training	✓	✓	✓	✓✓✓
	Options for respite care of home HD patients	✓✓✓	✓✓✓	–	–
Patient-Centered Considerations	Promotion of a culture of self-management	✓	✓✓	✓✓	✓✓✓
	Flexibility of training times	✓✓	✓✓	✓✓	✓✓✓
	Proximity to home	✓	✓✓	✓✓	✓✓✓
	Safety and security	✓✓✓	✓✓	✓✓	✓✓✓
	Homelike environment	✓	✓	✓✓	✓✓✓
	Options for patient peer support	✓✓✓	✓✓✓	✓✓✓	✓
Optional Considerations	Potential for shared staff and logistic infrastructure	✓✓✓	✓✓✓	–	–

✓✓✓ = Usually; ✓✓ = Sometimes; ✓ = Seldom; – = Usually Not. HD = hemodialysis.

Adapted from Fortnum et al. Kidney Health Australia: A model for home dialysis, Australia, 2012.[6]

the need for a home HD infrastructure; however, these cost savings may be offset by the expense of unnecessary home installations for patients who fail training.

Number of Home HD Training Stations to Support the Program

The required number of HD stations for the hub depends on several factors: (i) number of home HD patients who train each year, (ii) duration of training, (iii) number of days per week and hours per day during which the training facility operates, and (iv) whether the hub provides respite or "fallback" support for patients.

There is marked variation in service delivery among programs, although some general guidance can be provided:

- For new programs, it is typical to have modest training objectives for the first year, such as targeting only 5 to 10 patients. In contrast, larger programs may target up to 20 to 30 patients per year to maintain a census of approximately 100 trained home HD patients.
- In general, it is hard to predict the average duration of training for a cohort of patients, especially given individual patient variability and differing models of care. There is little evidence published on this topic, and what has been published requires careful interpretation before findings are extrapolated to different settings. The duration of training will vary according to patient-related factors, such as literacy, health literacy, general health, and level of functioning; service-related factors, including effectiveness of training, experience and confidence of trainers, and the clinical culture around patient safety and risk aversion; the ease of use and intuitiveness of the dialysis machinery; and whether patients have to learn to needle their fistula or graft, and how easy it is for them to do so.[7,8] In published reports and cumulative clinical experience, the number of sessions needed to complete training requirements is 20 to 40 sessions, but occasionally more may be needed (see the "Patient Selection and Training for Home Hemodialysis" module).[8–15] In the anecdotal experience of the authors, the duration of training tends to be consistent across countries: those with a lower prevalence of home HD, such as the United States, report a lower number of home HD training sessions (< 30) than countries with a higher prevalence of home HD patients, such as New Zealand (> 30). It is possible that this relates to the higher degree of patient selection in the United States (ie, only the most capable and motivated patients undergo home HD) and the reduced availability of "ideal patients" in New Zealand, where training needs to accommodate a more educationally and medically diverse home HD patient population.
- Respite or "fallback" support is provided for patients in the event of illness, technical problems, or home/social circumstances that require temporary support in a dependent-care HD facility.[16] Often, home HD training facilities rather than hospital or satellite facilities will manage respite support. In this way, a culture of self-management and consistency of patient care is maintained through the home-oriented training staff, with an explicit expectation of an eventual return to home HD as the long-term treatment modality. Where respite support is managed by the training facility, approximately 1 to 2 respite stations will be needed for every 3 to 4 training stations, depending on the size and comorbid burden of the home HD census.

A guide for determining the required number of training stations in a hub is provided in Table 2. Based on the estimated number of patients that the program plans to train and the approximate length of their training, the table indicates the required number of HD training stations (not including respite or fallback support) as a function of the operating days and hours of the training facility.

Of note, local reimbursement regulations may dictate a scale of economy such that an HD training facility needs to have a certain throughput to be viable. For instance, in the United States, it has

Table 2. Minimum Number of Home HD Training Stations Required for a Hub[a]

Training 3 Days per Week, 50 Weeks per Year					Training 5 Days per Week, 50 Weeks per Year				
A	**B**	**C**			**A**	**B**	**C**		
Home HD Patients Trained per Year	Home HD Training Shifts per Day[b]	Sessions Needed to Complete Training			Home HD Patients Trained per Year	Home HD Training Shifts per Day[a]	Sessions Needed to Complete Training		
		20 Sessions	**40 Sessions**	**60 Sessions**			**20 Sessions**	**40 Sessions**	**60 Sessions**
		Home HD Training Stations Needed (n)[c]					**Home HD Training Stations Needed (n)[d]**		
5	1	1	2	2	5	1	1	1	2
	2	1	1	1		2	1	1	1
15	1	2	4	6	15	1	2	3	4
	2	1	2	3		2	1	2	2
25	1	4	7	10	25	1	2	4	6
	2	2	3	5		2	1	2	3

HD = hemodialysis.

[a]Does not account for respite or "fallback" support.

[b]Either morning only (1) or morning and evening (2).

[c]Calculated as (A x C) / (3 x 50 x B). This number is rounded up, taking the ceiling value (the integer n such that [n-1] < [home HD training stations] < n).

[d]Calculated as (A x C) / (5 x 5 B). This number is rounded up, taking the ceiling value (the integer n such that [n-1] < [home HD training stations] < n).

been widely recommended that a successful unit should train at least 1 patient per month, with a goal of maintaining a census of 20 active patients.[17–19] Although no calculation is readily available to support these numbers, it is a consistent recommendation from opinion leaders from that country. Therefore, it is important to be aware of local factors that may dictate facility size in any given country and/or region.

Physical Requirements

General Principles

First and foremost, the hub should be fit for purpose. In smaller institutions, home HD and peritoneal dialysis programs may be colocated to provide functional integration of the 2 programs. This integration can allow for sharing of any or all of the following services: physical infrastructure (eg, training and clinical rooms), human resources (eg, cross-functional nursing and clinical dialysis technicians), and clinical services (shared clinics and drop-in services). If this is the case, then the physical setting should be suitable for both programs. Integrated home dialysis programs have been used in some programs to facilitate patients' awareness of both home dialysis modalities, and enable easier discussions of planned modality transitions that allow patients to remain independent.[20] At some institutions, however, there are sufficient numbers of patients for each program to exist separately, and a hub can be designed and orientated to purely home HD.

Whether colocated or stand-alone, there is no substitute for purposeful home HD infrastructure. The opportunistic location of home HD facilities in an unused space or corner of a hospital dialysis unit (colloquially known as the "one-room afterthought") will impede recruitment, training, and the growth of the program. The workspace should meet the needs of patients and their care partners in creating an optimal learning environment that is safe, private, and free of distractions. The workspace should also meet the needs of staff and minimize the time they spend handling logistics.

Ideally, the physical structure should showcase the program, as exemplified in Figure 3, and clearly establish that home HD is a priority and focus of the organization. A highly visible home HD hub will promote the program to both referring clinicians and patients.

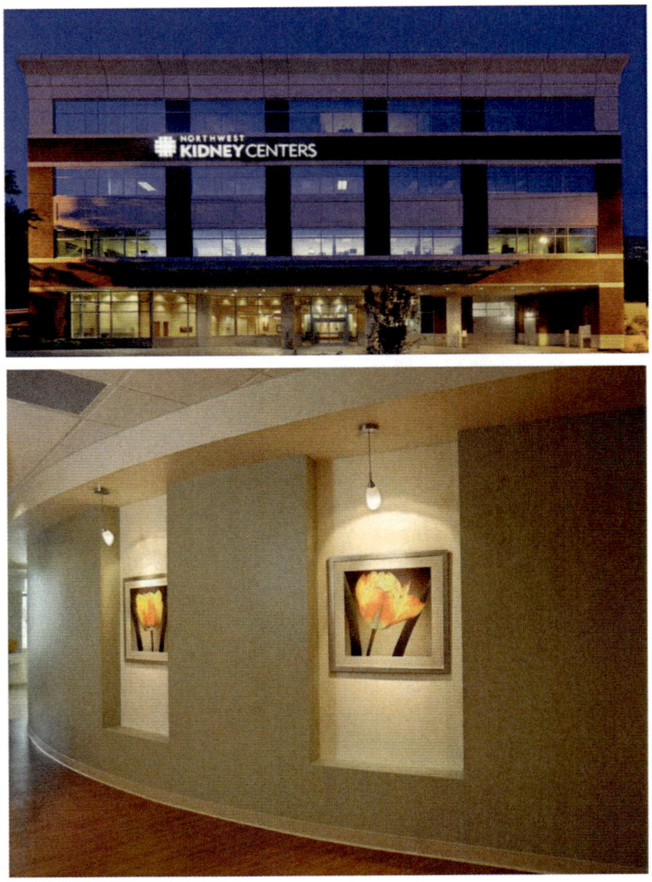

Figure 3. Showcasing your home hemodialysis hub: the Northwest Kidney Centers Home Dialysis Hub in Seattle (courtesy of Aaron Herold).

The generic components of a home HD hub are listed in Table 3, with key components discussed in the following subsections.

Patient Areas

Home HD training stations will generally have minimum sizes that are specified by local legislation, but should be large enough (eg, 5 × 4 m) to accommodate the dialysis equipment (machine, blood pressure machine, side table, and disposal facilities) as well as a guest chair and training aids. In general, home HD training stations

Table 3. Components of a Home HD Hub

Patient areas • Home HD training stations (options for solo and open-plan training are ideal) • Clinic rooms • Procedure room • Patient toilets with wheelchair access • Patient kitchenette/lounge areas	Soiled utility room Storage • Spare machines, wheelchairs, and equipment • Bulk storage for large deliveries • Clean supply (eg, solutions, disposables) • Secure chemical storage • Secure external storage for biohazard and recyclable waste
Staff areas • Office space for administrators, nurses, nephrologists • Meeting room • Staff toilets, showers, lockers • Staff kitchenette or common break areas	Vehicle Parking Home HD Machine Workshop Remote Monitoring Facilities
Reception area • Drop-off zone • Greeter desk • Seating area • Education and communication surfaces	
Clinical workstations for nurses and clinical dialysis technicians	
Clean utility and medication room(s)	

HD = hemodialysis.

have a "solo" arrangement, with a single HD station per room. Some programs, however, have very effective stations with open plans, similar to what might be found in a hospital HD facility. The advantages and disadvantages of solo and open-plan training are presented in Table 4. Whatever the configuration, training spaces should be able to accommodate educational resources, such as DVD players, television monitors, whiteboards, written materials, and a computer (ideally wall mounted) or mobile wireless computer workstation (Figure 4).

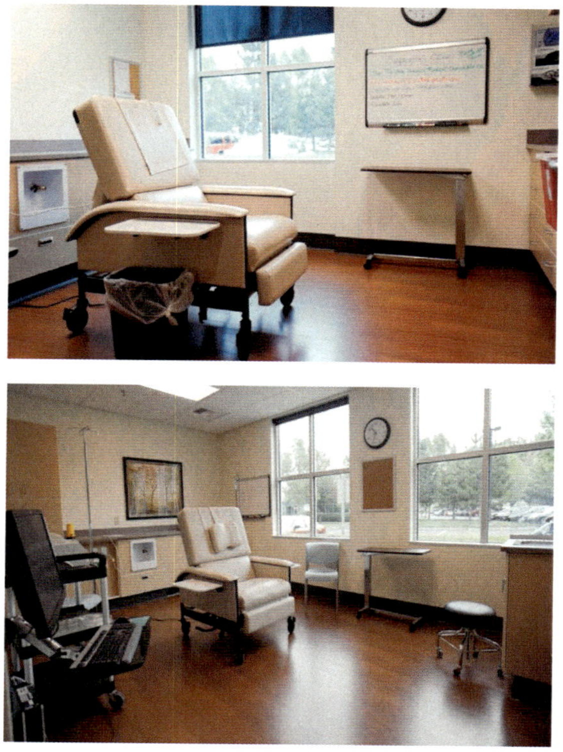

Figure 4. The Northwest Kidney Centers Home Dialysis Hub in Seattle: A home dialysis training station (courtesy of Aaron Herold).

Table 4. Solo vs Open-Plan Configurations for HD Training Stations

Solo Configuration	Open-Plan Configuration
Minimizes risk of cross-infection	Potential for increased risk of cross-infection
Potential for lack of monitoring during training	Easy monitoring during training
Potential social isolation	Socialization
Private	Potential lack of privacy
Quiet and conducive for learning	Potentially noisy and distracting
Only option is solitary training	Option for shared learning and group teaching
Isolated training experience	Peer support during training
Mimics the home HD treatment environment	

HD = hemodialysis.

Clinic rooms can be generic. A separate and specifically designated procedure room is sometimes desirable for home HD hubs that are not colocated with a hospital. This room can be equipped for minor procedures, such as tunneled central venous catheter removals and wound dressings, or for even more major procedures, such as central venous or peritoneal dialysis catheter insertions (if the home HD and peritoneal dialysis programs are integrated and colocated).

There are other special characteristics to consider, including the following:

- Safety systems should meet national and state licensing and regulatory requirements. Hubs should also be designed to include a resuscitation trolley ("crash cart") bay, and clearly marked and adequate thoroughfares for emergency ambulance access. Lighting, electrical systems, and plumbing should also meet national and state licensing and regulatory requirements.

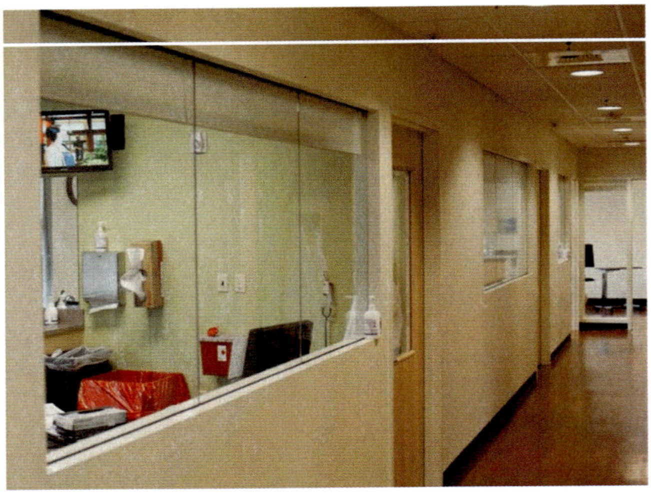

Figure 5. The Northwest Kidney Centers Home Dialysis Hub in Seattle: Large glass sections allow for patient monitoring during training (courtesy of Aaron Herold).

- Large glass sections should be used where appropriate to allow for monitoring (Figure 5).
- Rooms should include a counter with a sink, hand washing facilities, and a mirror (Figure 6).

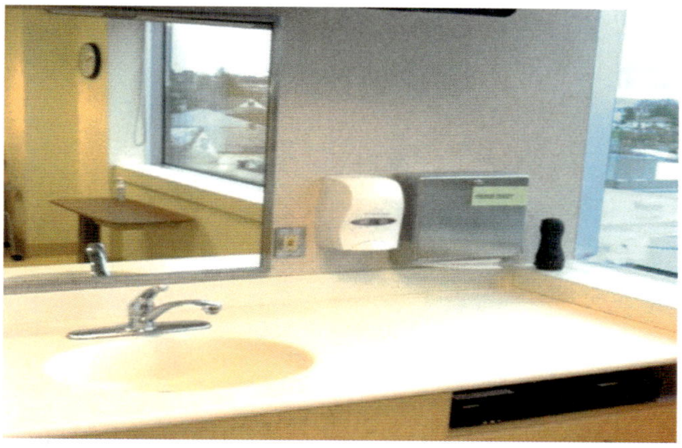

Figure 6. The Northwest Kidney Centers Home Dialysis Hub in Seattle: Rooms should include a counter with a sink, a faucet, and a mirror (courtesy of Aaron Herold).

- Patients should be kept comfortable through the use of appropriate furniture and climate controls.
- Home HD training spaces should be able to accommodate training for nocturnal dialysis, including flexible lighting, comfortable trundle beds, noise control, and blinds to allow privacy.

Staff Areas

Office space can be generic but should accommodate necessary staff and provisions for their required job functions. In most cases, separate offices are required for the nephrologist, manager, and charge nurse, with workstations for nurses and clinical dialysis technicians that have appropriate privacy options. An often overlooked but essential office space is an appropriately sized meeting room that can be used for clinical handover, continuing professional development, or business meetings.

The schedule of accommodation should account for the communication equipment used for clinical and business operations management. Office space should be designed with cabling and capacity for a sufficient number of telephones (all compatible with an after-hours forwarding service) and the means to receive patient treatment information, such as via fax. Other options for communication might be desirable, such as the use of e-mail through a secured patient portal and video conferencing, and these may require additional design considerations.

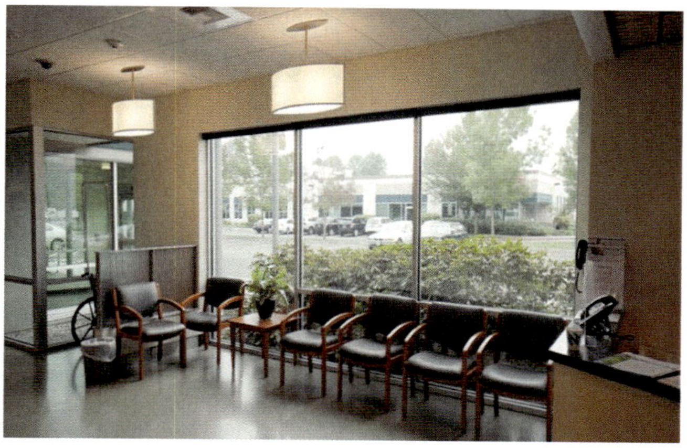

Figure 7. The Northwest Kidney Centers Home Dialysis Hub in Seattle: The reception area (courtesy of Aaron Herold).

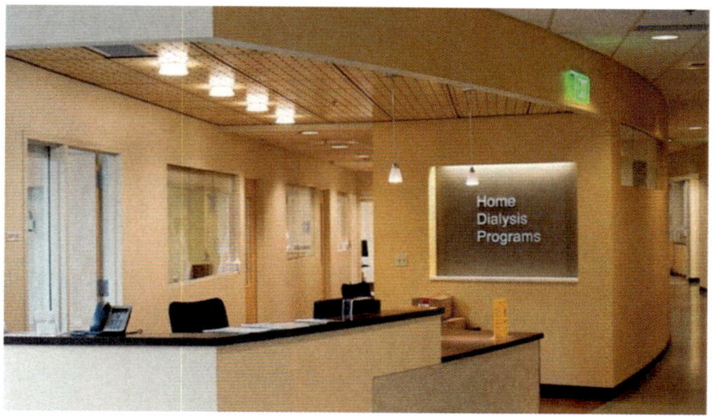

Figure 8. The Northwest Kidney Centers Home Dialysis Hub in Seattle: The greeter desk (courtesy of Aaron Herold).

Reception Area

Entry to the reception area should include a drop-off zone for patients that is adequately lit for security and safety and ideally covered for all-weather access. The building should have wheelchair access with a ramp and a wheelchair storage area near the exit in the reception area (Figure 7).

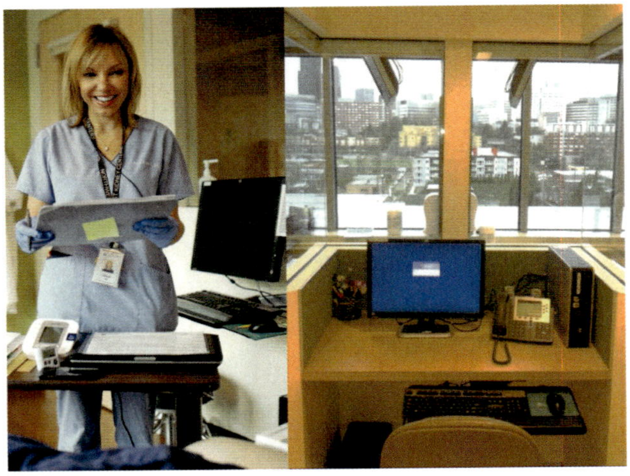

Figure 9. The Northwest Kidney Centers Home Dialysis Hub in Seattle: Clinical workstations for nurses and clinical dialysis technicians (courtesy of Aaron Herold).

The reception area itself should contain a seating area and a warm and welcoming greeter desk (Figure 8). A greeter telephone is highly recommended: when no one is attending the reception area, this telephone rings through to all other rooms. A worthwhile investment is to ensure that the greeter desk is set up to also serve as an additional workstation for staff should the need arise. The reception area should have surfaces for educational materials, pamphlet dispensers, and bulletin boards for information from local patient support and advocacy groups. It is common to have a refreshment bar or a water cooler as a pleasant, value-added extra.

Workstations for Nurses and Clinical Dialysis Technicians

Clinical workstations should provide adequate surface space and storage for training and case management materials (Figure 9). There should be the ability to monitor patient arrival and treatment, but with sufficient noise control and privacy options to permit sensitive activities (eg, having discussions with patients, calling physicians for orders, entering clinical data, and performing other maintenance-related activities). In most cases, this requires a separate room with individual cubicles or workspaces. An increasingly popular option for the management of home dialysis patients is through telemedicine. In this case, a separate room will be required with telepresence and other technical equipment to allow for noise control and privacy.

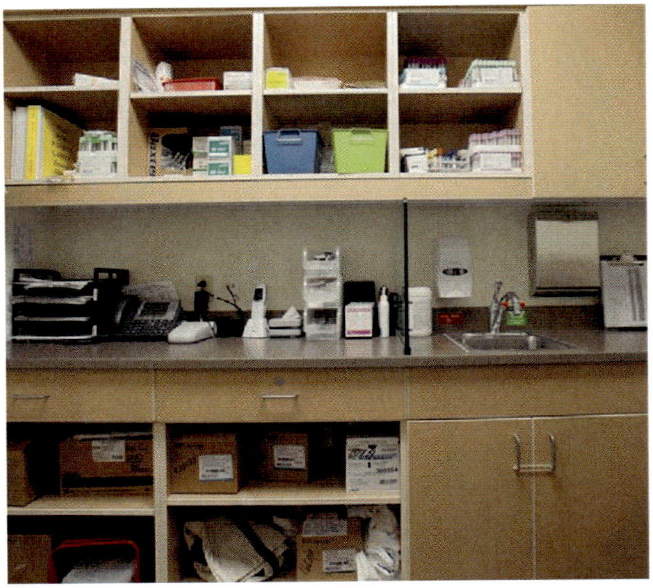

Figure 10. The Northwest Kidney Centers Home Dialysis Hub in Seattle: Clean utility bench space and shelving (courtesy of Aaron Herold).

Utility Rooms

The clean utility and medication room must have secure access and be able to store drugs and sterile consumables. There should be adequate bench space for drug preparation and shelving (Figure 10). The soiled utility room (sluice room) does not require secure access and should include a sink and hand washing facilities.

Storage

Storage facilities should comply with local regulations and accommodate the types of supplies listed in Table 3. The schedule of accommodation should also allow for the equipment necessary for stock management and equipment tracking. There should be external access for deliveries and easy access for staff from the training and clinic areas.

Vehicle Parking

Vehicle parking is frequently overlooked in facility planning and is important for those who are either training or attending clinic at the home HD hub. Unlike facility HD patients, most home HD patients drive and are ineligible for free transport options. In the spirit of promoting self-management and independence, allocated on-site parking should be readily available for patients and their care partners. Parking must also be allocated for visitors with disabilities.

Staff who perform patient home visits are an integral part of any home dialysis service, and there should also be adequate parking for the on-site staff vehicle pool.

Machine Workshop

Not every program requires a workshop, and many will arrange machine servicing and repairs off-site. If a workshop is required, there should be adequate bench space for repairs and floor space for machine storage, with external access to allow for easy transport.

Common Break Room

It is important to provide a lounge for staff that incorporates lockers, a table(s) and chairs, and a refrigerator or kitchenette. This allows space for staff to place their belongings, take breaks, and eat in a room separate from the clinical work areas. Showers are not a requirement, but they allow staff more flexibility, if available.

Remote Monitoring Facilities

There are different options for remote monitoring available to home HD units and their patients, although they all have the similarity of providing a means of communication between home HD staff (physicians, nurses, and clinical dialysis technicians) and patients.[21] Remote monitoring allows staff to review and assess patient's treatment, observations, recordings, and general health status remotely, allowing the patient to live as independently as possible on home HD away from the hospital setting while still receiving a high level of care and support. In addition to providing staff with up-to-date information on patients at home, remote monitoring can also assist in easing some of the fears and anxieties of patients and their families about performing HD away from the hub.[22] For some patients, this will help them feel supported in an independent environment.

It is important to acknowledge the negative features of remote monitoring systems. First, there is significant cost associated with the technical elements of monitoring and staffing. This can be a financial burden for providers and a disincentive to home HD uptake. Another issue is a negative perception among some patients, who often find monitoring intrusive. Finally, it is unlikely that remote monitoring prevents serious adverse events; however, it is plausible that more timely access to patient observations (eg, weight and blood pressure) may improve routine patient care.[21,23] In general, more research is needed to clarify the role of remote monitoring, and many programs do not routinely offer it in the modern era.

Integrated Governance Structure

Service Delivery and Patient Care

The concept of governance refers to the activities that direct, administer, and control an organization. A framework for the governance of home HD programs is suggested in Figure 11 and describes the groups that guide service delivery and patient care. A formalized governance structure is important for these programs—there must be transparent accountability and linkages around all the critical processes that impact clinical outcomes. Accountability, in turn, refers to personal responsibility for delivering on these processes.

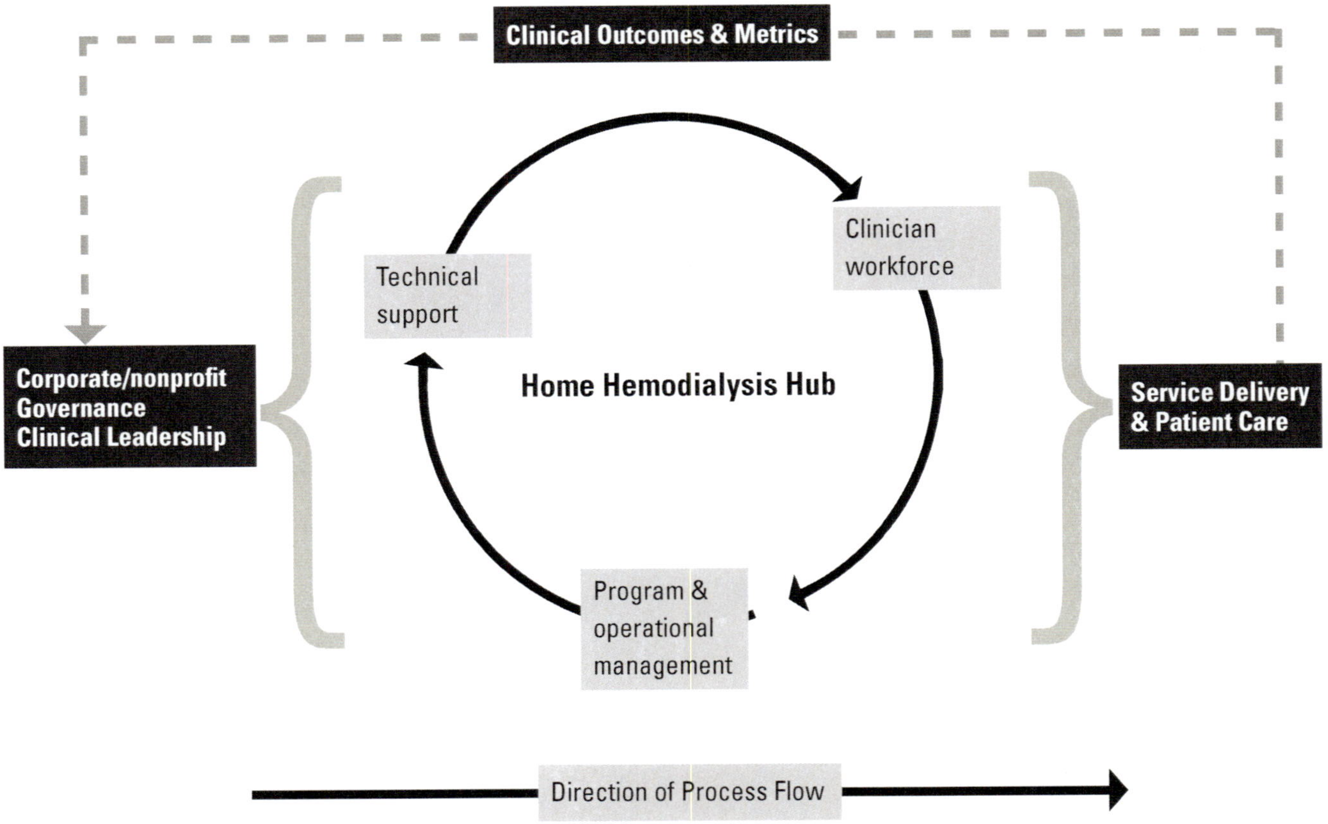

Figure 11. A framework for integrated governance of a home hemodialysis program or hub.

For every home HD program, there are either corporate or nonprofit bodies at the top of the governance structure that exercise ultimate authority. For corporate-governed programs, boards of directors (or their like) set policies that determine how the program runs to meet corporate goals and the nature of relationships among directors, management, and stakeholders (regulators, financiers, suppliers, employees, patients, the community at large, etc). For nonprofit-governed programs, boards of trustees or governmental groups set the policies instead. Whatever the structure, there are always normative and binding rules or standards that set overriding goals for the program and specify how the goals are met. Further discussion on governance options is outside the scope of this module, which instead focuses on the key accountabilities and linkages for those governance groups that function in the home HD program or hub: managers, clinicians, and technical staff. It is vital, however, that these individuals be aware of their organization's overriding strategic objectives and imperatives, and ensure that the processes for which they are accountable are aligned and compliant.

Clinicians play a key role in the governance of home HD programs. Management governance is usually "top-down" and related to business and regulatory concerns. Clinical governance is more distributive and relies on the expertise and engagement of healthcare professionals throughout the whole service. Ideally, management and clinical governance should coexist; this helps ensure that patient care and outcomes are the prime drivers in defining clinical service delivery

Table 5. Roles and Responsibilities of the Program (Strategic) and Operations (Tactical) Managers in a Home HD Program

Key Accountabilities	Linkages	Examples
Financial	Business or finance service unit and analysts	• Key performance indicators for cost-effectiveness (eg, weeks per patient trained, home HD technique survival) • Capital budget and expenditure (eg, dialysis machinery and reverse osmosis units) • Operating budget and expenditure (eg, staff and consumables) • Contracts and procurements
Administration	Business or finance service unit and analysts	• Billing • Stock supply chain (eg, dialysis machinery reverse osmosis units, consumables)
Staff Management	Human resources service	• Recruitment and retention
IT and Database	IT service	• Procurement and upkeep of software and hardware to ensure business and clinical continuity
Communications	IT service	• Supply of fax, telephone, secure patient e-mail services, after-hours on-call redirect
Risk Management	Quality service	• Quality and clinical performance indicators • Patient safety • Occupational health and safety • Incident and complaints system

HD = Hemodialysis; IT = information technology.

and decision-making. In any home HD program (and arguably healthcare in general), strategies for clinical engagement should be formalized and allow clinicians to have a voice in decision-making processes and to lead clinical initiatives.[24]

The roles and responsibilities of managers, clinicians, and technical staff are summarized in Tables 5 through 7, respectively. In larger programs, there is often division of labor among many; in a smaller program, many of these roles and responsibilities might fall to 1 or 2 people in each group. Nonetheless, it is necessary only to know that tasks are being accomplished and that appropriate persons are held accountable, as determined by their professional role assignment.

A particular area of importance and shared responsibility is that of disaster recovery planning. Disasters such as hurricanes and earthquakes often severely disrupt power, water, and sewage utilities; even if utilities are not interrupted, supply chain disruptions may limit how long HD can be sustained at home. Large-scale disasters may also damage local in-center dialysis facilities, and acute hospital facilities are in high demand due to acute kidney injuries, so many patients must be transferred to other nearby

Table 6. Roles and Responsibilities of the Clinical Leadership in a Home HD Program

Key Accountabilities	Linkages	Examples
Model of Care		• Care principles and organization of evidence-based, patient-focused interactions between clinicians and patients • Multidisciplinary team care (medical, nursing, technical, pharmacy, physiotherapy, occupational therapy, social work, health psychology) • Home visiting program
Clinic Performance Indicators, Clinical Audit, and Case Reviews	Quality service, IT service	• Training time and failure rate • Home HD technique survival and drop-out rates • Vascular access survival and complication rates • Program recruitment rate • Hospital admission rate • Patient survival rate • Key performance indicators on clinical processes (monthly labs, home visits)
Risk Management		• Patient Safety (eg, "near miss" case conferences) • Home HD dropout (eg, drop-out case conferences) • Incident and complaints system
Maintenance of Clinical Standards		• Clinical policies and standard operating procedures • Product and technology evaluation • Criteria and audit of acceptance to home HD program
Research		• Abide by protocols and collect trial data
IT and Database	IT service	• Clinical data entry to ensure clinical continuity
Staff Management	Human resources service	• Recruitment • Orientation and onboarding • Credentialing • Continuing professional development
Clinical Capital Evaluation	Business or finance service unit, analysts	• Contracts and procurement

HD = hemodialysis; IT = information technology.

Table 7. Roles and Responsibilities of Technical Support in a Home HD Program

Key Accountabilities	Linkages	Examples
Dialysis Machinery and Reverse Osmosis Units (see "Infrastructure, Water, and Machines in the Home" module)		• Stock management • Maintenance and servicing • Technical troubleshooting • Home installations, particularly in relation to a safe and reliable water supply
Clinical Capital Evaluation	Business or finance service unit/ analysts	• Contracts and procurements (dialysis machinery, reverse osmosis units)
Staff Management	Human resources service	• Recruitment • Orientation and onboarding • Credentialing • Continuing professional development
IT and Database	IT service	• Technical data entry to ensure business and clinical continuity
Risk Management	Quality service	• Key performance indicators for water quality • Key performance indicators for machinery maintenance and servicing • Occupational health and safety • Incident and complaints system • Key performance indicators for compliance with technical standards (eg, electrical and plumbing standards)

HD = Hemodialysis; IT = information technology.

programs. Evacuation of home HD patients during these events is typically the only feasible option. Establishment of organized disaster plans is recommended for all home HD programs. Managers, clinicians, and technical staff should identify alternative HD arrangements for their patients, educate patients about dietary restrictions, and establish evacuation procedures to allow the early transfer of home HD patients, along with their key documentation, out of the disaster area. Integration of the home HD disaster plans with those of local health authorities helps ensure alignment of transportation and logistics.[25] One such disaster plan has been published by NxStage Medical and is designed to facilitate emergency preparedness for home HD patients (available here).

Another disaster plan was published following the February 2011 Christchurch earthquake in New Zealand, and is aimed at facilitating disaster recovery and management for home HD providers and the teams helping them.[25] Both are useful references for those programs developing their own disaster plans.

Options for Outsourced Home HD from a Large Dialysis Organization

Large dialysis organizations have many options for governance of home dialysis patients if patient care needs to be outsourced. Several models of training could occur, including (i) outsource training to a local facility but retain the patient once the training has been completed, (ii) outsource training and subsequent follow-up of the patient to a local facility, and (iii) training in a central location with referral to local dialysis units ("hub-and-spoke" model). The benefits and challenges of each model are described in the following subsections.

Outsource Training

If a dialysis facility does not have the capacity to develop a home HD program owing to staffing or building constraints, potential patients can still be trained for home HD by outsourcing training to an established home HD program. Programs can then have the patient return to the main dialysis facility for maintenance of care and evaluation by clinical staff (physicians, nurses, and clinical dialysis technicians) on a regular schedule. An example of this type of model is the training of pediatric patients and families. In this example, the parent facility may not have sufficient experience or infrastructure for the task and may choose to outsource. Clinical staff at the parent program can be trained in the specifics of the home HD technique and related troubleshooting; however, the training itself, machine care, and standard maintenance are taken care of by the training dialysis program. Appropriate agreements for emergency issues, machine maintenance, and respite care must be in place for this model to be successful. The prime benefit to the parent dialysis program is that it can offer home HD but does not need to invest in the training infrastructure to maintain this modality.

Outsource Training and Follow-up

Another model that can be used to offer home HD is to outsource training and subsequent follow-up of home HD patients by partnering with a local established home HD program. In this model, patients are recruited by the parent dialysis program, but all home HD training and subsequent follow-up is performed by the outsourced organization. The benefits of this model are that it allows the parent dialysis program to offer home HD to all patients potentially closer to where patients live; however, it does not facilitate direct management of patients by the parent facility. Difficulties with this model are loss of control of management of dialysis patients and the need for a liaison for referral when issues arise with dialysis access or need for emergency dialysis. Quality metrics and oversight must be in place to ensure that referred dialysis patients are receiving quality dialysis care.

Hub-and-Spoke Model

Large dialysis facilities or health maintenance organizations that offer dialysis can potentially use a model that relies on regional training of home HD with subsequent follow-up in smaller units. This centralized hub-and-spoke model has been used in the US Veterans Health Administration for the evaluation and treatment of patients with spinal cord injury. Patients are referred to centralized regional centers of excellence but receive traditional care at smaller local centers. This model allows overall evaluation of all potential patients for home HD in a regionalized central location that can offer experience and long-term follow-up options. Challenges with this model are that local expertise is needed for daily emergencies and respite dialysis, and patients will need accommodations close to the regional center for the duration of their training. An example of this type of model would be to have a large centralized HD training center that refers patients to local, more rural spokes that can then take care of minor emergencies. All machine repairs and patient training are completed at the regional center of excellence, and all minor issues are dealt with closer to the patient's home.

Conclusion

A well-functioning home HD program critically depends on adequate hub facilities and support functions and transparent and accountable organizational processes. The likelihood of optimal service delivery and patient care will be enhanced by fit-for-purpose facilities and implementation of a well-considered governance structure.

References

1. Alhomayeed B, Lindsay RM. Technical aspects of home hemodialysis. Saudi J Kidney Dis Transpl. 2009;20:185-191.
2. Tonozuka Y, Liu J. Data on file. Baxter Healthcare Japan Ltd. 2014.
3. ANZDATA Registry. Summary of Australia and New Zealand Dialysis and Transplantation 2012. Adelaide, Australia. Clayton P, McDonald SP, Hurst K. Available at: http://www.anzdata.org.au/anzdata/AnzdataReport/36thReport/2012_Summary_v1.pdf. Accessed September 4, 2014.
4. McLaughlin R, Aupiu J, Colin M. Hemodialysis training in the home: a new experience. J Am Assoc Nephrol Nurses Tech. 1981;8:35-38.
5. Cocks J. Home dialysis: domiciliary training. Queens Nurs J. 1973;16:131-132.
6. Fortnum D, Mathew T, Johnson K. A model for home dialysis, Australia, 2012. Kidney Health Australia website. Available at: http://www.kidney.org.au/LinkClick.aspx?fileticket=BfYeuFvtJcl%3d&tabid=811&mid=1886. Accessed September 30, 2014.
7. Young BA, Chan C, Blagg C, et al. How to overcome barriers and establish a successful home HD program. Clin J Am Soc Nephrol. 2012;7:2023-2032.
8. Pipkin M, Eggers PW, Larive B, et al. Recruitment and training for home hemodialysis: experience and lessons from the Nocturnal Dialysis Trial. Clin J Am Soc Nephrol. 2010;5:1614-1620.
9. Schachter ME, Tennankore KK, Chan CT. Determinants of training and technique failure in home hemodialysis. Hemodial Int. 2013;17:421-426.
10. Tanaka H, Sakai R, Kita T, Okamoto K, Mikami M. Overnight home hemodialysis: eight patients and six years of experience in Sakairumi clinics. Contrib Nephrol. 2012;177:133-142.
11. McGregor D, Buttimore A, Robson R, Little P, Morton J, Lynn K. Thirty years of universal home dialysis in Christchurch. N Z Med J. 2000;113:27-29.
12. Kraus M, Burkart J, Hegeman R, Solomon R, Coplon N, Moran J. A comparison of center-based vs. home-based daily hemodialysis for patients with end-stage renal disease. Hemodial Int. 2007;11:468-477.
13. Honkanen E, Muroma-Karttunen R, Taponen RM, Grönhagen-Riska C. Starting a home hemodialysis program: single center experiences. Scand J Urol Nephrol. 2002;36:137-144.
14. Kumar VA, Ledezma ML, Rasgon SA. Daily home hemodialysis at a health maintenance organization: three-year experience. Hemodial Int. 2007;11:225-230.
15. Connaughton DM, Jamal A, McWilliams J, et al. Home haemodialysis in Ireland. Ir J Med Sci. 2013;182:91-96.
16. Agar JW. Home hemodialysis in Australia and New Zealand: practical problems and solutions. Hemodial Int. 2008;12(Suppl 1):S26-S32.
17. Moran J, Kraus M. Starting a home hemodialysis program. Semin Dial. 2007;20:35-39.
18. Blagg C. Some thoughts on the future of home hemodialysis. Dial Transplantation 2010;39:335-337.
19. Anderson C, Blagg CR, Mailloux LU. Organization and elements of a home hemodialysis program. In: Rose BD, ed. UpToDate website: http://www.uptodate.com/contents/organization-and-elements-of-a-home-hemodialysis-program. Wellesley, MA; Wolters Kluwer Health. 2001. Accessed September 30, 2014.
20. Golper TA, Schreiber MJ. The course of therapy – changing the paradigm. In: Fadem SZ, ed. Issues in Dialysis. Houston, TX: Nova Science Publishers; 2012.
21. Marshall MR, Pierratos A, Pauly RP. Delivering home hemodialysis: is there still a role for real-time treatment monitoring? Semin Dial. 2015;28:176-179.
22. Cafazzo JA, Leonard K, Easty AC, Rossos PG, Chan CT. Patient-perceived barriers to the adoption of nocturnal home hemodialysis. Clin J Am Soc Nephrol. 2009;4:784-789.

References (cont'd)

23. Hoy C. Remote monitoring in nocturnal home hemodialysis 2003. Hemodial Int. 2004;8:144-150.

24. Whitlock DJ, Stark R. Understanding physician engagement – and how to increase it. Physician Leadership J. 2014;5:8-12.

25. Irvine J, Buttimore A, Eastwood D, Kendrick-Jones J. The Christchurch earthquake: dialysis experience and emergency planning. Nephrology (Carlton). 2014;19:296-303.

2 Funding and Planning: What You Need to Know for Starting or Expanding a Home Hemodialysis Program

Kirsten Howard, PhD[1]
Phil A McFarlane, MD, PhD, FRCPC[2]
Mark R Marshall, MBChB, MPH, FRACP[3,4]
Debbie O Eastwood, BBus, PG Cert Health Sciences, MSc[5]
Rachael L Morton, PhD[1,6]

[1]The University of Sydney, School of Public Health, Sydney, Australia; [2]Division of Nephrology, St Michael's Hospital and Department of Medicine, University of Toronto, Toronto, Ontario, Canada; [3]Faculty of Medical and Health Sciences, University of Auckland, Auckland, New Zealand; [4]Department of Renal Medicine, Counties Manukau District Health Board, Auckland, New Zealand; [5]Department of Medicine and Health of Older People, Waitemata District Health Board, Auckland, New Zealand; [6]Nuffield Department of Population Health, Health Economics Research Centre, The University of Oxford, Headington, United Kingdom

Implementing Hemodialysis in the Home
A Global Perspective

ISHD
International Society for Hemodialysis

CONTENTS

Abstract

Planning and funding a home hemodialysis (HD) program requires a well-organized effort and close collaboration between clinicians and administrators. This resource provides guidance on the processes that are involved, including: a thorough situational analysis of the dialysis landscape, emphasizing the opportunity for a home HD program; careful consideration of the clinical and operational characteristics of a proposed home HD program at your institution; the development of a compelling business case, highlighting the clinical and organizational benefits of a home HD program; and careful construction and evaluation of a request for proposal.

Introduction

Making the correct fiscal case for change is a crucial step in developing a home hemodialysis (HD) program. Smaller programs or pilot projects can often be started and managed within existing hospital HD infrastructure with costs being absorbed into existing funding. Once programs grow to beyond 5-10 patients; however, there is often requirement for separate and specialized home HD infrastructure and staffing. Figure 1 compares the size of home HD programs between Japan and Australia/New Zealand.[1,2] In Japan, most home HD programs are small and located within hospital HD facilities.[1] In Australia/New Zealand, home HD programs are larger and, in most cases, enabled by specialized facilities and personnel.[2] Expanding a home HD program therefore requires substantial resources, and typically this requires a sound business case for financial investment.

Functionally, a proposal to start or expand a home HD program can be regarded as a 3-step process:

1. Development of an overarching clinical and strategic framework
2. Consolidation of these principles into a formal business case
3. Execution and handling of a request for proposal (RFP)

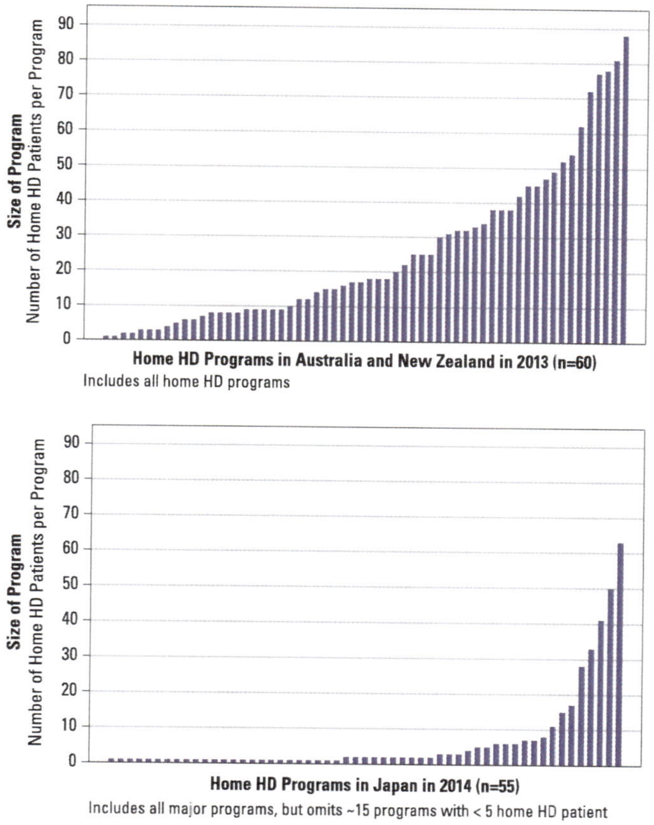

Figure 1. Size of Home HD Programs in Australia and New Zealand and Japan.[1,2]

It is vital that the framework and business case are credible and well supported: most providers and payers without experience of home HD programs perceive a high degree of clinical and financial risk in establishing a new home HD program, particularly when they are uncertain about the benefits to patients.[3] For those responsible for developing the business case, choosing an overarching framework and deciding on suitable content can be daunting. In order not to be overwhelmed, we recommend that clinicians and administrators work together to accomplish these goals. The importance of this relationship cannot be overemphasized—an individual nephrologist may be able to start a pilot home HD project, but only a team effort will ultimately result in a sustainable and sizeable program.

The medical literature is the best starting point for evidence to support the project. Where it has been evaluated, home HD is less expensive than in-center (facility) HD and is associated with better survival and health-related quality of life.[4,5] This has been demonstrated for both conventional short-hour, thrice-weekly HD, as well as frequent and/or extended-hour HD in the home setting.[6] In 2010, the United Kingdom's (UK's) National Health Service (NHS) Purchasing and Supply Agency published an economic report of home HD, using assumptions based on the most likely UK scenario at the time. In that report, home HD dominated satellite HD with a cost saving of approximately £17,000 and a quality-adjusted-life-year (QALY) gain of 0.38 over a 10-year time horizon.[7] Home HD also dominated hospital HD, with similar cost saving and QALY gain. The greater cost of satellite and hospital HD was mainly attributed to a greater number of dialysis staff employed and patients' travel-related costs. Despite the high initial (front-loaded) costs of home HD due to patient setup and training, the payback period (relative to facility HD) is typically estimated to be relatively short at approximately 14 months.[4, 7-9] When considering these economic evaluations, one must be aware that most are biased *against* home HD, as these evaluations yield intentionally conservative estimates of cost-effectiveness (eg, no survival benefit is used in base case scenarios, despite multiple observational studies reporting this benefit).[10]

To navigate this process more easily, the following resources have been developed by a group of clinicians and administrators with first-hand experience in home HD and can be used in the development of business cases and RFPs.

- A set of questions for consideration, which will help inform the business case in the areas of capital, staffing, maintenance, and stakeholder consultation
- Guidance on how to write a business case for a home HD program
- Practice tips for dealing with RFPs

The questions in the next section should be considered in detail, before starting or expanding a home HD program, or writing a business case. For each set of questions, we have indicated specific resources that are available to the reader for further information. The clinical and administrative leads of the project should be comfortable that the majority of these questions have been answered to their satisfaction. In most cases, however, there is no "correct" answer. Rather, we encourage readers to consider the options that are available to them, taking into account factors that are unique to their anticipated program structure and size, staffing sources, budget constraints, available equipment, local environment, and cultural practices. In some cases, we have clarified the question with additional considerations that are listed as bullet points.

Questions to Consider Before Starting a Home HD Program or Writing a Business Case

Clinical Models of Care and Availability of Supporting Services

Q: What mix of home HD therapies will be offered?

- Identify the types of HD that the program will offer (nocturnal, short daily, conventional)
- Identify the frequency of HD that the program will offer (conventional 3 sessions/week, short daily 4-6 sessions/week, daily 7 sessions/week)
- Determine a targeted number of HD hours per week (eg, 12-15 hours/week, 15-20 hours/week, > 20 hours/week)
- Determine the maximum or minimum standards for the frequency and/or duration of therapy, set either by local clinical standards of care or pragmatic/costing constraints
  - » For example, the program might offer a minimum 12 hours of dialysis per week (clinical standard), but no more than 5 treatments per week (budget constraint)

Q: Why will these types of treatments be offered?

- Conceptualize the expected benefits for your program and your patients

Q: Is there good support for starting this program at your center?

- Consider the level of support among local nephrologists, nursing and multidisciplinary teams, management and hospital administration, as well as the level of support from regional or national authorities
  - » For example, in Ontario, Canada, the province pays for dialysis and is strongly supporting an initiative to increase the availability of all forms of home dialysis

Q: What is the capacity of facility HD programs?

- Determine if home HD is being considered because of capacity limitations in the hospital or satellite dialysis facilities
- Determine if there is sufficient capacity in either the proposed home HD unit or in other dialysis facilities to allow for fallback/respite care for home HD patients?

Stakeholders

It is important to clearly identify internal and external stakeholders in relation to a proposed home HD program. These specific people or groups are those who will be required to support the program, either through mitigating clinical and financial risks or through promoting and/or directly contributing to it.

Q: In your wider dialysis program, have you assessed patients' levels of awareness and interest in home HD?

- The most important stakeholder is the patient. During the planning process, there should be wide-ranging consultation with patients and advocacy groups. This should be done to ascertain the general level of interest in home HD, and also performed in a manner that promotes awareness and potential demand for the modality. This can be accomplished via a survey with an introduction containing a précis of clinical benefits, or through focus groups with patients and their families

Q: In your local region, are there initiatives or policies directed to increase the proportion of patients on home HD?

- Identify or create home HD patient recruitment pathways (see "Systems to Cultivate Suitable Patients for Home Dialysis" module)

Q: What information is needed to approach the department of human services, government, or ministry payer for increased reimbursement and initial capital expenditure to fund a home HD program?

- Determine what their drivers are, and decide if it is possible to align with these entities to motivate home HD program development

Q: What factors will encourage administrators and clinical staff to become supportive and engaged?

- Those who are heavily invested in facility HD may see home dialysis programs as competition. It is important to have systems and strategies in place to promote your new home HD program to not only patients and families, but also to the members of your nephrology service as well

Q: How will home HD candidates be identified and made known to the home program?

- Many programs have found that it is difficult to move patients from facility to home HD. However, within most programs there are a small number of individual patients who will self-identify as candidates for home HD when informed of the availability of this modality, usually after a careful description of the advantages, disadvantages, expectations, etc. It is important to have systems and strategies in place to identify such patients, and motivated and informed staff to approach patients with information about the modality and reasons why they should choose it. It is essential to promote home HD as an integral part of the shared decision-making process, when patients are discussing modality choice with predialysis educators and clinicians (see "Systems to Cultivate Suitable Patients for Home Dialysis" module)

- Home HD has been offered as a modality for patients who are failing peritoneal dialysis (PD) and want to maintain dialysis in the home setting. Programs that already offer PD should consider how to ensure that candidates for home HD are able to make a smooth and timely transition, when appropriate

- Patient selection criteria for home HD should be defined. Any proposal for starting or expanding a program should include estimates of growth and demand, which will in turn be determined by the number of recruits and the criteria used to select them (patient selection is discussed in detail in the "Patient Selection and Training for Home Hemodialysis" module). Any patient who is physically and cognitively able and motivated can perform home HD. In addition, there are many patients with complex combinations of comorbidities who have better outcomes with more frequent or longer HD treatments that are more easily administered in the home setting (refractory volume overload, difficult to control hypertension, right heart failure or uncontrolled ascites, persistent hyperphosphatemia, etc.). Clearly identify the types of patients within your service who could benefit medically from a survival and/or quality-of-life standpoint, and provide an estimated number of patients in the business case

Q: How will the home HD program integrate with local dialysis services?

- Determine if your home HD program will offer training and/or ongoing care to patients (and their care partner, if appropriate) for other regional dialysis services that do not have this option?

Q: For patients identified as candidates for home HD, what resources are required to ensure that such patients can have a smooth and optimal dialysis start?

- In particular, emphasis needs to be given to ensure that patients initiate HD as an outpatient with a permanent vascular access if possible

- Determine if staff (eg, a nurse navigator) and procedures are in place to help ensure that home HD patients are not lost to facility dialysis
  - » Even after patients are identified as candidates for home HD, many patients may still start HD urgently in a hospital setting[11]

Budget

A key component to a successful launch of a new home HD program is to ensure that the program is financially sustainable. It is accepted that home HD is a cost-effective alternative to conventional facility HD and an attractive option from a health system and societal perspective. However, these "global" cost savings may not help a local program that has day-to-day costs that are more than their incoming funding. For example, reductions in the costs of hospital admissions and medications may be attractive to the payer (eg, in the case of the Provincial Ministry of Health in Ontario, Canada), but these costs are usually not borne by the dialysis program, so they do not contribute to financial sustainability at the program level.

An important consideration is modality mix, in terms of extended-hours or frequent HD. Longer treatments have very low marginal costs per dialysis hour, as the only additional costs are for extra utilities (ie, power and water) and dialysate. More frequent treatments have higher marginal costs per dialysis hour due to the need for new connectology, tubing sets, and dialysis membranes.

Q: How does the dialysis equipment affect these costs?

- Systems that make extended use of dialyzers and tubing, for example, may reduce the marginal cost of adding extra treatments (see "Infrastructure, Water, and Machines in the Home" module)

Q: How is home HD funded in your local region (ie, paid by modality type, per week, or per treatment)?

- Funding per unit of time (eg, weekly or monthly) will make more frequent treatments less attractive from a budget perspective. This should not be a barrier when treatments are funded by modality type (for example, when nocturnal home HD is funded differently than conventional home HD) or when funded per treatment (the cost per treatment is similar for short and long home HD sessions)

Q: What are the anticipated costs relative to the funding level?

- Consider costs reimbursed to the dialysis provider and those borne by the dialysis program
- Determine if other programs in your region find that funding is at an appropriate level
  - » Anticipate that costs relative to funding are going to be high when the program is first initiated. Costs related to staff, space, overheads, etc., are often fixed (eg, clinical space must be allocated for regardless of whether there are a small or large number of patients), and incoming funding will be low due to the small number of initial patients. As the program grows over time, the ability to balance costs should improve, as the marginal costs of adding new patients are lower
- Programs should plan for how they will balance costs, because during the initial start-up period incoming funding will be low, and likely lower than costs

Q: What are the potential resource impacts on other hospital programs?

- Supporting a larger number of home HD patients over time will subsequently impact other hospital services, such as laboratory, interventional radiology, and inpatient services
  - » Patients undergoing home HD often require treatments and care in the hospital for a variety of reasons (eg, to address access problems, to treat acute illness, to provide respite care). Treatment space in either the home HD training area, hospital, or satellite HD facilities needs to be available to care for patients during times when they are ill or are unable to perform home treatments themselves

Q: What should be done if the home HD program is running (or anticipated to run) a budgetary negative variance (ie, costs are higher than incoming funding)?

- Determine if payers provide "start-up" funds to cover the initial costs of starting the program
- Determine if the dialysis provider would be willing to lower costs in the initial phase of the program when patient numbers are low
- Determine if the home HD program can be administratively combined with programs running a budget with a positive variance (eg, combined with a PD program or a hospital/satellite HD program)

Home HD Training and Physical / Organizational Infrastructure

Q: Where will home HD training be performed, and where will the home HD hub be located?

- Possibilities include a purpose-built training and clinical support center; within an existing community health building, main hospital, or satellite HD facilities; or in another existing hospital space. For small programs, training can even be performed in the patient's home. There will, however, always be a requirement for some clinic space to accommodate additional functions that support the entire patient journey (eg, clinical support, respite HD for patients). In smaller institutions, home HD and PD programs are co-located to allow for shared physical and human resources. For some, there is sufficient scale for each program to exist independently, and the infrastructure can be dedicated and orientated to purely home HD (see "The Home Hemodialysis Hub - Physical Infrastructure and Integrated Governance Structure" module)

Q: When will training occur?

- Home HD is often attractive to patients who are still employed. They may prefer to train at nights or on weekends

Capital Equipment

Capital equipment is one cost category where home HD is more expensive than facility HD. For facilities, an item such as a HD machine is typically shared among 6 patients, and a water treatment plant would supply water to all of the patients in a dialysis unit. In the home setting, each patient needs his or her own HD machine and water treatment equipment. In addition, the patient's home may require moderate renovations to provide sufficient water, drainage, and electrical service to the room where the treatments will be performed (see "Infrastructure, Water, and Machines in the Home"). Additional items may be required for patient purchase, such as scales and blood pressure machines (see "Patient Borne Costs" section).

The major capital purchases for the home will include the HD machine and the water treatment system.

Q: How will this equipment be purchased or provided?

- Determine if the full amount will be required at the time of equipment acquisition, or verify if the vendor will allow for the capital costs to be incorporated into the ongoing supply costs, spreading the cost of purchasing the machines (lease model) over a period of time

Q: How many HD and water treatment machines are needed for the program?

- Consider expected patient enrollment as well as extra equipment, as discussed in the "**HD Machine** Maintenance and Delivery **of Supplies**" section
- Consider the expected duty-cycle (life expectancy) of the home equipment. When the equipment is due for retirement, determine what funding will be available for replacing it?
  - » Some programs are required to pay an annual amortization amount on capital equipment. This cost should be incorporated into budget planning. Often, these funds go into the global hospital capital budget. Firm commitments need to be in place so that when the existing equipment reaches the end of its life cycle, these amortization funds are available to the renal unit for purchase of new home HD equipment
- Those starting a new home HD program should be aware of capital cost thresholds in their region. For example, in Ontario, Canada, some funders allow capital requests up to $250,000 to be handled by the dialysis branch of the Ministry of Health. Beyond this level, the capital request must move to a higher level of governmental approval, where it may compete not only against other health-related applications, but against applications related to civic projects such as new roads, schools, etc. It may be beneficial to break a larger capital request into smaller requests dispersed over several years to stay within local capital threshold levels

Staffing

Q: How will nursing and other dialysis staff be hired?

- Possibilities include hiring staff from the PD unit, hospital unit, satellite HD unit, other areas of the health service, or new hires

Additional Resources

- Costs of starting and maintaining a home HD program:
  - » Komenda P, Copland M, Makwana J, Djurdjev O, Sood MM, Levin A. The cost of starting and maintaining a large home hemodialysis program. Kidney Int. 2010; 77:1039-1045.[12]
- Example of payer support for home HD:
  - » Nissenson AR, Moran J. A large dialysis provider committed to home modalities. Am J Kidney Dis. 2012; 59:739; author reply 739-740.[13]
- Example of a centralized home HD training model:
  - » Honkanen EO, Rauta VM. What happened in Finland to increase home hemodialysis? Hemodial Int. 2008; 12 Suppl 1:S11-15.[14]
- Example of home HD training in a Japanese HD facility:
  - » Tomita K. Practice of home hemodialysis in dialysis clinic. Contrib Nephrol. 2012; 177:143-150.[15]
- Home training support for patients in remote areas:
  - » Zacharias J, Komenda P, Olson J, Bourne A, Franklin D, Bernstein K. Home hemodialysis in the remote Canadian north: treatment in Manitoba fly-in communities. Semin Dial. 2011; 24:653-657.[16]

- In planning the number of required home HD training staff, it is important to consider how the home HD program will scale up from a small start-up to the full program

Q: How will technical support for home HD machines be provided?

- Possibilities include contracting with the dialysis HD machine provider or via hospital employees (biomedical engineers)

Q: What types of after-hours support will be provided to your home HD patients?

- Possibilities include 24/7 on-call renal nurses, dialysis machine technicians, hospital ward or emergency department staff, or none

Q: Will a nurse and/or technician home visiting service be provided?

- Most programs plan for periodic home visits by nurses and other health professionals. A number of issues that will impact program budgets and resources need to be considered:
  - » Determine how transportation will be provided for home visits (eg, taxi, hospital car, staff members' own vehicles, public transportation)
  - » For purposes of staff safety and security, many programs require at least 2 staff members perform a home visit. This off-site activity needs to be accounted for when planning staffing requirements

Q: How many staff and transportation vehicles are needed for home visits?

Q: How will new home HD staff be trained and developed? (See "Workforce Development and Models of Care" module)

HD Machine Maintenance and Delivery of Supplies

Q: What mechanism will be used for stock-take and delivery of supplies to patients' homes?

- Possibilities include an arrangement by the dialysis company or equipment vendor, or as an extension of hospital stores. Typically the dialysis company or equipment vendor provides this service

Q: Who will be in charge of ordering supplies?

- Typically it is the patient who tracks supply levels, orders when needed, and coordinates delivery times; however, this can lead to ordering an inappropriate number of supplies. Over-ordering may result in extra charges to the program for supplies that expire or go unused. Under-ordering can result in a patient not having essential items, necessitating urgent deliveries either by the vendor or the program

Q: In the case of using the dialysis vendor's systems, how will this be incorporated into the patient contract?

- Consider which party is liable for charges related to nonstandard deliveries (eg, special deliveries when a patient's dialysis prescription is changed, when a patient runs out of a particular item, or when a patient forgets to phone in their supply order)
- Similarly, determine who will be liable for extra delivery services for patients who require more frequent deliveries (eg, some patients need weekly deliveries of supplies due to highly restricted storage space in a small home)
- In the case of the home HD program providing this service, consideration should be given to the costs of stockpiling supplies and providing personnel and equipment to accept incoming orders from patients, and to coordinate the delivery service

Additional Resources

- Example of building a home HD unit from an existing PD unit:
  - » Borg DL, Keller JA, Faber MD. Adding home hemodialysis (HDD) to a peritoneal dialysis (PD) program. Nephrol Nurs J. 2007; 34:138.[17]
- Examples of resources required to start a new home HD program:
  - » Agar JW. Home hemodialysis in Australia and New Zealand: practical problems and solutions. Hemodial Int. 2008; 12 Suppl 1:S26-32.[18]
  - » Moran J, Kraus M. Starting a home hemodialysis program. Semin Dial. 2007; 20:35-39.[19]

Q: Waste management and disposal in the community: are there any local restrictions?

- If there are special disposal rules for used dialysis supplies, then the costs of recovering and disposing of waste items needs to be considered

Q: What are the arrangements for initial home HD power and water setup in patients' homes?

- Costs of setup will include modification of the home to provide adequate power and water for home HD. Some locales may require building permits prior to home modifications, which come at an additional cost
- Determine who will pay for this
  - » Some programs pay for all installation costs while others pay none of these costs. Some programs split the costs in some manner between the patient and program
  - » Determine if there will be an installation cost ceiling
- While some homes are modern and easily adapted for home HD, others require extensive retrofitting that can be costly. Determine at what point a home inspection will be performed
- Determine how contracts with plumbers, electricians, and other installation tradespeople will be managed
  - » One approach is to allocate a component of operational budgets for machine maintenance for each new patient setup
  - » Determine who will be responsible for ensuring the quality of the work
  - » It is important to remember that these modifications are being made in a patient's home, often in the bedroom. The installation of electrical and water services for a home HD system must not only meet technical and regulatory standards, but also be aesthetically pleasing. Patients will likely object to installations that are highly disruptive of the look of the home

Q: Who will pay for the home utilities including heating, power, and water?

- Possibilities include patients, local government, or patients with a subsidy from the government

Q: How will maintenance of the dialysis equipment be performed?

- Consider both routine and urgent maintenance (when equipment has failed). Determine if maintenance will be provided on-site in the patient's home, or will the equipment be swapped with a back-up machine
- If on-site maintenance is planned, determine if it will be provided by the equipment vendor or by the home HD program
  - » If provided by the vendor, then the terms of this service must be clear and incorporated into the contract
  - » If provided by the program, then the program needs to provide (1) sufficient technical personnel, (2) a stockpile of parts, and (3) a method of transporting both equipment and technicians to the patient's home
  - » Consider policies that limit the number of visits to the patient's home. Multiple visits to repair equipment can be very disruptive
- The program will need to maintain a pool of extra dialysis machines and water treatment systems to replace malfunctioning equipment that cannot be repaired in a timely manner
- If equipment is to be swapped for routine and urgent maintenance, several factors need to be considered
  - » Determine how equipment will be packaged and delivered. Consider both the replacement equipment being delivered to the patient, as well as the existing equipment being returned to the program
  - » Determine what types of delivery service guarantees will need to be in place (eg, timeliness of delivery, weekends and weekdays, care for fragile equipment)

- Consider how back-up equipment will be provided to those patients who live long distances from the dialysis program

Q: Who will provide periodic water monitoring, and what are the costs of this ongoing monitoring?

- It is important that the medical and administrative leads be familiar with local water quality regulations for the production of dialysate. These regulations will specify the standards for water quality, as well as the frequency and type of monitoring required (see "Infrastructure, Water, and Machines in the Home")
- A clear delineation of responsibility for water quality is required. Typically, this rests with the medical director of the program, even when water testing is performed by external agencies

Q: How will maintenance of the water system be performed?

- Examples include swapping of carbon tanks and replacement of reverse osmosis (RO) filters
- Programs can combine staff visits with other home-based activities (eg, routine maintenance, water sampling)

Q: Who will pay for any renovations to the home required for the patient to initiate home HD?

- See "Checklist for Costs Related to Infrastructure for HD in the Home" in the Appendix

Q: Many rented or leased homes require that any dialysis-related alterations made to the home will be removed and the home restored to predialysis condition when the patient moves.

- Determine who will cover these costs

Q: If the program is covering costs related to home renovations, is there any limit to the number of times a patient can change residence?

Q: Who will pay for assorted single-time purchases such as scales, blood pressure machines, tables to hold equipment and supplies, recliner chairs, and leak detectors, if appropriate?

Q: How will the increased cost of power and water be handled?

Patient-Specific Costs

In a home HD program, some cost categories are moved from the program to the patient, which can potentially offset the benefits of home HD for the patient through avoiding other costs related to, for example, transport and parking. For example, home HD is associated with an increased demand for power and water, which are often paid for by the patient. Consideration should be given to the costs that may be borne by the patient and how these would be handled if the patient did not have sufficient resources to pay for them. It is important to be clear from the start who bears the financial responsibility for what costs, if necessary, by legal agreement.

Additional Resources

- Published examples of the costs of a home HD program:
  - » McFarlane P, Komenda P. Economic considerations in frequent home hemodialysis. Semin Dial. 2011; 24:678-683.[20]
  - » Komenda P, Copland M, Makwana J, Djurdjev O, Sood MM, Levin A. The cost of starting and maintaining a large home hemodialysis program. Kidney Int. 2010; 77:1039-1045.[12]

Writing a Business Case for a Home HD Program

The next step in establishing a home HD program is to secure funding for capital and operational expenses and initiate the procurement of the necessary goods and services. To do so, most private and public payers require a business case: a document designed to justify expenditure of money and effort in order to make a decision on funding.

A compelling business case is a well-structured and logical document. It captures the expected clinical benefits of developing a viable home HD program for the patient, identifies the required resources, defines models of care, and determines the relative priority of the program in relation to competing initiatives.[21]

For the payer, the business case helps reassure that:

1. The program is a high-value opportunity with measurable and accountable clinical benefits
2. The nephrology service can deliver the purported benefits
3. Due consideration has been given to complex interdependencies with other services such as surgery, radiology, and information technology; and
4. Quality, patient safety, and incident management aspects of the program have been considered and incorporated

Occasionally, there will be payer templates available to use in preparing business cases; these should be followed strictly. More often, business cases are formal but unscripted, and should contain the key elements listed in Table 1.

Table 1. Key Requirements of a Business Case

Section	Key Requirements
Table of Contents	Display organization of the document and page numbers
Glossary	Define key terms
Executive Briefing or Summary	Convey to the audience what they can expect in the document. This section is an opportunity to have an immediate impact by presenting a succinct and compelling story around home HD
Introduction or Background	State the clinical need for home HD, include an opportunity statement (ie, the potential opportunities this service could provide), and establish a sense of urgency for the solution
Service Objectives and Critical Success Factors	Clearly explain how the home HD project outlined in the business case is connected to the strategic goals of the dialysis service, hospital, or provider
Approach or Methodology	Convey a deep understanding of the current clinical and financial landscapes using data and analyses—this is a crucial component of the business plan. If the payers do not understand or concur with the assessments in the business case, they will not be convinced enough to agree to its final recommendations around home HD
Overall Scenario Analysis or Justification	Provide high-level descriptions of the service options, tell how they fit within the existing organization, and note the key differences between service offerings so that the reader can quickly compare options. The financial analysis must answer the following key question: "Do the proposed options result in cost savings and/or avoidance of cost over an acceptable timeframe to the payer, or provide additional clinical effectiveness at an acceptable cost?"
Linkages and Stakeholder Summary	Identify any additional resources that may be needed, including the larger team required to make implementation a success
Implementation	Lay out a high-level plan for implementing the home HD program
Risks and Mitigation	Highlight the key risks to successful implementation

Glossary

- Provide a list of key terms used in the business case that may be unfamiliar to the payer (see Appendix)

Executive Briefing or Summary

- This should be succinct, and at most 1 to 2 pages long. The Briefing/Summary might start with foundational statements highlighting the limitations of facility HD (negative impact on clinical and patient-centered outcomes, high healthcare costs, etc.) and the benefits of home HD (clinical and patient-centered benefits, affordability)
- The Briefing/Summary should then:
    - » Summarize the clinical and financial data used for synthesis of recommendations
    - » Highlight, if appropriate, any unmet clinical need and the current difficulties with dialysis service provision (unsustainable growth in patient numbers, inadequate facility HD staff and infrastructure, unsustainable healthcare costs, etc.)
    - » Summarize recommendations contained in the business case
    - » State the recommended decision to be made by payers

Introduction or Background

- This section should contain the clinical and financial case for the home HD program relative to other competing options. This is an important section, because there is often a high degree of uncertainty about the possibility of financing home HD with payers. It is necessary, therefore, to highlight the clinical evidence supporting home HD to ensure a strong negotiating position with payers
- Provide necessary background for the reader by starting with a ***general description*** of conventional and frequent or extended-hour home HD, referencing national or international service trends around home HD use, and recommendations from local policies or clinical practice guidelines around optimal modality mix for services, or optimal modality selection for particular patient groups[22]
- Next, provide a subsection outlining the ***expected benefits of home HD*** compared with in-center (facility) HD.[23] The business case needs to include clinical benefits of frequent and/or extended-hour modalities, because the establishment of a home HD program offers this technique to everyone, whether or not they choose to use it. The key benefits are as follows:
    - » Patient
        - – Improved patient satisfaction and independence/empowerment[24-26]
        - – Improved quality of life[4, 5]
        - – Fewer dietary and fluid restrictions[27, 28]
        - – Added convenience[29]
        - – Reduced impact on family life[4]
        - – Improved maintenance of social functioning[4]
        - – Clinical benefits to the patient
            - › Reduced associated mortality risk compared with PD and other HD modalities[10, 30-33]
            - › Regression of left ventricular mass[34-35]
            - › Improved blood pressure control[36]
            - › Improved serum phosphate control[37]
            - › Greater chance of successful pregnancy[38, 39]
            - › Increased urea clearance[25, 40]
    - » Healthcare costs
        - – Reduced travel costs for patients[41]
        - – Reduced medication costs due to improved blood pressure control and improved mineral metabolism[34, 35, 40]
        - – Reduced dialysis staffing costs[41]
        - – Reduced costs from constrained facility HD infrastructure
- A ***situational analysis*** should be included that defines renal replacement therapy within the current dialysis service, provides growth projections in terms of dialysis populations and modality mix, provides geographical mapping, and offers a summary of the strategic direction and optimal clinical model for dialysis services within the organization. Ideally, this includes a patient segmentation exercise to determine the expected demand for home HD in the service. It is vital that the modeled demand for home HD patients is realistically aligned to the potential within the current patient population
- The situational analysis should also provide a ***gap analysis***. This analysis is a comparison between the current situation with respect to delivery of home HD vs the optimal or future situation
- It is vital that the business case considers a ***range of options*** as alternatives to home HD, as well as the option of doing nothing (that is, maintaining a similar patient distribution among the different modalities). It often helps to have a patient dialysis modality profile such as the one offered in Table 2. This is not a guide defining those who can perform home HD or derive benefit from this therapy: instead, it builds a portrait of potential patients for those in clinical governance and executive leadership groups who may have very little experience in dealing with renal patients in general and dialysis in particular. In our experience, this has been a very useful inclusion in business cases

Table 2. Patient Dialysis Modality Profiles

Patient Dialysis Modality	Key Characteristic	Location	Examples of *Typical* Demographic (needs to be localized to each service)	Specialist Clinical Support
Dependent stable +/- medically unstable	Model of care is provided by specialist clinical support	In-center or hospital HD facility	• Person aged > 75 years • Person with ≥ 3 comorbidities • Requires social or functional assistance at home • Not working	• Access to acute medical services • High nursing input (eg, dressings) • Requires specialist HCP review approximately weekly • Frequent hospital admissions
Self-care	Patients who are expected to perform a portion of their dialysis treatment	Satellite HD facility	• Person aged > 60 years • Person with 1-4 comorbidities • May require some social or functional assistance at home • < 50% working or full-time house duties	• Low nursing input • Specialist HCP review approximately monthly
Home HD	Patients who are expected to perform their dialysis procedure independently after training	Home setting	• Person aged < 70 years • Person with 1-4 comorbidities • Independent at home • > 50% working or full-time house duties	• Low nursing input • Monthly laboratory review • Self-manages dialysis at home • Primary contact is primary nurse • Specialist HCP review ≤ monthly
Peritoneal dialysis	Patients who are expected to perform their dialysis procedure independently after training	Home Setting	• Person aged < 70 years • Person with 1-4 comorbidities • May require some social or functional assistance at home • < 50% working or full-time house duties	• Low nursing input • Monthly laboratory review • Self-manages dialysis at home • Primary contact is primary nurse • Specialist HCP review ≤ monthly

HCP = healthcare provider.

Service Objectives and Critical Success Factors

- This section should contain definitions for service objectives, which are the anticipated benefits of starting or expanding the home HD program. These objectives can be used to compare the option of home HD with other dialysis modalities. Some examples of commonly used service objectives are provided in Table 3
- The ***critical success factors*** in Table 4 can be used to score the various options

Table 3. Commonly Used Service Objectives in Business Cases for Home HD

Service Objectives	Definition	Exemplary Considerations
Clinical Results	Optimizing clinical outcomes of the service	Do the proposed solutions improve patient outcomes (eg, mortality and health-related quality of life), increase patient safety, or decreased hospitalization?
Access to Optimal Care	Bringing the clinical and patient benefits of home HD to the service in an equitable manner	Do the proposed solutions increase the proportion of patients treated with home HD, especially frequent or extended-hours HD, including those in geographically remote areas?
Meeting Dialysis Demand	Ensuring sufficient service dialysis capacity to enable treatment to new patients	Do the proposed solutions provide adequate capacity for growth in patient numbers over the period of the proposal?
Constraining Facility HD Capacity	Providing an alternative to facility HD capacity investment, thereby using this resource more efficiently for the more dependent patient group that needs it most	Do the proposed solutions avoid significant investment in infrastructure through decreased relative utilization of facility HD, or improve access to care through community-based health service delivery?
Safety	Providing a clinically safe and sustainable service	Are the proposed solutions likely to result in excess patient mortality, hospitalization, or emergency care consultations?

Table 4. Commonly Used Service Objectives for Determining Critical Success Factors in Business Cases for Home HD

Objectives	Scoring
Service Objectives	The extent to which objectives of clinical care are realized by the proposed option
Strategic Fit	The extent to which the proposed solution meets the strategic objectives of the healthcare organization, as well as regional and national objectives
Achievability	The capacity and capability of the service to implement the proposed solution within required timelines
Scalability	The extent to which the proposed solution can be expanded or contracted to meet demand
Affordability	The ability of the payer to afford the capital and operating costs of the proposed solution

Approach or Methodology

- This section describes the research methods and sources of data used in the business case. Sufficient information around the approach and methodology used in this exercise will convince payers of the credibility and validity of the business case. For instance, if the scenario analysis uses prevalence and modeled growth data, then the source of those data and the methods for modelling should be described. If the analysis uses new data on qualitative issues that have been collected as part of business case, the method should also be described (focus groups, ethnography, stakeholder interviews, surveys)

Overall Scenario Analysis or Justification

- This section contains a description of the home HD program option and each alternative option, along with financial analyses for each. For payers, home HD is perceived to have high initial setup and training costs with an uncertain financial payback period. Therefore, it is essential to have a high degree of clarity around the implementation and cost models for home HD. Ambiguity may increase the likelihood that the payer will fail to consider new alternatives and default to facility HD
- Evidence should be provided for each option in an *overall scenario analysis*. In this analysis, there is a detailed description of each option within the business case, justifications for models of care, and robust financial evaluations. Each option should be assessed against the clinical objectives and scored using the critical success factors illustrated in Table 5
- A key part of the Overall Scenario Analysis section is *financial analysis*, which includes the costs and risks of inactivity. Although this is important, it is often impossible to precisely quantify costs until a preferred option is identified from the RFP. As such, costing is often based on a number of assumptions around the costs and outcomes of each option. The general method to perform a financial evaluation is as follows:
  - » Apply all calculations over an agreed timeframe (eg, 5 years)
  - » Determine expected growth rate of the dialysis population
  - » Create scenarios based on different patient distributions in the future across different modalities, considering local nuances such as self-care and satellite HD, because these may significantly alter estimates of cost and reimbursement. When modelling home HD, take into account dropouts to facility HD and transplantation. Depending on the setting, dropout from home HD may be on the order of 20% per year, mostly due to transplantation and illness resulting in a transfer to facility HD

» Perform the cost calculation on a per-year basis for each modality. Three considerations should be made:

1. It is important to break down the patient distribution to frequency per modality (eg, 4 sessions per week home HD), as the treatment schedule also affects the cost
2. Where possible, a full-cost accounting approach should be used, which takes into account all direct and indirect costs
3. An increase in home HD patients in the program leads to more home HD machines proportionally than a corresponding increase for facility HD, and, therefore, different capital costs

» Costs categories might include those related to:

- Staff (including departmental and administration overheads, direct and indirect nursing care, technical support)
- Facilities (including utilities and equipment)
- Dialysis machinery, consumables, and technical considerations (machine purchase or lease, technical support, water management and treatment, waste management)
- Additional miscellaneous costs (medication, transportation, training costs for home HD, utilities and home equipment for home HD, etc.)

» In dialysis services that are block-funded (ie, one funding source to be dispersed as the clinic sees appropriate), these cost calculations will suffice. For those that are revenue or activity-base funded, the operational margin per modality should be calculated to identify the difference between the reimbursement level and the costs for a specific modality

Table 5. Commonly Used Service Objectives and Sample Scoring Matrix for a Home HD Business Case

Dialysis Service Options	Critical Success Factor (score)				
	Service Objectives (1)	Strategic Fit (2)	Achievability (3)	Scalability (4)	Affordability (5)
Home HD	✓	✓	✓	✓ or × ?	✓
Option B	×	✓	✓	×	×
Option C ...n	...	...	...	...	...

Linkages and Stakeholder Summary

- Detail in this section any organizational changes expected to allow the home HD program to be implemented, and acknowledge the independent requirements from other clinical and logistic services. Consider including the following issues:
    - » New infrastructure and space requirements (eg, offices, space for patient training, patient waiting area, respite care)
    - » Modifications to existing infrastructure and spaces (eg, construction, plumbing, and electrical work)
    - » Clinical process changes and modified patient pathways
    - » Workforce development and new roles and responsibilities for the home HD program (new nursing and medical supervision requirements, new administrative roles)
    - » Impact, if any, of the home HD program on surgery and radiology
    - » Information technology (IT) system requirements
- Do not forget to identify or quantify any improvements in resource utilization arising from the home HD program (ie, freed capacity from constrained growth for facility HD)
- In this section, it is also useful to provide a list of the stakeholders who have been consulted in the development in the business case. This helps reassure the payer that complex requirements and relationships have been considered, and there is a low likelihood of unforeseen challenges that might derail or delay the implementation of the business case

Implementation

- This section defines timelines for the initiation of the first patient in the home HD program and serves as a checklist of milestones that should be achieved along the way

Risks and Mitigation

- Explain what might not go as planned and categorize the likelihood of the risks as high, moderate, or low. If there do not appear to be any foreseeable risks, it is important to ensure that the audience realizes that this is a considered position, and that this issues have been thought through
- The primary risks to be considered are to costs and schedule. For example:
    - » What if the costs or availability of home HD machinery changes?
    - » What if the project manager or team changes or leaves? What if the home HD champion or clinical lead changes or leaves?
    - » What if clinicians or patients struggle to adopt or adapt to the new home HD program?
    - » What if the home HD equipment or infrastructure does not perform as expected (eg, quality, performance)?
    - » What if vendors do not deliver on time?
    - » What if the cost of raw materials increases?
- In this section, propose strategies to mitigate these risks and identify any opportunities that might arise

Dealing with RFPs

When a large contract or capital proposal is being offered to vendors, most private and public payers require that a RFP or request for tender (RFT) process be followed. The RFP process is usually highly scripted, with many rules and regulations. In the case of publicly funded systems, the RFP process may be codified in law. In all cases, the RFP process *must* strictly adhere to the local rules and guidelines to protect the program from a variety of liabilities. As a result, it is in the interest of those starting a new home HD program to become familiar with their local RFP process.

Before embarking on an RFP for home HD equipment and service, it is important to become familiar with the strengths and weaknesses of various vendors. Once an RFP is open for tender, it usually cannot be altered. The RFP process is not the time to learn about what vendors are able to offer—this should be done before construction of the RFP. The RFP is best written by a multidisciplinary home HD program team, including an experienced dialysis nurse and technician. This team will research the following topics and consider the costs, where applicable.

The HD Machine

- Research and choose the best HD machines available for home use. From the short list of selected machines, the team will determine the best machine option by assessing the following questions:
  - » Is the machine appropriate for the home setting? Consider the size, noise level, ease of use, screens that can be accessed from the supine position for those patients undergoing nocturnal treatment
  - » Will it be easy to train patients on this system? For example, does the machine take the patient step by step through the procedures for starting and finishing dialysis?
  - » How long does it take to set up the machine and to disconnect from a treatment? How many steps are required to perform these tasks?
  - » Is the machine easy to maintain and repair?
  - » Is it flexible enough to provide a variety of forms of dialysis? For example, quotidian nocturnal HD with long treatment times using low blood and dialysate flows, and conventional HD with fast pump speeds?
  - » What safety features are provided (eg, blood leak/needle disconnect sensors, blood pressure monitors)?
  - » What language requirements are there in your home HD program, and does, or can, the dialysis machine support specific language requirements?
    - – What range of dialysate concentrates is available, and do these dialysates meet the various needs of your patients (eg, nocturnal HD often requires a higher calcium dialysate; patients performing extra hours of HD per week may not need a very high bicarbonate concentration or very low dialysate potassium)?
  - » How easy is it to "spike" the dialysate to customize the composition (eg, adding calcium or phosphate to the dialysate)?
  - » Home HD equipment is often located in less than ideal environments and may not be treated gently at all times. How robust is the equipment?
  - » What happens if the power fails during treatment? Can the machine recover from short power failures? What are the procedures for returning the blood after a power failure?
  - » How quickly can the equipment be ready to provide the next treatment?
  - » What are ongoing maintenance requirements for the machine, and how difficult will maintenance be for the patient to contend with?
  - » Modern HD machines offer a wide range of additional features, some of which may not be of particular value in the home setting; however, they may still be desired. The program team needs to decide if they value features such as online hematocrit monitoring, sodium profiling, etc., before investing in a machine that includes these features

The Water Treatment Equipment

- Is ultrapure dialysate desired, and if so, can the water system provide that?
- The RO unit is often the loudest part of the system. What is the volume level while operating the water treatment system?
- How can leaks be detected and how will leak status be communicated to the patient?
- Is the water treatment system integrated with the dialysis machine? Will it be provided by the same vendor?
- How easy is the machine to maintain and to clean?
- The patient will typically perform the routine cleaning. Will they also be doing tasks such as replacing RO cartridges?
- Will the vendor provide maintenance and/or supply delivery services? (See "Ongoing Maintenance and Supply Delivery" section)
- Will the vendor provide after-hours support, service, or maintenance? (See "HD Machine Maintenance and Delivery of Supplies" section.)
- Does the vendor already provide these services in your region? What is their reputation for reliability? Speaking to senior technicians from other home HD programs may be useful

Information Technology

- What IT systems will be requested from the vendor? These can range from simple systems that interface with the HD machines to full electronic medical records
- What are the purchase costs for the IT systems? Are there ongoing charges for the use of these systems?
- How will home equipment and patients interface with these systems? What equipment will be needed in the home for this? What type of IT connection will be required (eg, high-speed Internet)? Who will pay for the costs of connection?

Full-Service Provision Options

- Has due consideration been given for outsourcing of the home HD service, in terms of partnership with a large dialysis organization (LDO)? This is an emerging clinical and business model and is an arguably easier way to start a home HD program, where clinical and financial risks may be mitigated by an experienced LDO

Once the home HD program team has become familiar with the offerings of the various vendors active in their region, the RFP can then be constructed. It is crucial that the program team be clear about which features and services they expect from the vendor and their equipment. The program team should construct a "wish list" of desired features and rank them in terms of importance. Some features are critical and a vendor will be eliminated if they cannot deliver this feature. Others will be desirable, but will not necessarily be deal breakers if they are absent. Proper construction of the "wish list" is important because most RFP processes require not only a list of desired features, but the weighting applied to each of these features. The vendors will be asked to submit a list of services and equipment that will be provided, and a list of charges. The program team should understand its budgetary limitations before constructing the RFP and consider what weight will be applied to the budget component of the RFP.

It is extremely important that the RFP be constructed properly. The RFP should be written in a manner that ensures that the program team is able to select a vendor that will meet not only all of their needs but also the program's budgetary requirements as well. A vague and poorly written RFP may lead to selection of an inappropriate vendor.

Because the RFP process is highly regulated, the program team involved in creating the RFP should understand the local rules governing that process. For example, once the RFP is completed and open for vendors to review, changes to the contents of the RFP are usually not permitted. Interaction between the vendors and the team is usually highly restricted. For example, the program team may not be allowed to meet or communicate with members of a vendor company outside of the channels of communication that are part of the RFP process. Team members participating in developing the RFP should also be prepared to give a detailed list of potential conflicts of interest, based on previous involvement with the each vendor.

Conclusion

Planning and funding a home HD program requires a well-organized effort and close collaboration between clinicians and managers. Up to a year should be allocated for the following:

- A thorough situational analysis of the dialysis landscape, emphasizing the opportunity for a home HD program
- Careful consideration of the clinical and operational characteristics of a proposed home HD program at your institution
- The development of a compelling business case, highlighting the clinical and organizational benefits of a home HD program
- Careful construction and evaluation of an RFP

References

1. Data on file. Baxter Healthcare Japan Ltd. 2014.
2. ANZDATA Registry. Summary of Australia and New Zealand Dialysis and Transplantation 2012. Adelaide, Australia. Available at: http://www.anzdata.org.au/anzdata/AnzdataReport/36thReport/2012_Summary_v1.pdf. Accessed September 4, 2014.
3. Tong A, Palmer S, Manns B, et al. Clinician beliefs and attitudes about home haemodialysis: a multinational interview study. BMJ Open. 2012; 2:e002146.
4. Mowatt G, Vale L, Perez J, et al. Systematic review of the effectiveness and cost-effectiveness, and economic evaluation, of home versus hospital or satellite unit haemodialysis for people with end-stage renal failure. Health Technol Assess. 2003; 7:1-174.
5. Dale PL, Hutton J, Elgazzar H. Utility of health states in chronic kidney disease: a structured review of the literature. Curr Med Res Opin. 2008; 24:193-206.
6. Walker R, Marshall M, Morton RL, McFarlane P, Howard K. The cost effectiveness of contemporary home haemodialysis modalities compared to facility haemodialysis: a systematic review of full economic evaluations. Nephrology (Carlton). 2014; 19:459-470
7. Ananthapavan J, Lowin J, Bloomfield E. Economic report: home haemodialysis (CEP10063). London, UK: NHS Purchasing and Supply Agency; 2010. Available at: http://nhscep.useconnect.co.uk/CEPProducts/Catalogue.aspx?ReportType=Economic+report. Accessed June 10, 2014.
8. Mackenzie P, Mactier RA. Home haemodialysis in the 1990s. Nephrol Dial Transplant. 1998; 13:1944-1948.
9. Delano BG, Feinroth MV, Reinroth M, Friedman EA. Home and medical center hemodialysis. Dollar comparison and payback period. JAMA. 1982; 246:230-232.
10. Marshall MR, Hawley CM, Kerr PG, et al. Home hemodialysis and mortality risk in Australian and New Zealand populations. Am J Kidney Dis. 2011; 58:782-793.
11. Mendelssohn DC, Curtin B, Yeates K, et al. Suboptimal initiation of dialysis with and without early referral to a nephrologist. Nephrol Dial Transplant. 2011; 26:2959-2956.
12. Komenda P, Copland M, Makwana J, et al. The cost of starting and maintaining a large home hemodialysis program. Kidney Int. 2010; 77:1039-1045.
13. Nissenson AR, Moran J. A large dialysis provider committed to home modalities. Am J Kidney Dis. 2012; 59:739; author reply 739-740.
14. Honkanen EO, Rauta VM. What happened in Finland to increase home hemodialysis? Hemodial Int. 2008; 12 Suppl 1:S11-15.
15. Tomita K. Practice of home hemodialysis in dialysis clinic. Contrib Nephrol. 2012;177:143-150.
16. Zacharias J, Komenda P, Olson J, et al. Home hemodialysis in the remote Canadian north: treatment in Manitoba fly-in communities. Semin Dial. 2011; 24:653-657.
17. Borg DL, Keller JA, Faber MD. Adding home hemodialysis (HDD) to a peritoneal dialysis (PD) program. Nephrol Nurs J. 2007; 34:138.
18. Agar JW. Home hemodialysis in Australia and New Zealand: practical problems and solutions. Hemodial Int. 2008; 12 Suppl 1:S26-32.
19. Moran J, Kraus M. Starting a home hemodialysis program. Semin Dial. 2007;20:35-39.
20. McFarlane P, Komenda P. Economic considerations in frequent home hemodialysis. Semin Dial. 2011; 24:678-683.
21. Adams A. ABC MedTech Case. In: Sheen R, Gallo A, eds. HBR Guide to Building Your Business Case Ebook + Tools. Boston: Harvard Business Review Press. 2012; 1-23.

References (cont'd)

22. Technology Appraisal Guidance No. 48; Guidance on home compared with hospital haemodialysis for patients with end-stage renal failure. London: National Institute for Health and Care Excellence; 2005.

23. Masterson R. The advantages and disadvantages of home hemodialysis. Hemodial Int. 2008; 12 Suppl 1:S16-20.

24. Christensen AJ, Smith TW, Turner CW, Holman JM Jr, Gregory MC. Type of hemodialysis and preference for behavioral involvement: interactive effects on adherence in end-stage renal disease. Health Psychol. 1990; 9:225-236.

25. Polaschek N. Haemodialysing at home: the client experience of self-treatment. EDTNA ERCA J. 2005; 31:27-30.

26. Polaschek N. Client attitudes towards home dialysis therapy. J Ren Care. 2007; 33:20-24.

27. Schorr M, Manns BJ, Culleton B, et al. The effect of nocturnal and conventional hemodialysis on markers of nutritional status: results from a randomized trial. J Ren Nutr. 2011; 21:271-276.

28. Kraus M, Burkart J, Hegeman R, et al. A comparison of center-based vs. home-based daily hemodialysis for patients with end-stage renal disease. Hemodial Int. 2007; 11:468-477.

29. Levy J. Home dialysis can improve quality of life. Practitioner. 2007; 251:8,10-12, 14, 15.

30. Blagg CR, Kjellstrand CM, Ting GO, Young BA. Comparison of survival between short-daily hemodialysis and conventional hemodialysis using the standardized mortality ratio. Hemodial Int. 2006; 10:371-374.

31. Kjellstrand CM, Buoncristiani U, Ting G, et al. Short daily haemodialysis: survival in 415 patients treated for 1006 patient-years. Nephrol Dial Transplant. 2008; 23:3283-3289.

32. Nesrallah GE, Lindsay RM, Cuerden MS, et al. Intensive hemodialysis associates with improved survival compared with conventional hemodialysis. J Am Soc Nephrol. 2012; 23:696-705.

33. Johansen KL, Zhang R, Huang Y, et al. Survival and hospitalization among patients using nocturnal and short daily compared to conventional hemodialysis: a USRDS study. Kidney Int. 2009; 76:984-990.

34. Culleton BF, Walsh M, Klarenbach SW, et al. Effect of frequent nocturnal hemodialysis vs conventional hemodialysis on left ventricular mass and quality of life: a randomized controlled trial. JAMA. 2007; 298:1291-1299.

35. FHN Trial Group, Chertow GM, Levin NW, et al. In-center hemodialysis six times per week versus three times per week. N Engl J Med. 2010; 363:2287-2300.

36. Nesrallah G, Suri R, Moist L, Kortas C, Lindsay RM. Volume control and blood pressure management in patients undergoing quotidian hemodialysis. Am J Kidney Dis. 2003; 42:13-17.

37. Mucsi I, Hercz G, Uldall R, et al. Control of serum phosphate without any phosphate binders in patients treated with nocturnal hemodialysis. Kidney Int. 1998; 53:1399-1404.

38. Hladunewich MA, Hou S, Odutayo A, et al. Intensive hemodialysis associates with improved pregnancy outcomes: a Canadian and United States cohort comparison. J Am Soc Nephrol. 2014; 25:1103-1109.

39. Barua M, Hladunewich M, Keunen J, et al. Successful pregnancies on nocturnal home hemodialysis. Clin J Am Soc Nephrol. 2008; 3:392-396.

40. Rocco MV, Lockridge RS Jr, Beck GJ, et al. The effects of frequent nocturnal home hemodialysis: the Frequent Hemodialysis Network Nocturnal Trial. Kidney Int. 2011; 80:1080-1091.

41. Komenda P, Gavaghan MB, Garfield SS, Poret AW, Sood MM. An economic assessment model for in-center, conventional home, and more frequent home hemodialysis. Kidney Int. 2012; 81:307-313.

Appendix

Funding & Planning

Implementing Hemodialysis in the Home

A Global Perspective

ISHD

International Society for Hemodialysis

Table of Contents

Glossary

The following terms and definitions are specific to dialysis, as discussed in this module.

- Direct costs: Those directly attributable to the dialysis procedure, including capital costs and the portion of operating costs specific to the provision of dialysis. This will include the cost of dialysis machinery and consumables, and salaries for dialysis staff

- Dominant (health economics): The intervention costs less and is at least as effective as the alternative

- Indirect costs: Those costs are not directly attributable to the dialysis procedure, and include costs for overhead, management, insurance, taxes, maintenance, and accommodation

- Payer: The organization that pays for dialysis-related hospital or medical bills instead of the patient. This is often a government-contracted intermediary, an insurance carrier, or managed-care organization

- Provider: Hospitals, physician groups, commercial entities, or other healthcare agencies such as a large dialysis organization that are contracted for the direct delivery of dialysis to the patient

- Vendor: A commercial entity that is engaged by providers in the normal course of business. This is often a manufacturer of dialysis machinery or a reseller

Checklist for Costs Related to Infrastructure for HD in the Home

- ❑ Patient Training and Assessment
    - ❑ For example, training in the dialysis clinic, hospital, or patient's home
    - ❑ Staff visits to the home and associated travel costs
- ❑ The Patient Dwelling
    - ❑ Housing improvements/construction/retrofitting/repairs needed for dialysis-related alterations. Written instructions should be available concerning who is responsible for paying for dwelling alterations in connection with dialysis installation, and how often requirements are to be reassessed
        - Rental properties may have restrictions on what can be modified and whether the dwelling will need to be returned to its original condition if the patient relocates
    - ❑ Extra dialysis outlets (eg, weekend cottage)
    - ❑ The patient may choose to relocate at some point while undergoing home HD. What costs are required to restore home/rental unit to predialysis state? The economic consequences and responsibilities of this action should be outlined and planned for in all legal agreements
    - ❑ Tax considerations. Some dwelling modifications may be tax deductible for patients
- ❑ HD Machine
    - ❑ Rent or purchase
    - ❑ Repairs and maintenance
    - ❑ Replacement

Checklist for Costs Related to Infrastructure for HD in the Home (cont'd)

- ❑ Furnishing and Equipment
  - ❑ Chair
  - ❑ Scales
  - ❑ Cupboard
  - ❑ Lighting
  - ❑ Refrigerator
  - ❑ Leak detectors
  - ❑ Blood pressure equipment
- ❑ Water Supply
  - ❑ Installation and required modifications in the home
  - ❑ Water purification
  - ❑ Water consumption
    - Public water rates can be quite high due to local water shortages or environmental considerations
    - Consider reduction in flow rates to 200 mL/min for long dialysis regimens (eg, nocturnal HD)
    - Water supplied by dialysis vendors may be expensive
  - ❑ Maintenance
- ❑ Water Quality Testing
  - ❑ Cost of testing (eg, provided by the nephrology service or outsourced to a private company)
  - ❑ Frequency
  - ❑ Staff required to perform testing

Checklist for Costs Related to Infrastructure for HD in the Home (cont'd)

- ❑ Water Disposal
  - ❑ Local requirements
- ❑ Plumbing (see Water Supply)
- ❑ Electricity Supply
  - ❑ Installation and required modifications in the home
  - ❑ Safety considerations (eg, additional grounding of electrical wires)
  - ❑ Power surge protector
  - ❑ Backup supply (eg, generator)
  - ❑ Electricity consumption
  - ❑ Maintenance
- ❑ Waste Disposal
  - ❑ Requirement for extra waste bins
  - ❑ Local restrictions and special disposal
- ❑ Communications
  - ❑ Telephone
  - ❑ Internet

Checklist for Costs Related to Infrastructure for HD in the Home (cont'd)

- ❑ Disposables
  - ❑ Filters (single use or reusable)
  - ❑ Dialysis lines
  - ❑ Needles
  - ❑ Dressings and plaster
  - ❑ Disinfectants
  - ❑ Fluids
  - ❑ Delivery charges
- ❑ Medicines
  - ❑ Drugs associated with dialysis process (eg, erythropoietin, intravenous iron)
  - ❑ Fluids (sodium chloride)
- ❑ Assistance
  - ❑ Most dialysis programs expect the dialysis to be performed by the patient, with the possible assistance of an unpaid family member. If paid assistance in the home is considered, the cost of this also needs to be calculated in overall costs
  - ❑ Respite care for patient

3 Workforce Development and Models of Care in Home Hemodialysis

Sandip Mitra, MBBS, MD, FRCP[1]

Cherl Cress, RN, CNN[2]

Tony Goovaerts, RN[3]

[1]Central Manchester University Hospitals, Manchester, UK, [2]Washington University, St Louis, Missouri, USA, [3]University Hospital St Luc, Brussels, Belgium

Implementing Hemodialysis in the Home
A Global Perspective

ISHD
International Society for Hemodialysis

CONTENTS

Abstract

Creating and maintaining a successful home hemodialysis (HD) program is highly dependent on the workforce model and quality of staff. We describe the minimum staff required to start a home HD program (eg, a clinical champion and lead nurse) and detail what additional workforce (eg, renal technician, dietitian, psychologist and others) may be necessary as the program evolves and expands. The goal of the program and allied staff should be to provide a seamless patient journey, a process that requires consideration of a patient recruitment strategy, a patient training pathway, thoughtful initiation of home HD, and development of support systems for routine care and emergencies at home. This module describes how care models are implemented at centers of excellence in various locations around the world, highlights the importance of an integrated care pathway, and describes workforce challenges that programs may encounter.

Introduction

Successful launch and self-sustaining maintenance of an effective home hemodialysis (HD) program depends on a team of professionals with particular expertise and specific skill sets to ensure the best care for patients undergoing HD. Typically, large and successful centers have a well-defined care model delivered by dedicated staff skilled in patient training, monitoring, and support.[1,2] For a care model to be successful, active participation, collaboration, and willingness to be flexible in the face of change are all essential attributes of team members. Home programs can only succeed with a motivated and caring workforce. This module focuses on how to organize such a team to successfully deliver home HD therapies.

The team structure and organization typically develop in stages and evolve over time as the program expands and becomes more established. The profile of the workforce can change with respect to staff members, the variety of skills, and operational responsibilities. At the outset, however, the program has to be led by a clinical champion and a lead trainer, and supported by clinicians, technicians, social workers, community support staff, and an administrator. As the program grows, other key personnel may be required to support patient pathways. The attributes of individuals within these roles are fundamental to the program's success, and they consist of a combination of generic and specific skills for home HD.

Workforce Development

Phase 1

Clinical champion — is a key individual, often at the epicenter of a vibrant and successful home HD program. The program needs a designated individual in charge—from the outset—and can be any one of the following: a dialysis physician, nurse, technician, clinical director, or departmental head. The 2 essential attributes of this individual are: (i) a passion and strong belief in home HD and its benefits in patients with end-stage renal disease, and (ii) leadership skills, with a clear vision and strategy for developing a successful care model.

Sufficient knowledge of the local kidney disease network and its infrastructure is desirable. Other roles for this individual would include the development of a quality assurance and governance framework for care delivery. This individual is a key player in establishing the model, and is often instrumental in energizing the workforce through building confidence, morale, and support for both junior and senior members on the team

Lead trainer / home HD nurse lead — is responsible for setting up a patient training program in home HD. Essential attributes include:

- Sound practical knowledge of HD combined with a passion to teach and empower

- Strong belief in the philosophy of self-care and in the benefits of home HD
- Good communication skills, including an understanding of adult learning techniques and an ability to speak the local language(s)
- Leadership and organizational skills

This individual in this role often takes the lead in the development of policy, procedures, and training pathways, and engages in and promotes staff development opportunities for all team members, including nephrologists, primary care physicians, technicians, in-center staff, and chronic kidney disease (CKD) nurses and trainees. Knowledge and skills in both peritoneal dialysis (PD) and home HD could be particularly useful in integrating home therapies into the care model.[3] In the United States, the Centers for Medicare and Medicaid Services provide regulations for home HD nurses.

Physician/nephrologist — a dialysis physician with an interest in and passion for promoting home HD, with expertise and experience in clinical management of patients on dialysis. Other attributes include skills in quality improvement and the ability to work in an interdisciplinary environment. He or she does not have to be senior member or a newly appointed nephrologist.

Dialysis technician — is the lead in HD equipment and technical support, installation, and maintenance. Typically this individual is an HD technician or engineer with an understanding of the machines used in home HD. Specific skill sets include knowledge of equipment maintenance and water quality issues with home HD, participation in the on-call service rotation, and an ability to perform home assessments and modifications to patients' dwellings to accommodate home HD. The ability to interact with patients and work with interdisciplinary staff can have a positive impact on patients' experience with home HD. Close collaboration and liaison with equipment manufacturers is the key to successful machine maintenance programs. The home HD centers may have their own technician or have a contract with dialysis machine manufacturers for technical support.

Renal social worker — plays a key role as a patient advocate with experience and knowledge in dealing with complex social issues for dialysis patients. For patients and care partners considering home HD, as well as those already undertaking treatment, the renal social worker is a valuable resource. This role is unique in that it provides support and assistance necessary to address patients' practical, emotional, social, financial, and psychological needs. Individuals in this role will be part of an interdisciplinary team and should work closely with patients to address and resolve their specific issues. Renal social workers perform statutory duties and responsibilities in accordance with social care legislation and framework, including assessments for at-home risk, community care needs, and care partner needs. Renal social workers are specialist advisors who are in fact healthcare liaisons, representing patients with specific needs and referring them to organizations and professionals, health and local authority services, housing organizations, benefits organizations, education establishments, employers, and other specialist services. Members of the medical team often refer patients who need such support to enable them to pursue home HD as a treatment option.

Renal social workers also play a supporting role in locations where HD patients may have less contact with community resources, and where care partners may feel more isolated in their role. Care partners frequently contact renal social workers for support and are encouraged to do so at any time. Through the renal social worker, patients and their care partners can continue to access information, get advice, request assistance, and obtain further support as they develop different needs or circumstances change.

Patient care technicians/healthcare assistants/community nurses — are patient advocates with good practical knowledge of HD. Key attributes include the ability to work both independently or on a team, travel to patients' homes, and participate in remote helpline/support and on-call services for home HD patients. Staff must proactively support the use of home HD and have some understanding of the benefits of at-home treatment. The ability to deal with issues between patients and care partners with sensitivity is a desirable attribute. The role of non-nursing support staff is limited in many countries and therefore may have little impact on a home HD program.

Home HD administrative assistant/secretary or manager — is responsible for management of logistics (eg, clinic, supplies, deliveries), activity log, and billing. Often, he or she will act as the central coordinator of operations and therefore will need to communicate and maintain close links with staff, and may also have to liaise with patients at home.

Dietician — is a person knowledgeable in HD and nutritional issues, with an awareness of the benefits of home HD and its impact on nutritional management. Requisite skill sets should include the ability to adapt and adjust dietary requirements with patients' variable HD schedules at home.

Phase 2

As the program expands, the clinical outcomes and patient benefits are often sufficient incentive to keep the staff committed to the provision of home HD. The workload eases to some extent as staff gains experience, but workforce expansion is necessary to meet demand. The staff needs to have a greater understanding and ability to train, support, and engage with challenging HD patients, while at the same time addressing their complex training needs and directing them to the support available in the community.[3] Additional expertise in dealing with issues of treatment burden and its complications is of paramount importance to sustain and further develop the program. The 2 phases of workforce development should be in continuum and may require overlap for seamless growth and development of the program. In Phase 2, there may be a need to draw on additional skills and personnel such as:

- *Additional training and support nurses* — who can either be seasoned or younger/new nurses. These team members must meet the same criteria and specific skills to complement the program, such as demonstrating a practical knowledge of dialysis, assisting in cannulation training, performing assisted dialysis for those patients in need, and exhibiting a passion to teach and empower
- *Outreach link educator* — who develops an outreach model and clinical interface with other patients and treatment modalities such as those patients who are on PD or in-center HD, individuals failing transplant, and patients with CKD stage 4 or 5
- *Expert patients* — who provide peer support to other patients and staff, before, during, and after training (see "Psychosocial Issues and Support in Home HD" module)
- *Psychologist or counselor* — an important member of the interdisciplinary team who addresses psychosocial issues and patient burden in home HD patients and their care partners

Workforce Challenges

Given the general shortage of dialysis workforce available to meet demand, adequate staffing—particularly acquiring those with adequate home HD skills—can be a formidable challenge in care delivery. A successful strategy could be to integrate or restructure care teams in allied therapies by having the same individuals overlap between modalities, such as PD and home HD (ie, grouped home therapies), or even between in-center HD and home HD. However, it is important that this strategy reinforces rather than reduces the overall skill base of the team. Investing in a self-sufficient home HD team should be considered an essential first step before an integration or overlap with other modalities. The specific expertise relevant to the home HD program must also be well-defined at the outset and have dedicated time set aside for these overlapping positions, depending on the activity of the program. It may also be advisable to delineate the program activity in different areas and adjust staff time to match the workflow.

Expansion of the home HD program can lead to increasing demand in the support of vascular access and self-cannulation. Home access support needs to be carefully monitored so that adequate staff is available to continue with the development and care of patients in the program (see "The Care and Keeping of Vascular Access in Home HD Patients" module).

Almost certainly there will be geographical differences in staffing.[4] In many countries, registered nurses are employed extensively (eg, Canada, United Kingdom) and less so in others (eg, United States). The proportion of registered nurses with specific renal qualifications also varies by region.[5] Staff-to-patient ratios in dialysis units vary greatly by region and organization, especially where there is variation in the prevalence of home therapies. Typically, a caseload of 20 to 25 patients is managed per registered nurse for home HD patients, but support at home can be variable due to substantial challenges in scheduling and coverage arrangements. The need for other allied health professionals also varies between countries depending on local practice, care delivery patterns, and the specific duties performed within these positions. Activities such as water sampling are typically performed by the technician, but in some centers, nurses and patients may be trained to undertake some monitoring procedures. The type of machines used and arrangements with the dialysis provider and manufacturer determine the need for workforce such as renal technicians. Typically, 1 full time renal technician is required to fully manage a program of 50 home HD patients.

Another challenge includes the ability of staff to support patients who are not proficient in the local language. The program must allocate enough resources to allow staff to be equipped to communicate with such patients, either through outside training, use of translators, or hiring of multilingual staff.

As the program grows to a sizeable patient population, case mix and comorbidities are likely to increase, which will impact the staffing ratios required to care for home HD patients. Staff must be well-versed in dealing with issues of nonadherence, difficult home situations, and changes in social circumstances that impact treatment. It is possible to build such expertise over time; however, buddy schemes or links with mentor programs may help staff learn to address some of these challenges. An effective model could be developed to include a range of mature programs that partner with and support staff in newer programs, providing guidance and encouragement on the management of these challenges. A similar buddy or mentor approach can be used within a program for training new or junior staff members, including rotational training schemes within the workforce. Such initiatives can be the key to achieving and sustaining growth of home HD programs.

Important issues to consider during program growth are education, training, and management of workflow. Observing how patients benefit in terms of lifestyle and clinical goals can be a rewarding experience for the staff; however, achieving these results can be labor-intensive with regard to patient monitoring, unscheduled visits, and addressing patient challenges, including clinical issues that result from home and family circumstances. These challenges can lead to staff and patient stress and burnout, if adequate support and resources are not made available.

Lack of support in the community can also be an isolating experience for staff, as home therapies are less visible than in-center programs, and community members may not understand or be aware of the therapy. Rotational training programs, a mix of junior and senior staffing in home care teams, and integration with in-center program staff are methods that can be employed to integrate the workforce across modalities. It is crucial that senior members support junior members and make themselves available as mentors to answer queries, provide guidance, and help solve problems. The key domains of workforce challenges to consider are depicted in Figure 1.

Key Workforce Challenges

Home Support	Patient Training	Transitioning Patients	Technical Support	Staff Training
• Difficult or changing home, social, or family setting • Coordination with in-center program • Unscheduled visits • Nonadherence	• Language (non-native) • Complex training needed • Training comorbid or complex patients	• Training to home dialysis • PD to home HD • Home to in-center HD • Failing transplant to home HD	• Cannulation • Medical issues • Dialysis disruptions • Retraining issues • Clinical governance • Helpline	• Adequate knowledge • Resourcing and allocation • Confidence • Support

Figure 1. Domains for workforce challenges.
HD = hemodialysis ; PD = peritoneal dialysis.
See "Psychosocial Aspects in Home Hemodialysis: A Review," "The Care and Keeping of Vascular Access for Home Hemodialysis Patients," and "Patient Selection and Training for Home Hemodialysis" modules.

Models of Care at Home

A Typical Care Model in Home HD Center of Excellence

An efficient home HD care model should aim to provide a seamless patient journey that is personalized, evidence-based, safe, and effective. The essential steps to consider in the patient care pathway when developing a care model are[6]:

1. Recruitment strategy and treatment pathway for all patients with CKD stage 5, including those who are not on dialysis, are on other dialysis modalities, and those who have received a kidney transplant approaching end-stage renal disease (see "Cultivating Suitable Patients for Home Hemodialysis" module).
2. Training module and pathway (see "Patient Selection and Training for Home Hemodialysis" module).
3. Treatment commencement at home with continued clinical and nursing support while the patient is on home HD.
4. Patient support systems for routine care and for clinical and technical emergencies at home (see "Ensuring Patient Safety During Home Hemodialysis" module).

Typically, the dialysis provider will either provide home HD services or will arrange onward referral to another unit that offers such services.[7] The number of staff required, monitoring schedules, and interdisciplinary team meetings are determined by the scale of each service and its stage of development. The provider will manage referrals in line with any relevant national or local guidelines or recommendations. The regulations, requirements, and infrastructure will vary from country to country, as well as from state to state. Patient training may be provided through 1 of a variety of geographical location options including in-center care facilities, community house centers, stand-alone facilities, or in the patient's own home.[8] The infrastructural setup will also depend on existing capabilities, patient populations, local utilities, and service delivery arrangements (eg, single-center model, health network, or regional care models) (see "The Home Hemodialysis Hub: Physical Infrastructure and Integrated Governance" module). The following section describes exemplar care models and interlinked support structures used in 5 home HD centers of excellence, including the variances that exist (if any) between these successful and comparable care models (Table 1).

Large, successful programs are often based on an integrated interdisciplinary team responsible for all self-care modalities: PD, home HD, and a self-care HD satellite unit. The nurses are cross-trained for all treatment modalities.

The following describes a service configuration and practical considerations in a typical center of excellence, including patient support and follow-up, logistics, technical support, and advantages and disadvantages. It has been adapted from the model used at University Hospital St Luc in Belgium, which has a home HD prevalence of 50 patients.

Table 1. Comparative Care Models in Centers of Excellence

	Location				
Key Elements	**Brussels[a]**	**Manchester[b]**	**Geelong[c]**	**Hong Kong[d]**	**United States[e]**
Patient Visits					
Home Assessment (by whom)	Team approach (nurse/tech/patient)	Team approach (nurse/tech/patient)	Team approach (nurse/tech/patient)	Team approach (nurse/tech/patient)	Team approach (nurse/tech/patient)
Home Assessment (timing)	Start of training	At the time of modality decision	At the time of modality decision	Start of training	Varies. May be at time of modality decision to during training
Machine Location at Home	Decision in consultation with the patient and partner	Decision in consultation with the patient and partner	Decision in consultation with the patient and partner	Decision in consultation with the patient and partner	Decision in consultation with the patient and partner
Home Visits	Day 0, Month 1, then 3 visits per year, or as necessary	First week, month 1, then at least 3 visits per year, and then as necessary	At start of home HD and then as necessary	In the first 3 months, then as necessary	On first day home after training completed, and then as needed
Clinic Visits	Every 6-8 weeks	At 1 month and then every 3-6 months	Every 6-8 weeks	Every 6-8 weeks	Monthly

Table 1. Comparative Care Models in Centers of Excellence

	Location				
Key Elements	**Brussels**[a]	**Manchester**[b]	**Geelong**[c]	**Hong Kong**[d]	**United States**[e]
Patient Visits					
Respite and In-Center Backup (cannulation, retraining, complications, burnout, etc.)	Yes, facility based	Yes, in home training unit and in-center facility	Yes, in home therapies unit	Yes, facility based	Yes, in home training unit
Correspondence (communication, dialysis log sheets, and blood samples)	Monthly	Every 3 months (combined with a home visit/review), monthly in-center interdisciplinary team review	Monthly, blood samples every 6 weeks	Dialysis logs and blood samples monthly, biweekly case meeting	Dialysis logs monthly, laboratory evaluations monthly
Logistics					
Deliveries at Home	Monthly	Monthly	Every 1-2 months	Monthly	Monthly
Waste Disposal	Monthly collection with deliveries	Monthly in line with local council regulations and arrangements	Monthly collected by the local councils	Disposed of with regular household waste in well-sealed double plastic bags. Sharps in hospital sharp boxes sent back to unit for disposal	NA
Technical Support					
Installation (plumbing, electrical)	Own tech team	Own tech team includes buildings manager	Own tech team	Techs (supplier) and external contractor	Tech

Table 1. Comparative Care Models in Centers of Excellence

	Location				
Key Elements	**Brussels[a]**	**Manchester[b]**	**Geelong[c]**	**Hong Kong[d]**	**United States[e]**
Technical Support					
Equipment Maintenance (machine, reverse osmosis, water softener)	Own tech (assistance from company technicians)	Own tech (24/7 on-call for emergencies)	Own tech (aim to rectify issues within 24 hours)	Tech (supplier)	Tech or dialysis vendor
Water Sampling	Quarterly by the tech, delivery driver, or nurse during a home visit	Every 4 months by tech during a home visit	Every 6 weeks (water chlorine testing daily prior to dialysis)	Quarterly by the supplier's tech or patients.	AAMI water analysis prior to starting home HD treatment
On-Call Nursing and Technical Support	24/7	24/7	24/7	24/7	24/7

[a]University Hospital St. Luc, Brussels, Belgium; [b]Central Manchester University Hospitals NHS Foundation Trust, Manchester, UK; [c]The Geelong Hospital, Barwon Health, Geelong, Australia; [d]Queen Mary Hospital and Princess Margaret Hospital, Hong Kong, Special Administrative Region of the People's Republic of China; [e]Barnes-Jewish Dialysis Center, St Louis, Missouri, USA.
Tech = technician; HD = hemodialysis; NA = not applicable; AAMI = Association for the Advancement of Medical Instrumentation.

Patient Support and Follow-Up

- *In-center dialysis backup.* Backup dialysis sessions in the unit are often necessary due to burnout, cannulation problems, medical complications, technical issues, retraining requirements, and other concerns. A minimum of 1 machine per 20 patients at home may be necessary for in-center dialysis as backup

- *On-call service.* On-call nursing support is mandatory and can be provided 24 hours a day, 7 days per week. Internet communication and telemedicine tools (eg, Skype) can also be used to communicate with patients

- *Outpatient clinics.* Every 6 to 8 weeks, the patients come to the clinic to be seen by the nephrologists, nurses, and, if needed, by the dietician and social assistant/social worker

- *Home visits.* A home visit is organized for the start of the first HD session and after 1 month of home treatment. Later visits are scheduled according to the wishes or needs of the patients with an average of 3 per year. During the visit, emergency procedures are reviewed and patients are retrained, if necessary

- *Correspondence.* On a monthly basis, patients send in their dialysis log sheets (per mail, email, or fax) and pre- and post-dialysis blood samples for testing (patients are provided with a centrifuge for home use and special envelopes to protect the vials). Overall frequency of communication and clinic visits can vary depending on the patient's level of experience and overall health

Logistics

- *Supply deliveries.* Monthly delivery of disposables, disinfectants, and salt for the water softeners are made to patients' homes. The packages of supplies for individual patients are prepared in the center's own home dialysis warehouse
- *Waste disposal.* The collection of the dialysis waste in special, sealed containers is picked up at the same time monthly deliveries are made. The delivery van is adapted with 2 compartments to separate the delivery materials from the waste products

Technical Support

- *Assessment of the home.* This is performed by nurse and technician before or at the start of the patient's training. In consultation with the patient and care partner, the decision of where the dialysis machine will be installed is made
- *Plumbing and electrical changes.* All plumbing and electrical wiring needed for dialysis is installed and managed by the technician
- *Equipment maintenance and repair.* The dialysis machine, reverse osmosis device, and water softener are maintained and repaired by the technician. On weekdays, technical problems are resolved within 24 hours. Assistance from dialysis company technicians is used as needed
- *Water sampling.* Performed quarterly by the technician, delivery driver, or nurse during a home visit

Key Advantages

- Nurses become real experts in training patients for self-care dialysis
- Less staff and space needed
- Only 1 on-call service is needed (1 nurse is on-call for both home HD and PD patients)
- Home visits of HD and PD patients can be combined
- Outpatient clinics can be combined
- Patients who change dialysis modality (ie, PD to home HD) are still in partnership with the same interdisciplinary team in a collaborative care model

Disadvantage

- Longer time is needed to train new nurses to become "expert" HD and PD nurses; however, this is easily compensated for by the care model's several advantages

Table 2. Allied Services in Home HD Care Model

Independent Services	Related Services
Medical and nursing coverage for emergencies	General practitioners and community services
Support at home by the community team	Specialist transplant teams
Technical support for equipment	Patient transport and delivery services
Surgery and interventional radiology	Estates and utilities
Psychosocial support	Environmental waste service
Pharmacy services and pathology	
Vascular access support services	
Nutrition and dietetic services	
Anemia management team	

Integrated Care Pathway

An integrated, multidimensional care model, fit for purpose with strong and well-defined links and interfaces with other existing modalities, can provide solid foundations for sustaining a large home HD program. Table 2 identifies key allied and interdependent services that may be involved in the care delivery. All models of care should develop links to transitional care (on a temporary or permanent basis) such as respite care, a vascular access management pathway, transplant program, and in-center HD support structures. Traditional segregation of these care processes has hindered growth of home programs.

Figure 2 demonstrates patients' journeys from early education and training to effective patient care delivered at 3 levels, each with clearly defined roles:

- Community- or home-based support led by a team of nurses
- Clinic review process that defines management plans
- In-center support dealing with emergencies that is responsive, immediate, and aimed at restoring patient's dialysis and home-based treatment needs at the earliest opportunity with minimum disruption to the patient's lifestyle

This care pathway is achieved by a team supported by an efficient administrative structure with appropriate links and pathways at transition points. The program must undergo a regular audit and quality assurance assessment of the pathway and its care indices to ensure best clinical practices and high standards within a defined care model.

Other Considerations

The workforce and infrastructure vary considerably in structure and working patterns between centers. The best practice would be to identify and implement the most productive ways to deliver an efficient model at the outset, and perform subsequent service design review at agreed intervals. Innovative care models focus attention on high-risk touch points in the care pathway. Slowly introducing incremental innovations when the program is doing well can help consolidate success in the care model.

The American Society of Nephrology Accountable Care Organization Task Force developed a set of principles for an integrated nephrology care delivery model.[9] Integrating complex dialysis care models will require incorporation of such holistic concepts in future care delivery. Specialty education for nurses is fundamental and needs to be effective in the practice of home HD.[10] Consideration should also be given to training an adequate number of nephrologists, accredited in the set up and practice of home therapies, to drive and sustain high-quality home HD programs in the future.

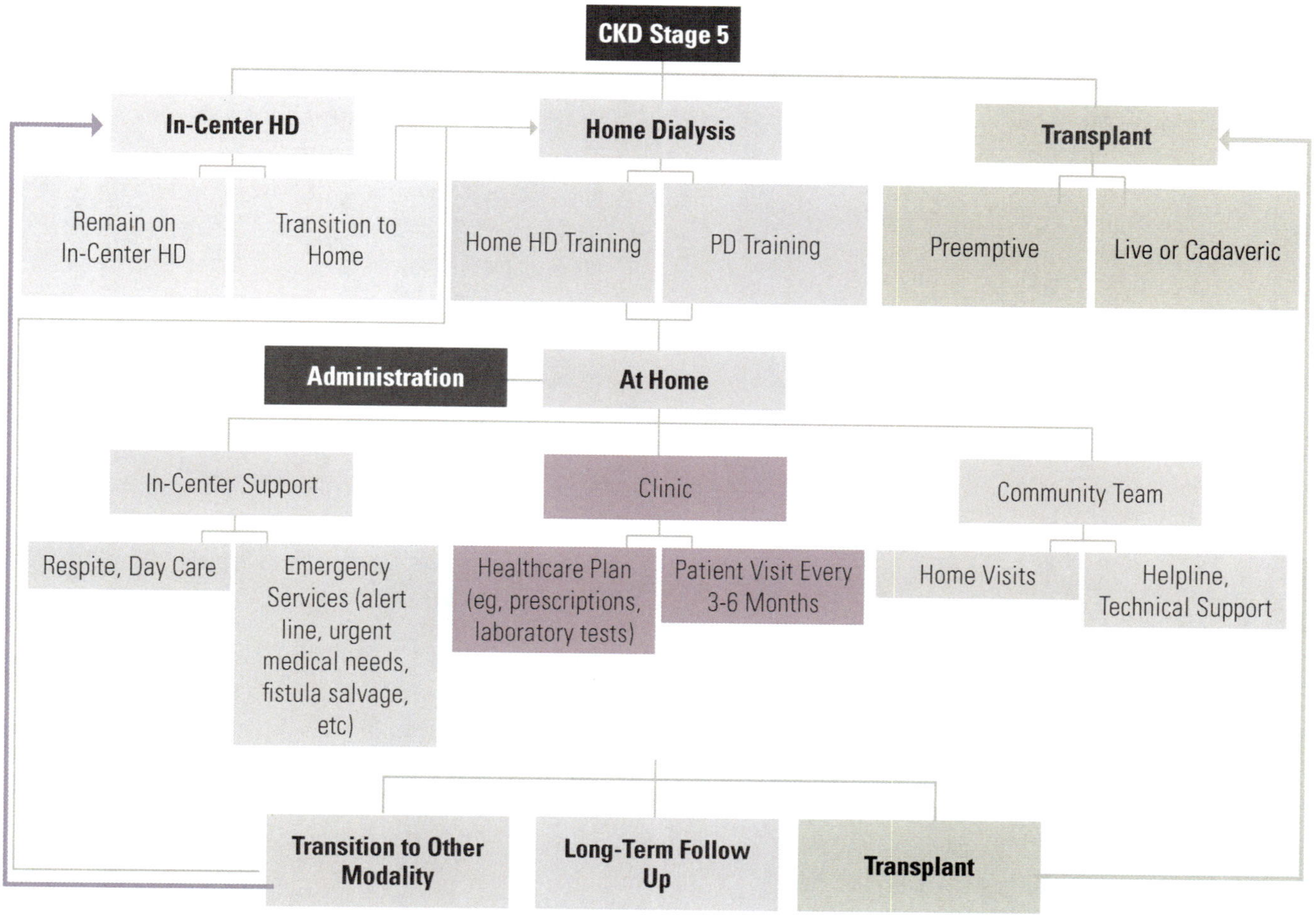

Figure 2. Integrated patient care pathway in home dialysis. CKD = chronic kidney disease; HD = hemodialysis; PD = peritoneal dialysis. Figure adapted from Greater Manchester East Sector Renal Network, UK.

References

1. Moran J, Kraus M. Starting a home hemodialysis program. Semin Dial. 2007;20:35-39.
2. National Institute for Clinical Excellence. Guideline TA48. Guidance on home compared with hospital haemodialysis for patients with end-stage renal failure. September 2002. Available at: http://guidance.nice.org.uk/TA48. Accessed June 20, 2014.
3. Peters A. Supporting and retaining nephrology nurses new to the peritoneal dialysis specialty. Nephrol Nurs J. 2013;40:21-23.
4. Murphy-Burke D, Haskett S, Sondrup B. Provincial organization: local implementation. (abstract) Hemodial Int. 2009;13:129-130.
5. Chow J, San Miguel S. Evaluation of the implementation of assistant in nursing workforce in haemodialysis units. Int J Nurs Pract. 2010;16:484-491.
6. National Health Service. Kidney Care. Improving choice for kidney patients: five STEPS toolkit to home haemodialysis. February 2010. Available at: http://www.wmrn.co.uk/admin/resources/uploads/TOOLKIT:%20Improving%20Choice%20for%20Kidney%20Patients:%205%20steps%20toolkit%20to%20Home%20Haemodialysis.pdf. Accessed October 14, 2014.
7. Mactier R, Mitra S, Boakes, S, et al. Renal Association Working Party on Home Haemodialysis final draft report 02.12.09. 2009. Available at: http://www.wmrn.co.uk/admin/resources/uploads/TOOLKIT:%20Improving%20Choice%20for%20Kidney%20Patients:%205%20steps%20toolkit%20to%20Home%20Haemodialysis.pdf. Accessed June 20, 2014.
8. Kidney Health Australia. A Model for Home Dialysis, Australia – 2012. Available at: http://www.kidney.org.au/LinkClick.aspx?fileticket=BfYeuFvtJcI=&tabid=811&mid=1886. Accessed June 20, 2014.
9. Hamm LL, Hostetter TH, Shaffer RN, ASN Accountable Care Organization Task Force. Considering an integrated nephrology care delivery model: six principles for quality. Clin J Am Soc Nephrol. 2013;8:682-686.
10. Polaschek N, Bennett PN, McNeil L. The Australian and New Zealand dialysis workforce survey in the international context. J Ren Care. 2009;35:170-175.

4 Systems to Cultivate Suitable Patients for Home Dialysis

Rachael C Walker, MN[1,2]

Christopher Blagg, MD[3]

David C Mendelssohn, MD[4]

[1]Renal Department, Hawke's Bay District Health Board, Hastings, New Zealand; [2]School of Public Health, University of Sydney, Australia; [3]Northwest Kidney Centers, University of Washington, Seattle, Washington; [4]Humber River Regional Hospital, Toronto, Ontario, Canada

Implementing Hemodialysis in the Home
A Global Perspective

iSHD
International Society for Hemodialysis

CONTENTS

Abstract

The key to developing, initiating, and maintaining a strong home dialysis program is a fundamental commitment by the entire team to identify and cultivate patients who are suitable candidates to perform home dialysis. This process must start as early as possible in the disease trajectory, and must include a passionate and daily focus by physicians, nurses, social workers, and other members of the multidisciplinary team. This effort must be constant and sustained over months, with active promotion of home dialysis for suitable patients at every opportunity. Cultivation of suitable patients must become a defining and overarching mission for the entire program. This website reviews some of the components involved in this worthwhile effort and provides practical tips and links to resources.

Introduction

There are 2 common pathways that lead a patient with severe chronic kidney disease (CKD) to successful home dialysis, which includes home hemodialysis (HD) or peritoneal dialysis (PD) therapy. By far, the easiest and preferred pathway is to identify suitable candidates months or years before they reach end-stage renal disease (ESRD) and start with a home dialysis modality when initiation of renal replacement therapy (RRT) is required. A second but more difficult pathway is to identify potential candidates who are on other forms of RRT and then switch them to home dialysis.

Optimal initiation of dialysis has been defined as starting dialysis electively as an outpatient and using an arteriovenous fistula (AVF), AV graft (AVG) (unless contraindicated), or PD catheter. In contrast, a suboptimal start is defined as hospitalized patients undergoing acute RRT and/or patients in whom a central venous catheter (CVC) has been placed. A suboptimal start is often associated with patients whose initial treatment uses a modality that is not his or her preferred choice and those who have not had the benefit of predialysis education.

This module primarily addresses issues regarding the first pathway; however, potential solutions to overcome suboptimal starts will also be briefly discussed.

Referral to a Nephrology Program

Screening the general population for CKD is not cost-effective and is not recommended. Instead, screening high-risk patient groups using blood and urine tests is recommended. Serum creatinine has been the standard test to assess kidney function, but an increasing number of countries have introduced estimated glomerular filtration rate (eGFR) reporting as a way of identifying patients at high risk of progressive kidney disease and encouraging earlier referral of those patients to nephrologists. In 2013, Kidney Disease Improving Global Outcomes (KDIGO) guidelines introduced a more nuanced staging CKD system that considers the cause of kidney disease, eGFR, and degree of albuminuria as a way to confer risk in a given patient.[1] Once fully implemented, this modified approach may prevent the unnecessary referral of patients with reduced GFR who are not at risk of progression, particularly elderly patients without microalbuminuria. One chapter of the KDIGO publication provides information on when to refer patients with CKD for specialized services. For full details, please see the full KDIGO guidelines section "5.1 Referral to Specialist Services".[1]

Preparation for RRT

Despite specific and nonspecific approaches to reverse or slow the rate of progression of CKD, far too many patients with CKD progress toward ESRD. It is a clinical challenge for patients and providers alike to shift focus and accept that preparation for RRT is required. For providers, this means accepting that therapy has failed to prevent progression. For patients and families, this means overcoming denial and other defense mechanisms, and considering information and choices that may be frightening and perhaps months or years away.

There is considerable evidence that offering a formal predialysis program is beneficial to patient outcomes and increases the uptake of home PD or home HD.[2-6] Indeed, international guidelines highlight that a model of multidisciplinary, team-based predialysis care (ie, a team consisting of nephrologists, nurses, dietitians, social workers, etc) is superior to the care provided by a solo nephrologist and is strongly recommended.[1,7]

Ideally, 1 year or longer is required to complete all the tasks required of the care team to educate patients and families, and to achieve timely decisions about modality of choice and optimal vascular access (Figure 1).[8,9]

One modern paradigm involves an eGFR-based approach to steps in the process of preparing patients for ESRD. We support the use of the approach described in the Canadian Society of Nephrology Vascular Access Working Group report, as follows:[10]

Figure 1: Ideal Predialysis Patient Flow

STEP 1	Identify patients likely to progress to dialysis in the next 12-18 months, and those who have started urgently without predialysis education
STEP 2	Early and frequent education on renal replacement therapy options to patients and family
STEP 3	Offer decision support
STEP 4	Home visit to assess environment Tour of training unit
STEP 5	Create vascular access 6 months before dialysis initiation
STEP 6	Planned commencement of home training upon dialysis initiation

- Set specific targets for tasks during management of CKD Stages 3, 4, and 5 according to the rate of decline of eGFR:

    1. Based on rate of decline of 2 – 5 mL/min/year, begin the predialysis modality education program when eGFR reaches approximately 30 mL/min. Patient and physician decisions regarding dialysis modality should be finalized when eGFR reaches 20 mL/min.
    Patients who choose HD should be referred for consideration/evaluation of AVF and AVG placement when eGFR reaches 15 – 20 mL/min.

    2. Patients who experience a rate of decline in eGFR more than 5 mL/min/year should begin the education and modality selection processes earlier, if possible.

    3. These task targets may be irrelevant for those patients who are elderly or are stable with non-progressive CKD and are not expected to require HD.

Comprehensive modality education should be provided to all patients, and to interested family members. Education should usually be provided by a nurse clinician/teacher, either individually or to small groups. Ideally, the nurse clinician/teacher will have previous experience with dialysis and a positive attitude toward home-based therapies. It is extremely important to provide all patients with excellent and timely information to allow them to make an informed decision regarding modality. The education program should also include meetings with training staff from both the home HD and PD programs and current patients and their families who are successfully undergoing home dialysis.

Patients who have received the most current, detailed information and are able to make informed decisions are much more likely to choose home dialysis than those patients who are never offered instruction or take part in an education program. There is general acceptance of patient autonomy as a part of the shared decision-making process around modality choice.[11, 12] A tenet embodied in the National Institute of Clinical Excellence (NICE) recommendations around dialysis modality choice states that the most appropriate modality is that which aligns to patients' lifestyles and personal circumstances alongside their clinical requirements.[13]

Predialysis education includes:

- Education about normal and impaired kidney function
- Education about treatment options available, including advantages of each treatment
    - » Transplant (live and cadaveric kidneys), including preemptive live donor transplant before dialysis is required
    - » Home HD
    - » Peritoneal dialysis
    - » Facility-based dialysis
    - » Conservative care and trial of dialysis

Practice Tip

A home dialysis program will not thrive without an energetic and proactive predialysis multidisciplinary team. The team needs to champion home dialysis, and be a credible resource and support to patients and clinical staff alike who will then in turn respect and support patients' decisions.

Overcoming Service-Level Barriers to Home Dialysis

The major barriers to greater use of home dialysis (both home HD and PD) at a service level relate to inadequate provision of information and education of patients, dialysis unit staff, and nephrologists, as well as to inadequate organizational or structural program support for home dialysis training and care.[14] A strong clinician recommendation that actively promotes home dialysis for suitable patients is a key element and requires optimal education about home dialysis in the course of physician training, and exposure to the local home dialysis program when these physicians enter practice.

Successful home dialysis programs should include (1) a medical director who is a champion of home dialysis and has the support of the physicians, social workers, and dietitians on the team, and (2) experienced nurses who are strong proponents of home dialysis and are good teachers. The program should be busy, supporting a home dialysis population of at least 12 to 20 patients and training 10 or more patients per year, thereby maintaining staff experience and cost-effectiveness. Often, the best approach is regionalization of home dialysis training, rather like transplant programs, with referral of suitable patients to the program for training and home support.

Links to Health Professional Resources*

- Baxter Healthcare, Healthcare Professionals Education Resources
- British Renal Society, Educational Resources
- DaVita
- The Kidney Foundation of Canada
- Kidney Health Australia, Health Professionals
- Life Options, How to Have a Good Future with Kidney Disease. Free downloadable CKD patient education toolkit for professionals
- National Kidney Foundation

Practice Tip

For a detailed discussion of the issues related to developing a successful home HD program, please refer to the report by Young et al, "How to Overcome Barriers and Establish a Successful Home HD Program", a paper developed on behalf of the American Society of Nephrology Dialysis Advisory Group.[14]

Links to Patient Education Resources*

- American Association of Kidney Patients, Understanding the Role of a Renal Social Worker
- British Renal Society, Educational Resources
- DaVita, Treatment Options
- Home Dialysis Central, Patient Education
- The Kidney Foundation of Canada
- Kidney Health Australia, For Patients
- HomeDialysis.org, Am I Ready to Choose?
- Kidney School Module 2, Treatment Options for Kidney Failure
- Life Options
- Life Options, How to Have a Good Future with Kidney Disease videos (set of 6)
- My Life, My Dialysis Choice
- National Kidney Foundation, Patient Resources
- RenalWEB, Patient Education

*Please see Web version of this manual on ISHD.org for hyperlinks.

Additional Approaches to Educate Patients

A valuable way to augment the education provided by the multidisciplinary team is to connect potential home dialysis patients and their family members with those who are already achieving success on home dialysis (sometimes called a home "champion"). This can be done on a one-on-one basis (ie, peer-to-peer) or in group settings. Peers can provide the additional context and support for ambivalent and frightened potential patients and their families in a way that catalyzes decision making in favor of attempting home dialysis. For more information, see the "Psychosocial Guide for Healthcare Professionals" module with its segment on peer support.

Suitability for Home Dialysis

There is astonishing variability in the prevalence of home dialysis (home HD and PD) both between and within nations, and the larger part of this variability is not explained by patient age and comorbidity.[15-17] The literature shows clearly that many more patients are eligible for home dialysis than are currently receiving it in most regions in the world.

Perhaps the most widely recognized tool for assessment of suitability is the MATCH-D tool (Method to Assess Treatment Choices for Home Dialysis), which starts at the default position of home dialysis, escalates to solving for any barriers, and then defaults to facility hemodialysis if the barriers prove insurmountable.[18] As both a practical and philosophical framework, the MATCH-D tool works to identify and maximize opportunities for patients to be offered and accept home dialysis (Table 1).

Table 1. Key Attributes of the Ideal Home HD Patient

Patients	• Motivated and committed toward home HD • Clinically stable • Well educated • Modality chosen to suit lifestyle • Good dexterity and sight • Literate
Home Setting	• Suitable storage and space • Adequate and stable water and electricity supply • Access to phone • Approval of landlord, if appropriate
Family Support	• Family support • Caregiver support, if required • Access to respite care, if appropriate

Adapted from Schatell 2007[18] and NICE Guidelines 2002.[13]

Practice Tip

The medical director should be a champion of home HD with the support of both nurses and doctors alike. The cultivation of patients, either directly or by proxy, requires interprofessional solidarity, as patients are not likely to follow inconsistent recommendations or mixed messages received from a divided professional front.

Seeking Home Hemodialysis Patients from Overlooked Populations

Failed PD patients

Unfortunately, technique failure is a common cause of PD transition to in-center HD. Because these are patients who previously selected and maintained themselves on PD, many would be suitable for a planned transition to home HD. Timing of these discussions is important, because ideally these patients would have an AVF or AVG created before the PD failure occurred; therefore, elective transfer to home HD could happen without the need for placing a CVC.

Failed transplant patients

Graft loss is another pathway often leading patients to in-center HD. Given that transplanted patients are a highly selected group, younger and more robust than an in-center population, this subgroup would also be potentially suitable candidates for a home dialysis option, either PD or home HD. Once again, timely education and early modality decision making would allow for effective transition to home HD. Shared care models and a multidisciplinary approach, involving both the transplant and home dialysis teams, might improve planning for this transition and avoid late referrals to in-center or to home programs.

Overcoming Suboptimal Initiation of Dialysis

Right Start Approach

Suboptimal initiation of dialysis, which includes initiating dialysis while the patient is hospitalized and/or via a CVC, can result in negative consequences; these negative consequences can occur with either early or late referral.[5] Fresenius and DaVita have published experiences with such a case-managed approach to the critical first few months of in-center hemodialysis.[7, 19, 20] The mechanics of this approach are variable and can be applied by a dedicated nurse, and/or in a segregated area where incident patients are clustered. One variation of case management involves forming a therapeutic relationship with hospital nephrologists, promoting home dialysis, while incident HD patients are still hospitalized, as has been described previously.[12]

Transition Care

One approach to optimizing uptake of home dialysis employs the philosophy that if at all possible, patients who are potentially suitable for home dialysis should be informed of and offered those modalities before beginning dialysis, and completely avoid exposure to an in-center HD unit.[12, 21] Patients who are undecided about which modality to choose, or those new and uneducated patients who start HD under suboptimal conditions may be dialyzed in a community-based facility or in a dedicated room adjacent to a home dialysis training area. Specialized nurses provide emotional support and gently teach patients the benefits of home dialysis in these areas, and actively encourage patients to choose a final modality that consists of either PD or home HD. A detailed discussion of the advantages and disadvantages of home dialysis should be provided. This discussion should include a thorough exploration of patient apprehensions and misapprehensions.[12, 21] This support should be available to undecided patients for at least a month before they are considered as in-center HD patients.

Even among patients who do start on in-center HD, it is often possible to promote future consideration of home dialysis. Education to all patients, therefore, must be comprehensive and demonstrate the benefits of home HD. Whenever possible, patients should be encouraged to participate in some level of self-care. Success in these activities can boost a patient's confidence to progress to independent home dialysis and allow for a fresh and more serious consideration of home dialysis.

Table 2. Key Strategies and Recommendations to Increase Home HD

Strategy	Recommendation
Individualized Patient Education	• Creation of a predialysis program or referral process to an established predialysis program • Criteria for patient referral to predialysis education • Established case management approach • Key performance indicator of patient education at defined eGFR
Patient Education Tools	• One-on-one individualized education • Educational materials clearly delineating and promoting the benefits of home dialysis • Written and audio-visual patient education materials • Group education sessions • Peer support groups or "expert home patients" • Tour of training centers
Staff Education	• Predialysis educator experienced in home dialysis • Established predialysis patient pathway • Physicians educated about home dialysis • Clinicians aware of the benefits of home dialysis and willingness to promote home dialysis • Education to other clinical staff within region of home dialysis benefits
Service	• Established "home-first" philosophy • Adequate resourcing of predialysis educators and predialysis multidisciplinary team members • Adequate patient resources and promotional materials • Adequate training resources (staff and facility) • Available respite resources • 24-hour on-call service • Accessible patient database for benchmarking and screening • Annual audit of predialysis program (inclusion in quality improvement program) • Established multidisciplinary team reviews
Promote Patient Self-Management	• Provision of patient decision support tools • Individualized patient time lines/checklists for key milestones: » Patient education received » Patient modality decision made » Modality sign off » Home visit and assessment » Home issues identified and addressed » Referral access » Tour of home training unit, meet staff » Patient buddy linkage » Access established » Tentative training date

eGFR = estimated glomerular filtration rate

Approaches to Remote Patient Populations

Patients living in remote areas should have equal access to renal services, including dialysis. Home dialysis is particularly suited to this patient group. Patients trained in home dialysis are able to return to their homes and continue in their normal activities with the least interruption to their lives and their families. There are many novel approaches to enable home dialysis. One example includes shared dialysis community facilities to accommodate those patients without a home deemed suitable for home HD. Patients who can perform unsupervised home HD can complete their HD within these shared settings. Approximately 7 of these community facilities now exist across Australia and New Zealand.[22-25] More information about the Australian facilities can be found **here.**

Selecting the First Patients for a New Home HD Program

To set up a new home HD program, it is important to initially select those patients who will most likely achieve success to train and then return home (Table 2). Below is a list of ideal characteristics your first patients should have.

- No comorbidities and no serious complications of kidney failure
- Life expectancy > 2 years
- Motivated and committed to go home
- Have a home suitable to accommodate home HD
- Literate with good self-management skills
- Physically fit and able to dialyze independently
- Established and reliable vascular access

Conclusion

A successful home dialysis program requires the commitment of the entire multidisciplinary team. The key to a successful home dialysis program is the identification and cultivation of patients who are suitable candidates to perform home dialysis. This process must start as early as possible using established guidelines and a multidisciplinary team approach to active promotion of home dialysis for suitable patients.

References

1. Kidney Disease: Improving Global Outcomes (KDIGO) CKD Work Group. KDIGO 2012 Clinical Practice Guideline for the Evaluation and Management of Chronic Kidney Disease. Kidney Int Suppl. 2013;3:1-150
2. Goovaerts T, Jadoul M, Goffin E. Influence of a pre-dialysis education programme (PDEP) on the mode of renal replacement therapy. Nephrol Dial Transplant. 2005;20:1842-1847.
3. Goovaerts T, Jadoul M, Goffin E. Influence of a predialysis education program on the choice of renal replacement therapy. Am J Kidney Dis. 2012;60:499-500.
4. Key SM. Optimizing dialysis modality choices around the world: a review of literature concerning the role of enhanced early pre-ESRD education in choice of renal replacement therapy modality. Nephrol Nurs J. 2008;35:387-395.
5. Mendelssohn DC, Curtis B, Yeates K, et al. Suboptimal initiation of dialysis with and without early referral to a nephrologist. Nephrol Dial Transplant. 2011;26:2959-2965.
6. Levin A, Lewis M, Mortiboy P, et al. Multidisciplinary predialysis programs: quantification and limitations of their impact on patient outcomes in two Canadian settings. Am J Kidney Dis. 1997;29:533-540.
7. Wilson SM, Robertson JA, Chen G, et al. The IMPACT (Incident Management of Patients, Actions Centered on Treatment) program: a quality improvement approach for caring for patients initiating long-term hemodialysis. Am J Kidney Dis. 2012;60:435-443.
8. Thomas MC, Caring for Australians with Renal Impairment (CARI). The CARI guidelines. Prevention of progression of kidney disease: pre-dialysis education for patients with chronic kidney disease. Nephrology (Carlton). 2007;12 (Suppl 1):S46-48.
9. Mendelssohn DC, Toffelmire EB, Levin A. Attitudes of Canadian nephrologists toward multidisciplinary team-based CKD clinic care. Am J Kidney Dis. 2006;47:277-284.
10. Canadian Society of Nephrology. Report of the Canadian society of nephrology vascular access working group. Semin Dial. 2012;25:22-25.
11. Lewis AL, Stabler KA, Welch JL. Perceived informational needs, problems, or concerns among patients with stage 4 chronic kidney disease. Nephrol Nurs J. 2010;37:143-149.
12. Porter E, Watson D, Bargman JM. Education for patients with progressive CKD and acute-start dialysis. Adv Chronic Kidney Dis. 2013;20:302-310.
13. National Institute for Clinical Excellence. Guideline TA48. Guidance on home compared with hospital haemodialysis for patients with end-stage renal failure. 2002.
14. Young BA, Chan C, Blagg C, et al. How to overcome barriers and establish a successful home HD program. Clin J Am Soc Nephrol. 2012;7:2023-2032.
15. Khawar O, Kalantar-Zadeh K, Lo WK, et al. Is the declining use of long-term peritoneal dialysis justified by outcome data? Clin J Am Soc Nephrol. 2007;2:1317-1328.
16. Mehrotra R, Kermah D, Fried L, et al. Chronic peritoneal dialysis in the United States: declining utilization despite improving outcomes. J Am Soc Nephrol. 2007;18:2781-2788.
17. Marshall MR, Walker RC, Polkinghome KR, et al. Survival on home dialysis in New Zealand. PLoS One 2014;9 (5):e96847.
18. Schatell D. MATCH-D: a roadmap to home dialysis therapy. Nephrol News Issues. 2007;21:41-44.
19. Wingard RL, Pupim LB, Krishnan M, et al. Early intervention improves mortality and hospitalization rates in incident hemodialysis patients: RightStart program. Clin J Am Soc Nephrol. 2007;2:1170-1175.
20. Lacson E, Wang W, DeVries C, et al. Effects of a nationwide predialysis educational program on modality choice, vascular access, and patient outcomes. Am J Kidney Dis. 2011;58:235-242.

References (cont'd)

21. Watson D. Acute start-chronic needs: education and support for adults who have had acute start dialysis. Semin Dial. 2013;26:184-187.

22. Marley JV, Dent HK, Wearne M, et al. Haemodialysis outcomes of Aboriginal and Torres Strait Islander patients of remote Kimberley region origin. Med J Aust. 2010;193:516-520.

23. Villarba A, Warr K. Home haemodialysis in remote Australia. Nephrology (Carlton). 2004;9 (Suppl 4):S134-137.

24. Kneipp E, Murray R, Warr K, et al. Bring me home: renal dialysis in the Kimberley. Nephrology (Carlton). 2004;9 (Suppl 4):S121-125.

25. Marshall MR, van der Schrieck N, Lilley D, et al. Independent community house   as a novel dialysis setting: an observational cohort study. Am J Kidney Dis. 2013;61:598-607.

5 Patient Safety in Home Hemodialysis: Quality Assurance and Serious Adverse Events in the Home Setting

Robert P Pauly, MD, MSc, FRCPC[1]
Deborah O Eastwood, BBus, PG Cert Health Sciences, MSc[2]
Mark R Marshall, MBChB, MPH, FRACP[3,4]

[1]Division of Nephrology and Transplant Immunology, University of Alberta, Edmonton, Alberta, Canada; [2]Department of Medicine and Health of Older People, Waitemata District Health Board, Auckland, New Zealand; [3]Faculty of Medical and Health Sciences, University of Auckland, Auckland, New Zealand; [4]Department of Renal Medicine, Counties Manukau District Health Board, Auckland, New Zealand

Implementing Hemodialysis in the Home
A Global Perspective

iSHD
International Society for Hemodialysis

CONTENTS

Abstract

Interest in home hemodialysis (HD) is high because of the reported benefits and its excellent safety record. However, the potential for serious adverse events (AEs) exists when patients perform HD in their homes without supervision. We review the epidemiology and literature on dialysis-related emergencies during home HD, and present a conceptual and practical framework for the prevention and management of serious AEs for those patients performing home HD. In addition, we recommend and describe a formal monitored and iterative quality assurance program, and make suggestions for the future development of safety strategies to mitigate the risk of AEs in home HD.

Introduction

Patients and their care partners acknowledge the benefits of home hemodialysis (HD) compared with traditional facility-based dialysis. However, as home HD training progresses, the initial positive attitudes expressed by patients and their care partners about home HD oftentimes change to an increasing apprehension about accepting responsibility for independently performing this complex medical therapy, and fear about managing potentially life-threatening dialysis-related emergencies alone.[1] Clinicians at facility-based dialysis centers who do not have experience working with home HD often share similar concerns about patient safety.[2]

Despite these fears, serious adverse events (AEs) during home HD are uncommon. Experienced home HD clinics have safeguards in place to mitigate serious AEs and, if they do occur, to manage them effectively. New home HD programs will benefit from these lessons and must instill a culture of safety – without inciting alarm or undermining assurances – that home HD is a generally safe therapy. To maintain a good safety record, vigilance by patients, care partners, and center personnel is paramount in avoiding and managing emergencies experienced in home HD programs.[3]

In this module, we describe a conceptual and practical framework for dialysis healthcare providers to help them address preventable serious AEs for patients during home HD, emphasizing those AEs that result from technical error with the potential to be life-threatening and/or have the capability to derail a home HD program. We highlight the life-threatening emergencies described in the literature, suggest a quality assurance process, and provide specific strategies to facilitate expeditious care in emergency situations.

Epidemiology of Dialysis-Related Emergencies in Home HD

There is little published literature of the epidemiology of dialysis-related emergencies. Notwithstanding, it can be assumed that relatively minor and common complications of HD seen in facility-based dialysis still occur to some degree when this treatment is administered at home. More concerning is the paucity of literature regarding dialysis-related emergencies with the potential to cause death. For the purpose of this module, such life-threatening emergencies include: blood loss (either from needle dislodgement or disconnection from a central venous catheter, bleeding *from* the dialysis circuit, or bleeding *into* the dialysis circuit), air embolism, hemodynamic compromise from aggressive ultrafiltration or dialysate leak, hemolysis, and acute electrolyte abnormalities associated with the treatment. While these complications are not unique to home HD, there is an inherently greater risk when they occur in a setting where trained staff cannot administer immediate emergency interventions. Infectious complications are not considered further but are addressed within a separate module (see "Increased Risk of Infection with Buttonhole Cannulation" in the "Care and Keeping of Vascular Access for Home Hemodiaysis Patients" module)

A 2013 quality-improvement study involving 2 home HD programs in Canada evaluated the frequency of these AEs, and reported 1 death and 6 potentially fatal AEs in their programs over 12 years.[4] This translates into a crude death rate of 2 per 1000 patient-years and a cumulative life-threatening procedure-related AE rate (ie, death plus potentially lethal AEs) of approximately 14 events per 1000 patient-years.[4] These findings are in line with a more detailed single-center analysis also from Canada, which reported a corresponding life-threatening, procedure-related AE rate of 9 per 1000 patient-years.[5]

The only direct comparison between home and facility HD comes from a cohort study from New Zealand, which posed the question: "For those on HD in New Zealand, does HD in the home setting result in a higher mortality risk from angioaccess bleeding or infection than HD in the facility setting, over a 15-year time frame?"[6] In this analysis, there were 11 such events recorded over 8755 patient-years for those patients undergoing facility HD (1.2 events per 1000 patient-years) and 1 per 2571 patient-years for those patients undergoing home HD (0.4 events per 1000 patient-years). After multivariate adjustment, the relative risk of angioaccess bleeding or infection in home vs facility HD patients was 0.30 (0.09-0.84).[6] While both the Canadian and New Zealand studies have limitations (retrospective, observational, registry-based, etc), they provide a reassuring signal that home HD is a safe therapy. Indeed, administrative data from the Scottish Renal Registry of conventional in-center hemodialysis recipients yielded a population incidence of death due directly to renal replacement therapy complications of 1.35 deaths/1000 renal replacement therapy patients per year; hyperkalemia was the most commonly attributable cause of death.[7] This indirectly suggests that home HD is no more risky than in-center hemodialysis though the nature of AEs is different.

Take-Home Messages

- Serious AEs during home HD are rare due to the use of patient safety heuristics within experienced home HD programs.
- Ongoing vigilance is paramount to avoid and manage emergencies experienced in home HD programs.

Conceptual Framework for Patient Safety in Home HD

As defined by the Institute of Medicine (IOM), "Patient safety is the prevention of harm to patients".[8] This definition is further expanded by the United States Agency for Healthcare Research and Quality (AHRQ) to include, "[Fundamentally] patient safety refers to freedom from accidental or preventable injuries produced by medical care".[9] However, these concepts require modification when referring to home HD. While traditional patient safety focuses on the care provided by healthcare professionals, safety in home HD involves patient vigilance in partnership with their care partners *and* healthcare professionals, with discrete safety practices specific to each group. In addition, traditional patient safety doctrine emphasizes almost exclusively the prevention of error. Patient safety during home HD must also include a proactive stance to minimize patient injury in the event that such an error does occur.

A formally monitored and iterative quality assurance program is strongly recommended to enhance patient safety, as illustrated in Figure 1. This framework will be most effective if it can be implemented as a formally monitored and iterative quality assurance program, emphasizing systems of care that (1) prevent procedure-related AEs; (2) minimize harm from those events that do occur; (3) provide a means to learn from the events that have already occurred; and (4) build a culture of safety among healthcare professionals, patients, and their care partners.

In the next sections, we discuss serious AEs reported in the home HD literature, outline strategies for their mitigation and management, and provide guidance on how to close the loop from serious AEs and continue ongoing quality improvement.

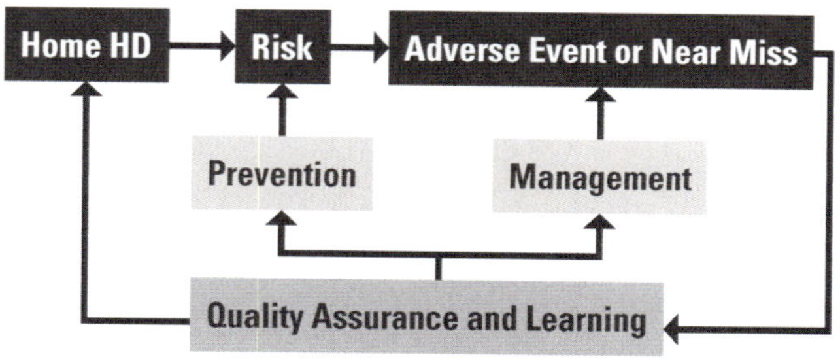

Figure 1. Patient Safety Quality Assurance Framework

Types of Procedure-Related Serious Adverse Events During Home HD

While patients dialyzing at home are subject to many of the same complications as those dialyzing in-center (eg, experiencing vascular access complications, infections, chloramine contamination), the current discussion is limited to emergencies that are unique to the home setting, either because such events cannot happen in a facility-based unit or are less likely to escape notice from trained personnel and escalate into a serious AE. The literature describes 9 cases of fatal or life-threatening AEs in home HD (Table 1), and several of these events are depicted in Figures 2 through 7.[4,10,11] Blood loss was the most common cause: 7 in total. Three episodes of bleeding from the circuit (due to poor connections between tubing and dialyzers, or the incorrect attachment of a heparin syringe to the circuit), 2 episodes of bleeding from central venous catheters due to poor connections or clamping, and 2 episodes of bleeding into the dialysis circuit (bleeding into drain bags during priming at the start of HD or during rinse-back at the end) were reported. Murlidharan et al report a case of near fatal hypercalcemia in a patient due to the inadvertent reversal of the reverse osmosis machine product water and drain solution lines, with the product water being inappropriately discarded while the drain solution (having a very high calcium concentration) being used to generate dialysate.[11]

Table 1. Severe Procedure-Related Adverse Events in Home Hemodialysis Described in Published Literature

	Patient Age, year	Year of Event	Experience with Home HD (mo)	Home Alone[b]	Adverse Event	Human Error	Details
1	65	2007	7	No	Blood loss	Yes	Multiple contributing factors including ignoring alarms, misthreading of arterial tubing to dialyzer head, and incorrect placement of wetness detectors. (See Figure 7)
2	40	2007	<12	No	Air embolism	Yes	Unclamped central venous catheter
3	46	2011	48	No	Blood loss	Possible	Possible misthreading of dialysis tubing to the central venous catheter. Possible closed connector device malfunction.
4	59	2011	<1	Yes	Blood loss	Possible	Possible failed integrity of closed connector device. Improper clamp placement.
5	50	2012	35	Yes	Blood loss	Yes	Incorrect machine setup. Failure to use wetness detectors.
6	35	2012	<24	No	Blood loss	Yes	Misthreading of venous tubing to dialyzer header. Inappropriate placement of wetness detectors. (See Figure 7)
7	59	2012	24	No	Blood loss	Yes	Failure to adhere to machine setup protocol as instructed. (See Figures 2-4)
8	67	2010	<1	Yes	Blood loss	Yes	Connecting the venous (instead of arterial) tubing to a saline rinse bag during rinse-back procedure. (See Figures 5 and 6)
9	46	2011	72	No	Hypercalcemia	Yes	Reverse osmosis waste water hooked incorrectly to dialysis machine to generate dialysate and product water to drain.

[a]Table adapted from the following publications: Cases 1-7 from Wong et al[4]; Case 8 from Allcock et al[10]; Case 9 from Murlidharan et al.[11]
[b]Home Alone indicates whether a patient was dialyzing with an attendant care partner present at the time of the adverse event.

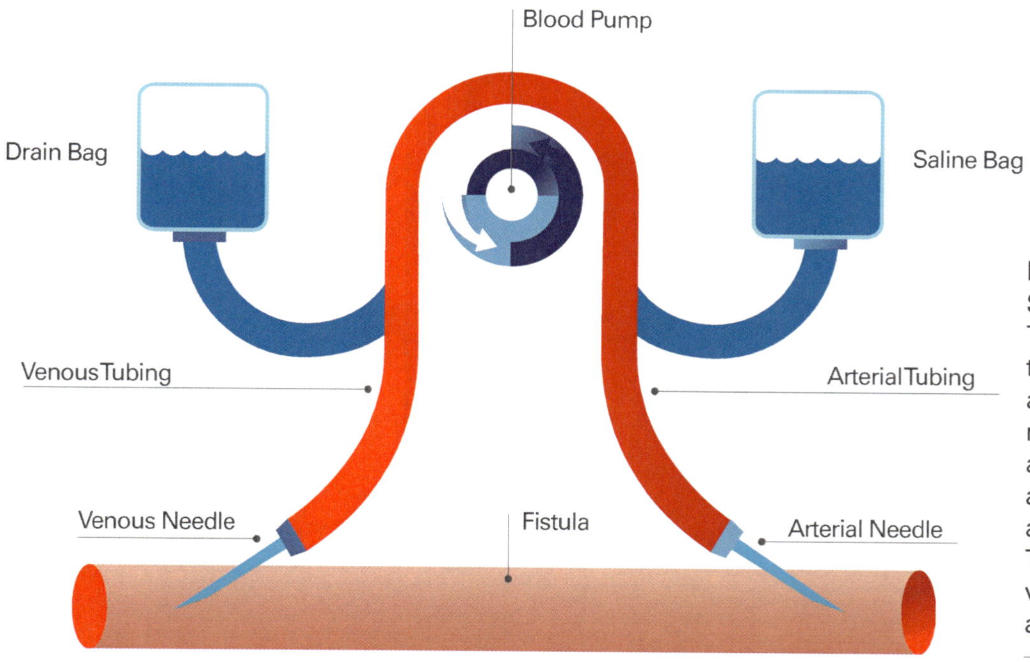

Figure 2. Generic Hemodialysis Setup
This figure depicts dialysis tubing connected to a patient's arteriovenous fistula by an arterial needle, with tubing passing around a standard pump, through a dialyzer, and returning through a venous needle into the fistula. The saline and drain bags are used variably during the saline priming and rinse-back procedures.

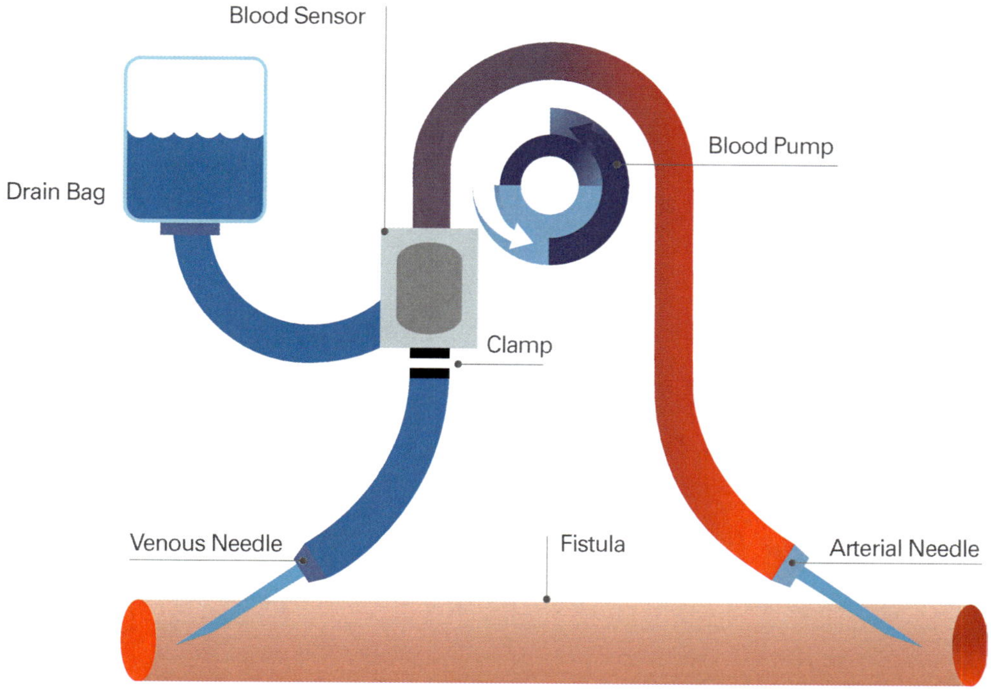

Figure 3A. Routine Blood Priming of the Hemodialysis Circuit
After the hemodialysis circuit has been primed with saline, the circuit must then be primed with blood before dialysis can commence. To do so, the arterial needle is connected to the patient's fistula, the pump is engaged, and blood is drawn out of the fistula into the tubing, around the pump, and through the dialyzer, pushing the saline ahead of it. In a typical priming protocol, the saline is diverted into a drain bag (and not infused into the patient) until blood is detected by the blood sensor.

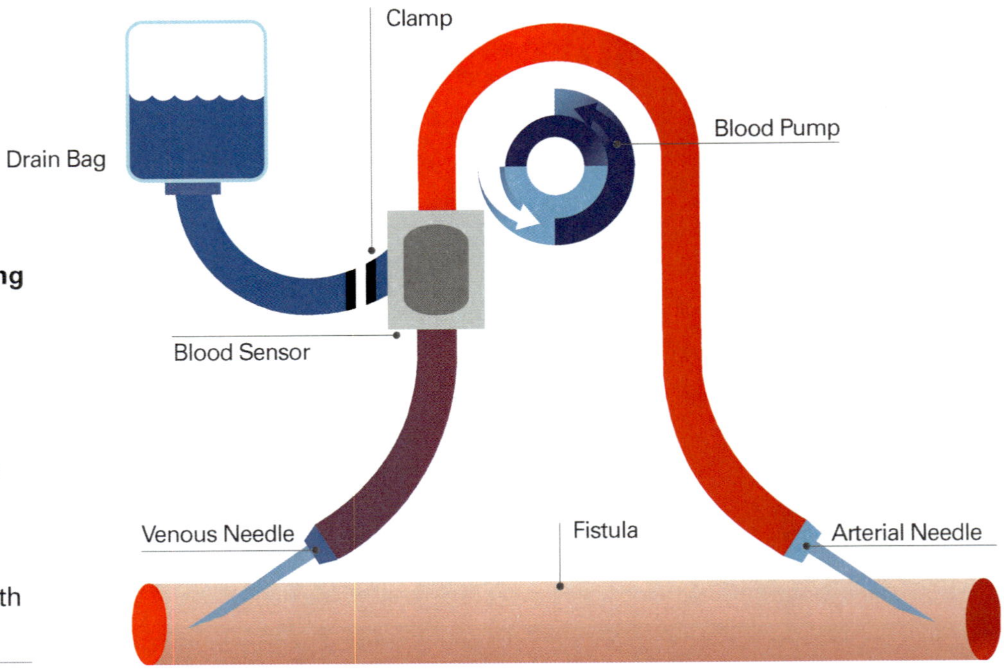

Figure 3B. Routine Blood Priming of the Hemodialysis Circuit
Once blood is detected by the sensor, the patient is cued by the machine to temporarily stop the pump, clamp the tubing to the drain bag, and open the clamp to his or her venous tubing to have blood flow through the venous needle into the fistula, thereby completing the circuit priming with blood.

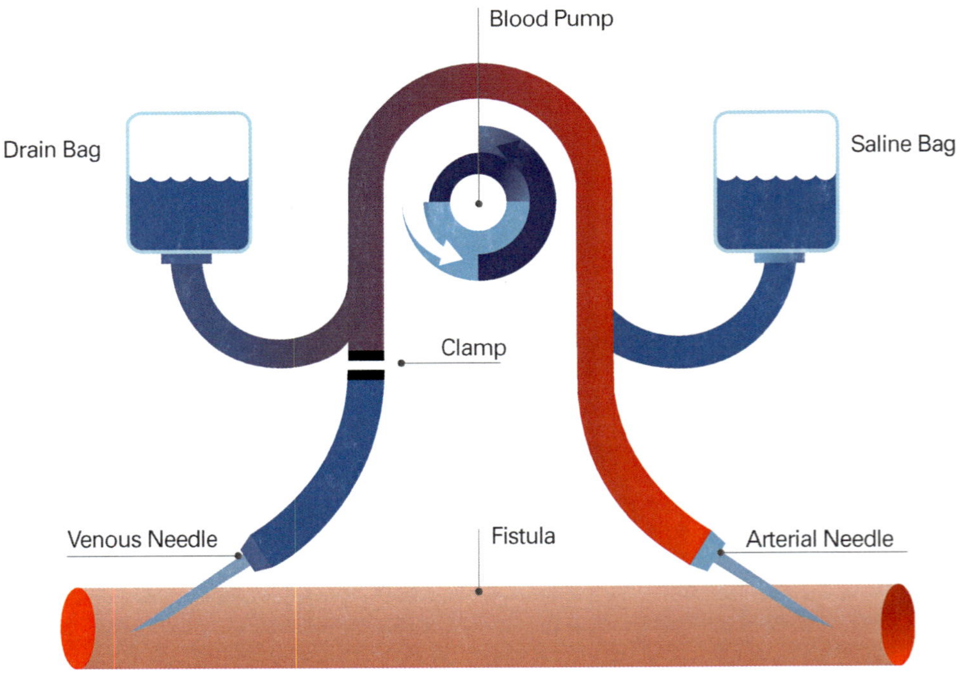

Figure 4. Variation of Blood Priming Without a Blood Sensor
If a patient is performing the same blood priming procedure as depicted in Figure 2 in the absence of a blood sensor, blood could enter the drain bag if the patient is not vigilantly watching the tubing as there is no automated cue signaling the patient to clamp the tubing to the drain bag and open the circuit to the fistula. Given the speed of the pump during priming, a patient losing concentration for even a minute or two can result in significant blood loss into the drain bag.

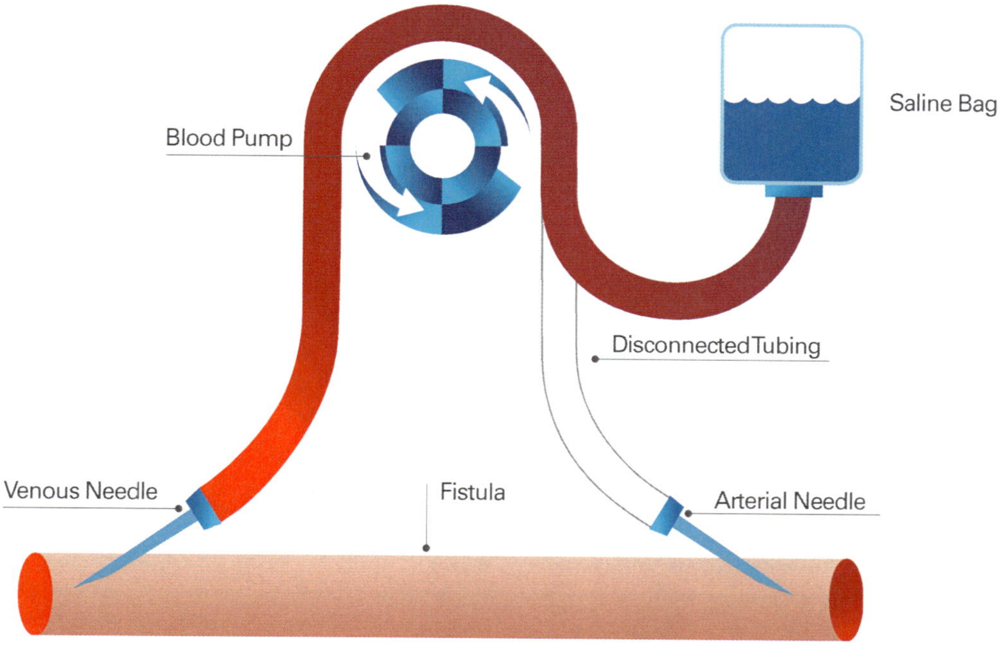

Figure 5. Routine Rinse-back After Dialysis Completion
After the hemodialysis treatment is completed, the tubing must be cleared of blood by rinsing it with saline. To do this, the patient disconnects the arterial tubing from the arterial needle and then connects the arterial tubing to a saline bag. The pump is then engaged and saline is drawn out of the saline bag through the circuit thereby pushing the blood ahead of it back into the venous side of the fistula ("returning blood to the patient").

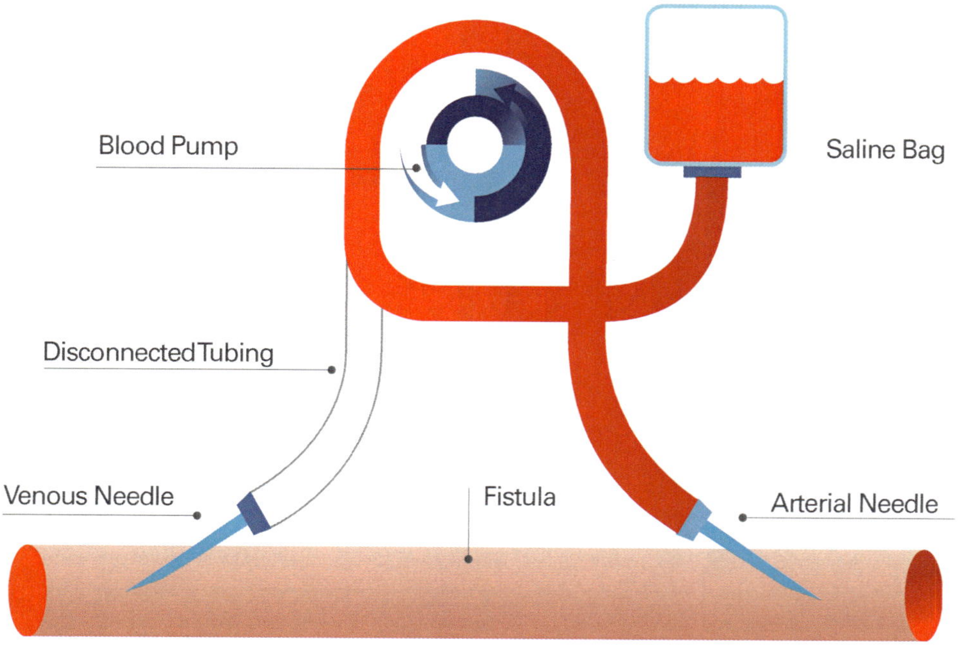

Figure 6. Rinse-back Procedure With Inadvertent Disconnection/ Connection Errors
The usual rinse-back procedure requires the patient to disconnect the arterial tubing and connect it to the saline bag (see Figure 4). However, if the patient inadvertently disconnects the venous tubing from the fistula and connects it to the saline bag instead, blood will be drawn incorrectly from the arterial line, pushing it into the saline bag. Blood will not be returned to the patient when the pump is engaged.

Figure 7. Dialyzer
The threaded connections between the arterial and venous tubing to the arterial and venous dialyzer headers, respectively (a), and the connections between the dialyzer and the dialysate tubing (b), may be problem areas. When threading is not carefully performed and verified by the patient, significant blood loss may occur from such misconnections. Likewise, dialysate may leak from a misconnection at the dialysate inflow or outflow ports if the tubing is not properly secured.

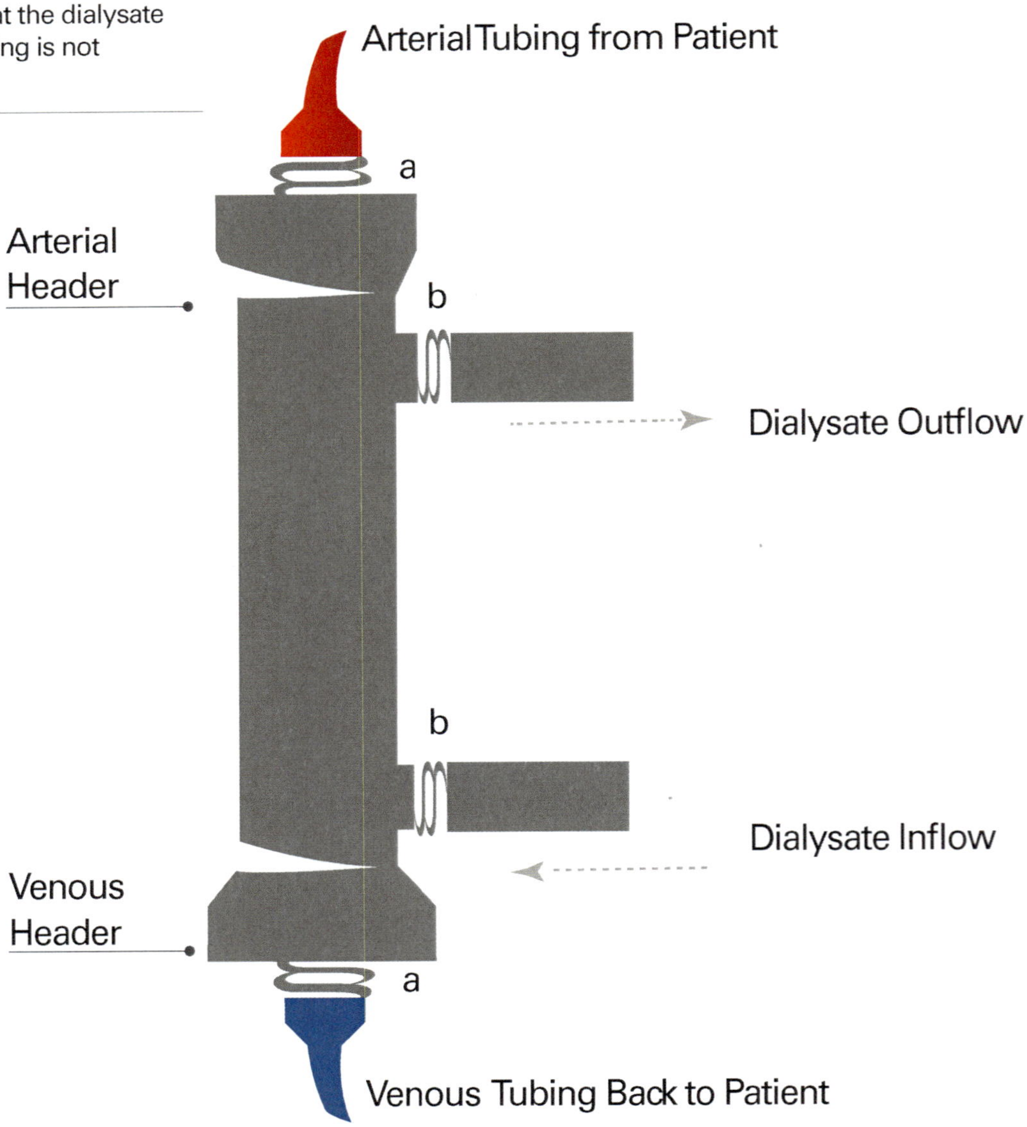

Wong et al describe a single case of air embolism in a patient occurring during disconnection from a central venous catheter.[4] No episodes of hemolysis or profound hemodynamic collapse from ultrafiltration or dialysate leaks have been described, even though such events are conceivable and, in the case of hypotension, are likely underreported.

A number of key themes emerge from these cases. First, blood loss from a variety of mechanisms is most often the cause of life-threatening AEs, as outlined above. Second, human error was implicated in 7 of 9 cases and probable in the other 2. Indeed, the reported home HD-related AEs did not occur because of an absence of safety measures, rather, they occurred because patients failed to follow prescribed procedures; for example, ignoring machine alarms or neglecting to appropriately use wetness detectors (see "Fistula Hemorrhage" in "The Care and Keeping of Vascular Access for Home Hemodialysis Patients" module). This underscores the importance of human error and the observation that patients will find a multitude of unpredictable ways to modify their dialysis that contravene standard operating procedures (SOPs) specifically designed to mitigate the risk of accidents. Third, there may be a lack of patient awareness that even small, seemingly insignificant changes in a procedure may lead to serious consequences. Fourth, Wong et al note in their case series that there does not seem to be a relationship between the experience of the program and the occurrence of a catastrophic event. The majority of their reported cases occurred in the last 2 years, even though the programs had been in existence for over a decade.[4] Fifth, there is no clear correlation between AE and patient experience with home HD. Four of the 8 relevant cases in the literature occurred in individuals having more than 1 year of independent dialysis experience at the time of their event. Finally, the presence of a care partner did not prevent the AE from occurring, although care partner presence may have prevented a fatality: 2 of the 3 events that occurred while patients were alone ended in death, while none of the 6 events that occurred while a care partner was present resulted in a fatal outcome.

Take-Home Messages

- The most frequently reported serious AEs during home HD involve blood loss, although air embolism, catastrophic electrolyte abnormalities, hemolysis, profound hemodynamic collapse from ultrafiltration, or dialysate leaks are also possible.
- Most reported serious AEs arise in part from human error, and have occurred as a result of some degree of nonadherence to SOPs.

Prevention of Procedure-Related Serious Adverse Events

Prevention is key in avoiding serious AEs, and there are technological, patient, and system factors that not only contribute to AEs, but by extension can also lead to their prevention.

Technological and Environmental Factors

At the present time, there are few home HD machines on the market that are specifically designed for home use, and most are in-center machines that are adapted for self-care at home; however, it is likely that future advances in home HD technology will provide increasing layers of safety features. In the meantime, there are still some programmatic measures that can be implemented.

Current home HD machines can and should be preset to preclude any erroneous actions or lack of actions. For instance, ultrafiltration rates for conventional home HD (short hours thrice weekly) might be set to avoid excessive fluid removal (eg, maximum of 1 L/hr) as determined by the care team. Various alarm parameters might also be preset to appropriate levels to detect deviation from SOPs, although care should be taken not to do so in a manner that causes excessive machine alarming and desensitization of the patient. The dialysis equipment should also permit rapid adjustment in therapy as required by an emergent situation (eg, rapid administration of fluid boluses, adjustments in ultrafiltration rates). Some renal programs may wish to implement real-time remote monitoring (ie, of vital signs, treatment parameters, or physiological markers such as hematocrit, etc), the advantages and disadvantages of which are discussed below and elsewhere.[12] Though not yet on the market, venous disconnect devices that automatically stop the blood pump if a needle is dislodged will likely be available soon and should also be considered as a possible safety mechanism.

The treatment environment, too, should be designed with safety and comfort in mind: a patient must have a direct line-of-sight to all screens and monitoring devices, wetness detectors should be placed around the access site and under the dialysis machine, and seating should be ergonomic for long treatment duration yet still permit rapid adjustment to a supine position in case of symptomatic hypotension (see "Infrastructure" in the "Infrastructure, Water, and Machines in the Home" module).

Patient Factors

Patient selection and training are perhaps the key elements in preventing serious AEs. We recommend that home HD programs develop an explicit policy for patient selection (see "Patient Selection and Training" module). For the staff, a policy is essential for driving program recruitment, and also for implementing a timely transition of patients to alternative modalities if and when home HD becomes inappropriate. For the patients, a policy makes explicit the medical requirements for home HD. It facilitates recognition that the therapy is more than simply a lifestyle choice and that there might be situations in which harm may outweigh benefits.

In general, patients should be physically and intellectually able and motivated to perform home HD and its related activities, including following the treatment prescription, maintaining equipment, monitoring water and blood work, and correctly executing procedures/protocols related to troubleshooting. Patients with skill barriers will require extra training or additional support at home to ensure their safety, or support to transition to an alternative modality if no solution offsets their increased risk. Communication plays a key role in the avoidance of error. Training staff should provide clear messages around safe practices and clear communication and demarcation of responsibility between patients and care partners around procedures/protocols, while emphasizing the final objective for training: technically excellent dialysis performed in the home, without compromise to safety. Depending on the patient, training may be an ongoing process to achieve this end result, with either formal or informal recertification of patients on an annual or biannual basis. Recertification is particularly important in those patients who are deemed at risk for a procedure-related AE but for whom this modality cannot reasonably be denied a priori.

Systems for Support of Patients at Home

Well-defined systems for technical support are essential for maintaining patient safety once patients have completed training. These systems will vary between programs and according to the needs of their home HD patients. In general, it is adequate

Useful Resources*

- National Institute for Health and Care Excellence, Guidance on home compared to hospital haemodialysis for patients with end-stage renal failure (TA48)
- Method to Assess Treatment Choices for Home Dialysis (MATCH-D)

* See Web version of Manual on ISHD.org for hyperlinks.

Practice Tip

- Appropriate patient selection and training are the cornerstones of ensuring patient safety.
- Patients with identified risks for AEs (eg, skill barriers, attitudinal barriers, nonadherence) should have individualized training with recertification at specified intervals, as appropriate.

to support patients through patient- or provider-initiated contact rather than by routine real-time telemetry monitoring of dialysis. While certainly not standard of care, some may see a role for real-time monitoring in assuaging anxieties in patients transitioning to home HD.[13] In our experience, however, lack of real-time monitoring is not borne out as a meaningful barrier to home HD. Clinical and technical assistance for patients and their care partners should be easily accessible 24 hours a day. An automatic alarm contact to the local paramedic unit is an option for high-risk patients. Assistance by either means may detect warning signs of impending problems, and can facilitate transfer of patients to emergency departments or respite facilities for diagnostic and therapeutic measures before an AE arises.

An important tool for maintaining patient safety is regular clinical review in the form of outpatient or home visits or telephone/ telemetric assessments. The frequency of follow-up is variable, but in Canada and New Zealand, the interval between clinic appointments is typically every 3 and 6 months, respectively, while blood work is monitored monthly. Whatever the arrangement, clinical review should include careful questioning regarding patient safety. Proper protocols and procedures should be reinforced at each visit, and appropriate reeducation given when gaps are identified.

One important area for inquiry is around near misses—those events that did not cause serious harm but had the potential to do so. Inquiries should be made in a manner that avoids undue criticism of the patient or instills a culture of blame (eg, "Have you had any accidents that we should tell people about who are training at the moment?"). Open disclosure by patients is important to identify opportunities for program development, and allows near misses to be used in a constructive fashion as a teachable moment. As noted elsewhere, home HD patients may find risky improvisations to simplify or speed up their treatments. Although not described in the original case report, 1 patient who died was using a self-built home HD station, which the patient designed and customized without the knowledge of his treating team. His setup did not allow him to have a direct line of sight to his saline bag, which almost certainly contributed to the AE.[10]

Nurse- or care partner–assisted home HD may be a helpful option to enable patients with worsening disability or frailty to continue dialysis at home.[14,15] Nurse-assisted home HD is typically performed for residents of extended-care facilities, although this can also involve nurses attending patients in their own houses if allowed/facilitated by the local healthcare system. This initiative is useful to extend technique survival. However, assisted home HD can be counterproductive in some circumstances: there may be a tendency for patients to not take full responsibility for their care by consciously or unconsciously limiting their understanding and competence of the equipment and the HD process if they know there is someone available to assist them in their home HD care.

The requirement for a care partner at home varies by program and by patient. Some centers require that the patient have a care partner routinely present during the entire treatment; other programs may require that the care partner be present only at specific times during a treatment, if at all. Care partners are useful for those patients needing a high degree of support, either for performing routine tasks such as initiating or discontinuing a treatment, or for emergencies that patients are not able to manage on their own. In the extreme, a care partner may perform the entire treatment for a patient who is otherwise incapable of doing so. In general, such arrangements have been shown to be safe.[14] However, the same scrupulous attention is required for training and maintaining competence of care partners as it is for the patients themselves. The best care partners are those who can provide reliable long-term assistance to the patient, and this is correlated with a stable social environment and a lack of concurrent medical problems. Notwithstanding, all care partners should be routinely monitored for burnout, which can compromise the quality of the support and consequently patient safety.

Finally, support for patients undergoing machine-based home HD should include a procedure for their timely transition to an alternative modality, either peritoneal dialysis (PD) or facility-based HD, if machine-based home HD is no longer feasible. This decision should be motivated by changes in medical, technical, or social circumstances that might impact patient safety and should be guided by the same principles used for patient selection. This transition should be made compassionately, and only after all other avenues of support have been exhausted.

Patient Access to Emergency Services for Advice and Care

When and how patients should access emergency care should be explicitly outlined before they complete home training. At minimum, patients should be clear about how to contact emergency medical services (EMS) and know the location and contact details for their nearest hospital emergency department. This may be self-evident in many jurisdictions (eg, by simply telephoning 9-1-1), but not so elsewhere (eg, remote locations or jurisdictions without centralized activation of EMS). Patients who subscribe to a personal medical alert system (a Lifeline®- or Alert 1®-type system) should be aware of how to activate that system. Patients should also know where to go for urgent respite dialysis in the event they cannot care for themselves (eg, as a result of acute illness, power outage, natural disaster). The primary center or associated hospital HD facility will usually be the unit providing respite dialysis for those patients living near the training center. For those living remotely, emergency care may be provided at satellite or local hospital facilities. Previous arrangements should be made with healthcare professionals at those sites to broker emergency care for patients, should it become necessary.

Communicating Risk to Patients

Because until very recently there has been no published empiric data concerning absolute risk of home HD, our communication of risk to patients has been largely predicated on the fact we have successfully managed patients self-administering home HD for decades. The conversation we have with patients aims to balance the benefits of home HD (ie, the flexibility of self-treatment and modality-specific benefits such as reduced dietary restrictions and pill burden with intensive home HD therapies like short-daily or nocturnal HD) with the risks and increased burden of independent home HD (ie, responsibility for one's own treatments/machine maintenance/water quality/supply ordering, rare and unforeseen procedure-related accidents, and risk of social isolation). It is not our practice to quote a specific procedure-related serious AE rate explicitly. Rather, all potentially life-threatening violations of SOPs are discussed in detail at the relevant point in patients' training. While the risk for home HD will never be zero, patients are reminded that home HD is very safe and that great care has been taken to design resources, policies, and procedures specifically aimed to minimize risk, where possible.

Emergency Management of Procedure-Related Adverse Events

Our experience with fatal and near-fatal procedure-related catastrophic events has taught us that despite the best-intentioned prevention strategies, a serious AE will eventually occur in a program. Thus, it is paramount to educate patients on emergency procedures and practice these as part of routine training and recertification. We advocate a simple "clamp-and-call" plan that should be initiated as soon as patients or care partners notice significant blood loss, air entry into the access, deteriorating level of consciousness, or any other atypical symptom while the patient is undergoing dialysis (Figure 8). This necessitates access to a personalized medical alert system or telephone that is within reach at all times. Clamping will stop the blood pump and prevent further blood loss (the most common cause of procedure-related events) and give patients time to call for help. For patients who dialyze with someone else in the home, the patient should call that person into the room where the dialysis is taking place to either activate the personalized medical alert system or call EMS if the patient's situation deteriorates. If no one else is present, patients are asked to activate their personalized medical alert system or call EMS themselves if there are atypical symptoms that may suggest a potential impending emergency (eg, presyncope, palpitations, chest pressure, focal neurological symptoms, deteriorating level of consciousness). In the absence of such symptoms, patients should contact their center-based on-call home HD staff (eg, the training unit directly or the after-hours on-call service) to discuss and appropriately manage problems. The on-call nurses or technologists should have a low threshold to initiate EMS on behalf of a reluctant or deteriorating patient.

We encourage all patients to have a preemptive emergency kit readily available and prominently positioned near their home HD machine. At the very least, kits should contain:

- Emergency contact information for the EMS, the home HD training unit, and the nephrologist
- A copy of the patient's medical history, including an up-to-date medication list
- An open letter addressed to EMS staff and hospital emergency department personnel (Table 2)

This open letter should communicate basic instructions to disconnect a patient from a hemodialysis machine (relevant for EMS crews who may be called to attend an unconscious subject still connected to a dialysis machine), contact information for home HD on-call services and the patient's nephrologist, and a request to contact the home

Practice Tip

- Telephone or Internet monitoring of dialysis function has been done by some centers, but is not generally warranted.
- Regular clinical review provides an opportunity for careful questioning regarding patient safety. Proper protocols and procedures should be reinforced at each visit, and appropriate reeducation given when gaps are identified.
- Care partners are useful for those patients who require a high degree of support, either for performing routine tasks or for emergencies that patients are not able to manage on their own.

Table 2. Open Letter to Emergency Medical Service (EMS) and Emergency Room Personnel

To EMS Personnel:	To Emergency Room Personnel:
The patient bearing this letter has end-stage kidney disease and undergoes home hemodialysis. If the subject is found connected to the hemodialysis machine and is not capable of disconnecting him/herself, please do the following: **INSERT SIMPLE MINIMUM INSTRUCTIONS TO REMOVE PATIENT FROM MACHINE.** **Perhaps include a diagram** This Emergency Kit/Envelope contains a medical history, a medication list, and contact information for the home hemodialysis unit. Please take this documentation with you when transporting the patient to hospital.	The patient bearing this letter has end-stage kidney disease and undergoes home hemodialysis. Please find included a patient history, medication list, and contact information for the home hemodialysis on-call service and/nephrologist. Once stabilized, please contact the home hemodialysis on-call service to discuss whether the patient's presentation to the hospital is related to the home hemodialysis procedure.

HD on-call service if the AE occurred while the patient was actively dialyzing. This latter issue is important because home HD equipment may need to be inspected and interrogated in a timely manner if an AE is potentially linked to hardware malfunction. More elaborate kits can be individualized and incorporate bridging therapy to stabilize patients while definitive treatment is being sought or accessed (eg, may contain blood culture sets and empiric antibiotics for likely blood stream infection).

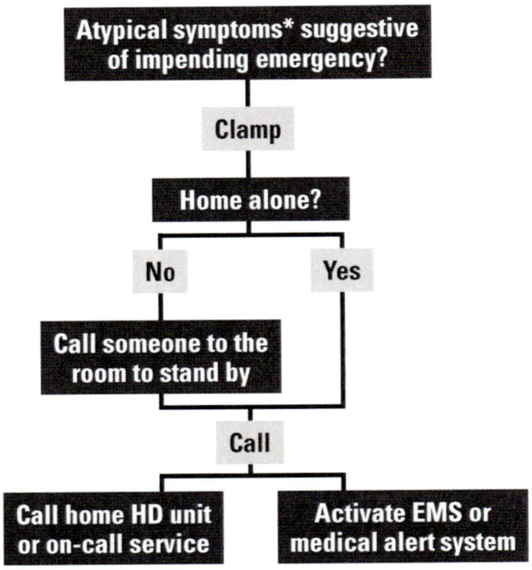

Figure 8. Home Hemodialysis "Clamp and Call" Emergency Management Algorithm
*Atypical symptoms include but are not limited to presyncope, heart palpitations, chest pressure, focal neurological symptoms, or deteriorating level of consciousness.
EMS = emergency medical services.

Quality Assurance Process

Central to any patient safety framework is an iterative quality assurance loop intended to prevent or minimize the occurrence or recurrence of an AE for an individual patient, and also for other patients within the same program.

The first step in developing a quality assurance process is certification and/or accreditation. In some parts of the world, it may be appropriate or required to have certification and/or accreditation of the home HD program itself. Irrespective of local standards, we recommend that new programs undergo a regular review by an external, experienced home HD training unit for a certain period after new program inception, if at all possible. There should be a robust training program for trainers, with regular credentialing of staff.

The second step in the development of the quality assurance loop is the establishment of robust SOPs for home HD. Quality assurance will be defined by variability of practice in relation to these procedures. SOPs need to be thoroughly understood by the staff as well as patients, and they should be individualized to meet local requirements. The importance of having SOPs cannot be overemphasized—ensuring quality assurance is not possible without them.

The third step is the documentation of process measures related to outcomes and safety. Process measures should include a key performance indicator of near misses. In addition, regular near-miss conferences should be held among the clinical staff within the training unit. Where possible, lessons learned from near misses and serious AEs should be incorporated into the home HD patient teaching curriculum. Existing patients within the program should be made aware of changes in policies and procedures during follow-up visits or by use of periodic communication from the program (eg, patient newsletters).

If a serious AE does occur, a specific Adverse Event SOP should be initiated (processes for consideration in creating such an SOP are outlined in Table 3). The purpose of this SOP is to provide guidelines in how to direct the investigation so that the appropriate parties can learn from the event. The Adverse Event SOP also provides guidance in how to disseminate the results of the investigation to appropriate stakeholders.

We feel there is potential benefit in 2 initiatives that do not yet exist but may provide the opportunity for knowledge discovery and enhancement of patient safety. The first is a global registry of serious AEs experienced by patients performing home HD, which could be set up and funded on a membership basis with information sharing among members. The second is a Web-based self-reporting system of AEs and near misses for home HD patients. This could ensure timely and comprehensive logging of events and yield valuable insight into patient-perceived concerns. Both of these initiatives are worth exploring as value-added components within a quality assurance process.

Table 3. Processes to Initiate After a Serious Adverse Event or Near Miss
The machine and consumables should be impounded as is from the patient's home, without being stripped or cleaned, and stored for examination in the home hemodialysis training unit.
All documentation resulting from the treatment should be impounded as is. We recommend that copies be made, and that the originals are stored securely to prevent inadvertent loss of key paperwork.
The sequence of events and context of the event should be ascertained as clearly as possible, from those present at the scene and through the liberal use of photography of the scene and machine.
Depending on the nature of the event, the machine should be interrogated for any stored information (eg, blood pressure measures, alarms, alarm overrides).
Depending on the nature of the event, hemodialysis technical staff (ideally from an external, independent home HD training unit) should ensure that the machine meets standard operational checks.
There should be immediate communication of the potential for the specific error in question to the home hemodialysis training staff and existing home hemodialysis patients.
Depending on the nature and severity of the event, there might be an external review of the home hemodialysis training program and its resources by the quality improvement team of the parent hospital or another home hemodialysis training unit with more experience. The review may involve root cause analysis or failure mode and effects analysis (ie, techniques for delineating errors that are usually beyond the capabilities of clinical staff).
Depending on the nature of the event, there might be communication with the manufacturer of the dialysis machinery to ascertain whether the event has occurred previously, and whether a technical solution is available to prevent similar events.
Depending on the nature of the event, consideration might be given to publication in an open-source medical journal, since this is likely the best method of communicating widely with clinicians.
Depending on the nature of the event, consideration might be given to communication of the event on a reputable Web-based patient discussion forum, in conjunction with a patient advocacy group.
We recommend that each unit keep a registry of serious adverse events, and communicate these events and near misses to other providers in the region to share experience.

References

1. Tong A, Palmer S, Manns B, et al. The beliefs and expectations of patients and caregivers about home haemodialysis: an interview study. BMJ Open. 2013;3:e002148.
2. Tong A, Palmer S, Manns B, et al. Clinician beliefs and attitudes about home haemodialysis: a multinational interview study. BMJ Open. 2012;2:e002146.
3. Hawley CM, Jeffries J, Nearhos J, Van Eps C. Complications of home hemodialysis. Hemodial Int. 2008;12(Suppl 1):S21-25.
4. Wong B, Zimmerman D, Reintjes F, et al. Procedure-related serious adverse events among home hemodialysis patients: a quality assurance perspective. Am J Kidney Dis. 2014;63:251-258.
5. Tennankore KK, D'Gama C, Faratro R, Fung S, Wong E, Chan CT. Adverse technical events in home hemodialysis. Am J Kidney Dis. 2014 (in press).
6. Marshall MR, Eastwood DO. Mortality risk from angioaccess bleeding or infection on facility versus home HD in New Zealand (abstract). J Am Soc Nephrol. 2014 (in press).
7. Bray BD, Boyd J, Daly C, et al. How safe is renal replacement therapy? A national study of mortality and adverse events contributing to the death of renal replacement therapy recipients. Nephrol Dial Transplant, 2014; 29:681-687.
8. Aspden P, Corrigan JM, Wolcott J, Erickson SM. Patient Safety. Achieving a New Standard of Care. Washington, DC: The National Academies Press; 2004.
9. AHRQ PSNet Patient Safety Network. Patient safety. Available at: http://psnet.ahrq.gov/glossary.aspx?indexLetter=P. Accessed September 2, 2013.
10. Allcock K, Jagannathan B, Hood CJ, Marshall MR. Exsanguination of a home hemodialysis patient as a result of misconnected blood-lines during the wash back procedure: a case report. BMC Nephrol. 2012;13:28.
11. Murlidharan P, Chan CT, Bargman JM. Catastrophic hypercalcemia as a technical complication in home hemodialysis. NDT Plus. 2011;4:251-252.
12. Marshall MR, Pierratos A, Pauly RP. Delivering home hemodialysis: is there still a role for real-time monitoring? Semin Dialysis. 2014 Nov 30. doi: 10.1111/sdi.12327. [Epub ahead of print].
13. Cafazzo JA, Leonard K, Easty AC, Rossos PG, Chan CT. Patient perceptions of remote monitoring for nocturnal home hemodialysis. Hemodial Int. 2010;14:471-477.
14. Tennankore KK, Kim SJ, Chan CT. The feasibility of caregiver-assisted home nocturnal hemodialysis. Nephron Clin Pract. 2012;122:17-23.
15. Cornelis T, Kotanko P, Goffin E, van der Sande FM, Kooman JP, Chan CT. Intensive hemodialysis in the (nursing) home: the bright side of geriatric ESRD care? Semin Dial. 2012;25:605-610.

6 Patient Selection and Training for Home Hemodialysis

Jean-Philippe Rioux, MD, FRCPC[1]
Mark R Marshall, MBChB, MPH, FRACP[2, 3]
Rose Faratro, RN, CNephC[4]
Raymond Hakim, MD[5]
Rosemary Simmonds, NP, MN[6]
Christopher T Chan, MD, FRCCP[4]

[1]Hôpital du Sacré-Cœur de Montréal, Quebec, Canada; [2]Faculty of Medical and Health Sciences, University of Auckland, Auckland, New Zealand; [3]Department of Renal Medicine, Counties Manukau District Health Board, Auckland, New Zealand; [4]Division of Nephrology, Department of Medicine, University Health Network, Toronto, Ontario, Canada; [5]Division of Nephrology and Hypertension, Department of Medicine, Vanderbilt University, Nashville, TN, USA; [6]Barwon Health, Geelong, Victoria, Australia.

Implementing Hemodialysis in the Home
A Global Perspective

iSHD
International Society for Hemodialysis

CONTENTS

Abstract

Patient selection and training is arguably the most important step towards building a successful home hemodialysis program. We present a step-by-step account of home hemodialysis (HD) training to guide providers who are developing home HD programs. Although home HD training is an important step in allowing patients to undergo dialysis in the home, there is a surprising lack of systematic research in this field. Innovations and research in this area will be pivotal in further promoting a higher acceptance rate of home HD as the renal replacement therapy of choice.

Introduction

Home hemodialysis (HD) has been associated with several clinical benefits compared with conventional thrice-weekly, in-center HD. To date, few resources have focused on the importance of patient selection, training, and education of a complex medical procedure such as home HD. In this module, we describe guiding principles for implementation of a home HD program with an emphasis on (1) patients' selection, assessments, and training, and (2) challenges of adult education. Future challenges in education research and the importance of quality assurance in home HD education delivery will also be discussed.

Patient Selection for Home HD

Guidance for patient selection has been provided by the National Institute for Health and Care Excellence (NICE)[1] and the MATCH-D initiative.[2] Primarily, the patient should be physically and intellectually able and, most importantly, motivated to perform home HD and its related activities. As noted by others, most patients are medically suitable candidates for home HD.[2,3] Our own programs have enrolled patients with complex combinations of comorbidities, and we have discovered that many of our patients do better with more frequent or longer treatments that are more easily implemented in the home setting.[4] Indications for and relative contraindications against home HD are listed in Table 1. At our centers, we have implemented, to various extents, a "home-dialysis-first" policy, which prioritizes proactive education to all patients with chronic kidney disease.[5] Policies such as these are important change agents, and help healthcare professionals facilitate a clinical culture of promoting home dialysis to appropriate patients.

Optimal patient selection for home HD involves a balance between enthusiastic program recruitment and careful shared decision-making to avoid recruiting patients who are either physically or mentally unsuitable for home HD, and those who face insurmountable social challenges. As a starting point, home HD programs should aim to engage with and recruit all appropriate patients in their wider dialysis program who would be potentially capable of performing home HD and benefiting from this therapy. Renal units that have a systematic practice in patient education and decision-making practices tend to have a significantly higher adoption rate toward independent dialysis[6] (see "Systems to Cultivate Suitable Patients for Home Dialysis").

Table 1. Considerations for Patient Selection for Home HD

Potential Candidates for Home HD
• Patients who are able to physically and cognitively manage the tasks of care (or have a support person who can) • Patients who are motivated and willing to learn the technique • Patients who wish to continue to work or continue schooling • Patients who have failed peritoneal dialysis and wish to continue therapy at home • Patients with the following medical conditions: » Severe sleep apnea » Persistent hyperphosphatemia » Right heart failure » Uncontrolled ascites » Refractory volume overload » Difficult-to-control hypertension » Symptomatic hypotension, cramps, or nausea on conventional HD » Inadequate control of uremic symptoms on conventional HD » Excessive recovery time after conventional HD • Women who are pregnant or planning to conceive
Contraindications to Home HD
• Unstable medical conditions (eg, uncontrolled arrhythmia, seizure disorders) • Lack of suitable vascular access • Unstable behavioral problems (eg, uncontrolled psychosis or anxiety, ongoing injection drug use and alcohol abuse) • Contraindication to anticoagulant use during dialysis • Conditions that may cause abrupt loss of consciousness (eg, severe and unstable intradialytic hypotension)

Adapted from Rioux et al.[4]

There are a number of tools to promote home HD to patients, which can be integrated into patient education programs (see "Home Hemodialysis Needs YOU!").

It is important for home HD programs to develop an explicit patient selection policy, which includes medical and social criteria for defining appropriate patients. A policy is crucial for driving program recruitment, and also for the timely transition of patients to alternative modalities if and when home HD becomes inappropriate. For the patients, a policy makes explicit the requirements for home HD and ensures they recognize that the therapy is more than simply a lifestyle choice.

It is ideal that an interdisciplinary team, which should include home dialysis nurses, technicians, and physicians, sees all interested patients (see the module, "Workforce Development and Models of Care in Home Hemodialysis").

Open discussions taking into consideration patient expectations and fears and the perspectives of care providers should be encouraged. Tests that assess hearing, vision, strength, and manual dexterity are helpful when evaluating patient suitability for home HD, and results from these tests should be documented accordingly; however, alterations from the norm in the majority of these assessments should not be considered absolute deterrents for home HD. Many of the initially perceived barriers to home HD can be overcome, often with the assistance of a care partner (see Table 2). A critical role for the interdisciplinary team is not only to identify patient barriers, but also solve them as well.

Another important issue to consider is that of nonadherence, which is a threat to patient safety as well as program credibility and longevity. Nonadherence in the setting of home dialysis is not well understood, although there are some general observations that are relevant to patient selection. One red flag is the case of the "unwilling" patient. Patients who lack control over modality selection have worse outcomes, probably due to resistance to training and nonadherence to treatment.[7,8] Those who are less motivated, therefore, are likely to require extra training to successfully make the transition to home HD. Another key determinant of adherence is patient attentional and coping style. For patients undergoing a complex, self-directed home-based treatment such as home HD, a more vigilant and active coping

Table 2. Potential Barriers to Home HD and Possible Interventions

Factor	Possible Intervention
Unkempt/poor personal hygiene	Hygiene education, dialysis partner
Frail/nonambulatory/ bedridden	Physiotherapy, occupational therapy, dialysis care partner
Illiterate	Pictures to train, return demonstration to verify learning, tape recorders for patient reports
Hearing impaired	Light/vibration for alarms
Brain damage, dementia, or poor short-term memory	Dialysis care partner
No use of either hand	Dialysis care partner
Severely visually impaired or blind	Change to peritoneal dialysis, dialysis care partner
Reduced awareness/ability to report bodily symptoms	Dialysis care partner

Adapted from Schatell et al.[2]

style is associated with more favorable adherence.[9,10] A general classification for nonadherence can be adapted to the home HD setting, and is shown in Table 3.[11] At-risk patients can still be trained, but they need to be managed carefully. This is one situation where support from health psychology is invaluable, especially during the selection process to identify at-risk patients, and also during the training period to mitigate the causal factors that underlie their predisposition.

Once there is agreement from the team that the patient is a suitable candidate and the patient himself has expressed interest in proceeding with home HD, a home inspection can then be scheduled.

For start-up home HD programs, appropriate selection of the first few patients is important to ensure a confident and successful training program in the future. These patients will, in general, be recruited from dialysis facilities, and should be highly motivated, have excellent social support, demonstrate a desire to learn and, most importantly, should have a good rapport with the wider clinical team. Successful home HD patients are a catalyst for program growth. Inviting patients to share their experience and stories to their dialysis peers either in person or by creating video footage is a powerful tool to improve uptake of home HD among others.

Useful Resources*

- » National Institute for Health and Care Excellence, Guidance on home compared to hospital haemodialysis for patients with end-stage renal failure (TA48)
- » Method to Assess Treatment Choices for Home Dialysis (MATCH-D)

*For hyperlinks see Web version of Manual on ISHD.org

Table 3. Risk Factors for Nonadherence and Possible Interventions

Category	Examples	Possible Intervention
Procedure-related factors	• Needle phobia • Burden of schedule/tasks • Unpalatable physical effects of treatment	• Health psychology, anesthetic cream • Dialysis care partner • Change to extended hours or frequent hemodialysis
Psychosocial factors	• Overwhelming situation/self-esteem issues • Lack of trust in health professionals • Unsupported home life • Drug or alcohol abuse	• Health psychology • Patient-to-patient peer support • Social work, community house hemodialysis • Rehabilitation
Deliberate nonadherence	• Depression, psychosis, or anxiety • Attention seeking • "Infallible" attitude • Risk-taking behavior (eg, adolescents)	• Health psychology, psychiatry • Health psychology, dialysis care partner • Health psychology, patient contract • Health psychology, patient contract

Adapted from Bullington.[11]

Training and Education for Home HD

Adult Learning and Home HD

Teaching an adult to perform HD at home may be challenging, and there is a paucity of published literature validating any specific training paradigm or program.

The personnel involved in training and supporting the patients and their care partners are important to ensure success of a program. Home HD nurses should be skilled practitioners, typically having a sound practical knowledge of dialysis with at least 12 months' experience in managing patients with chronic kidney disease. However, above all, nurses involved in training people for home HD must strongly believe that patients are capable of caring for themselves, and have a passion to promote the benefits of home dialysis to their patients. They must enjoy teaching and understand the principles of adult learning, and have the ability to invoke followership.

The principles of adult learning presume that adults are actively involved in the learning process and wish to be treated as equals to the teacher. The home dialysis learning process will benefit from having a staff that is informed of patients' and care partners' backgrounds, knowledge, and experience levels before these individuals enter the training program. A training program can then be tailored to allow patients to learn using styles and speeds at which they feel comfortable. Adults are motivated to learn things that they perceive will help them cope with real life issues; therefore, the ability to design active learning lessons that will help them to maintain their dialysis safety and long-term health are always best.

Adult learning is also motivated by a sense of self-esteem, and it is important to establish a friendly and open atmosphere, ideally in an informal, relaxed environment. The input of patients and their care partners should be respected and encouraged, and there should be frequent positive feedback given to patients as they progress through the training process.

Other unique considerations include the perceptions and reactions of the learners making errors—adults often blame themselves for their errors but do not always learn from their mistakes and make corrections accordingly. Finally, it is important to adapt to patients' different learning styles by using complementary visual, auditory, or kinesthetic techniques. Practically, a good start for any program is the use of training aids that are strong visually, with step-by-step photography to demonstrate the dialysis procedure with a minimal amount of text. These can be very easily developed and tailored for individual patient's needs by enthusiastic HD dialysis training staff.

Depending on learning style, aids such as DVDs, slide presentations, and/or websites may also be useful for patients and their care partners to peruse at home, and this approach has been used successfully in other settings.[12-13] Patients with very low literacy may benefit from the use of more elaborate audiovisual training aids (developed at low literacy levels).

The Training Program

Typically, patients are trained at the main home HD facility (ie, the home HD hub), although it is possible to train at a hospital or satellite HD unit, or even in patients' own homes. No matter the venue, it is important to involve care partners early in the process of planning for home HD and in the training of patients. The objectives of the training program are to (1) provide the appropriate amount of information to ensure that the patient will be able to dialyze safely at home; (2) enable the patient to monitor and manage other elements of his or her chronic kidney disease, such as obtaining samples for lab work and maintaining appropriate nutrition and diet; and (3) help the patient and his or her care partner(s) cope with barriers and fears associated with home HD (see the module, "Psychosocial Aspects in Home Hemodialysis").[13] During training, the patient will also receive technical education on the operations and maintenance of the water treatment system.

During training, the ideal nurse trainer-to-patient ratio is typically 1:1. An idealized schedule of training is described in Table 4,

Table 4. Weekly Education and Training for Home HD

Training Week	Education and Training Focus	Learning Objectives
1	• General operations of the dialysis unit • Learn new vocabulary • Proper hand washing technique • Self-assessment (blood pressure, weight) • Access care • Introduction to dialysis manual	• Understand concepts behind HD • Learn self-assessment
2	• Observation of the trainer doing tasks • Interpretation of the concepts of self-assessment and dialysis • Setup of the HD machine	• Set up the HD machine using the manual
3	• Equipment preparation • Disconnect procedure • Alarms management • Self-cannulation • Perform tasks under the supervision of the trainer	• Set up the HD machine without using the manual
4	• Alarms management • Complications management • Meet with technician to learn water management • Recirculation procedure	• Self-cannulation (may require additional time) • Manage complications and alarms
5	• Patient performing dialysis alone in absence of nurse	• Achieve total independent self-care
6-8	• Self-dialyze in the unit until ready for home HD • Challenge with alarms and potential complications • Formal examination	• Complete independence • Begin home HD

Adapted from Rioux et al.[4]

with weekly areas of focus and training objectives. In practice, however, training is individualized to address any identified learning barriers or risks for failure. The frequency and duration of actual HD training sessions are also variable, as shown in Table 5. Typically, approximately 6 weeks is necessary to complete training, although this training period tends to be shorter in counties with a low prevalence of patients who complete home HD, such as in the United States, and longer is countries with a higher prevalence of patients who complete home HD, such as in New Zealand. This may be related to the higher degree of patient selection in the United States (ie, only the most capable and motivated patients undergo home HD), and the reduced availability of "low-hanging fruit" for quick training in New Zealand, where training needs to accommodate a more educationally and medically diverse home HD patient population. Before training begins, dialysis professionals and patients should agree on and set an appropriate timeline for training, including incremental milestones that can be used to recognize difficulties in the training process and serve as markers of success.

At the end of each HD training session, there should be discussions with the patient to ensure that learning objectives have been met. Key points should be reiterated, as necessary, and patient understanding should be reaffirmed. At the end of training, the patient should be examined on his or her competency, usually through a written or some other formalized testing system (eg, a practical examination). In our programs, there are home visits made by training staff before and after training. They verify that the home is safe and suitable for home HD, and ensure that set-up and procedures used for training align with the particular physical arrangements that the patient

Table 5. Training Program Parameters for Home HD

Program*	Frequency of HD Training Sessions (per week)	Number of Training Sessions Required for Completion	Training Duration (weeks)	Proportion of Dialysis Patients on Home Dialysis, Nationally (2011)[14]	Proportion of Dialysis Patients on Home HD, Nationally (2011)[14]
Edmonton, Alberta, Canada	4	~24	6	21	3.9
Monash, Victoria, Australia	3	18-24	6-8	27.6	8.8
Geelong, Victoria, Australia	4	16-24	4-6	27.6	8.8
Toronto, Ontario, Canada[15]	3	18-24	6-8	21	3.9
Los Angeles, CA, USA[16]	5	15-30	3-6	8.7	1.3
Helsinki, Finland[17]	4-5	10-34	2-8	22.8	4.2
Lynchburg, VA, USA[18]	5	25-30	5-6	8.7	1.3
Christchurch, New Zealand[19]	4	~43	8-12	51.4	18.2
Auckland, New Zealand	3-4	26-48	12-16	51.4	18.2
FHN trial Group, USA/Canada[20]	3-5	11-59	3-12	3.1/21	1.3/3.9
Dublin, Republic of Ireland[21,22]	3-5	16-30	4-6	10.8	0.9
Kobe, Japan[23]	1-5	~45	8-28	3.2	0.1

FHN = Frequent Hemodialysis Network.

*Personal communications between July 17-21, 2014, with Robert Pauly (Edmonton, Alberta, Canada), Peter Kerr (Monash, Victoria, Australia), John Agar (Geelong, Victoria, Australia), Christopher Chan (Toronto, Ontario, Canada), Victoria Kumar (Los Angeles, CA, USA), Eero Honkanen (Helsinki, Finland), Virpi Rauta (Helsinki, Finland), Robert Lockridge (Lynchburg, VA, USA), David McGregor (Christchurch, New Zealand), and Mark Marshall (Auckland, New Zealand).

has at home (eg, placement of machinery in relation to patient, location of supplies, etc). Our programs also have home HD nurses present at the patient's home for the first treatment to alleviate patient anxiety and ensure proper techniques and procedures are used.

Various programs have adopted the use of simulation training in the context of nursing and medical education.[24] To date, there is a paucity of patient-based simulation education research data available, but some sort of patient-based simulation activity may be of interest and helpful to validate patients' readiness to launch home HD.

Training Failure

To understand the determinants of training failure, Schachter et al conducted a retrospective cohort study including consecutive patients who began training for home HD at their facility between 2003 to 2011.[25] Of the 167 patients who started training for home HD, 32 were classified as "failure," a term which included any discontinuation of home HD during the first year. The most common reasons for training failure are listed in Table 6; the strongest predictors of "failure" were patients with concomitant diabetes and those living in rental housing.

Vascular Access Training in Home HD Patients

The optimal form of vascular access is undetermined in home HD, but all forms (ie, arteriovenous fistulas and grafts, central venous catheters) have been used. A detailed discussion of vascular access in the context of home HD is discussed in the module entitled, "The Care and Keeping of Vascular Access for Home HD Patients".

Table 6. Reasons for Failure to Graduate from Home HD Training

Rank	Reason	Proportion of Patients (%)
1	Home is inappropriate or cannot be modified for home HD	17
2	Deterioration in medical status	13
2	Cannot cope with burden of home HD	13
2	Patient nonadherence	13
2	Failed training tests	13
3	Insurmountable language barrier	8
3	Inadequate family support	8
3	Imminent renal transplant, decided not to invest further in home HD training	8
3	Financial barriers	8
4	Patient anxiety/nervousness about home HD	4
4	Care partner anxiety about home HD for dependent patient	4
4	Inadequate manual dexterity	4
4	Insurmountable visual impairment	4

Adapted from Schacter et al.[25]

One of the biggest concerns of performing home HD is the fear of system disconnection. To this aim, multiple prevention and management strategies have been proposed, including the use of wetness detectors (situated proximal to the cannulation sites and/or on the floor), needle taping/fixing strategies, and single-needle dialysis.[5,15] Clearly, further technical innovations are needed to improve the safety of vascular access use in home HD, although the cornerstone of patient safety will always be thorough education and training. Safety is discussed in greater detail in the module entitled, "Ensuring Patient Safety During Home HD".

An equally important concern is the fear of cannulation itself. Different cannulation techniques have been advocated for home HD and are discussed in detail in the module entitled, "The Care and Keeping of Vascular Access for Home HD Patients". The provision of experienced home HD staff and a relaxed, informal, and supportive training environment will assist in alleviating some of the fears patients associate with cannulation. In addition, complementary use of psychotherapy and cognitive therapy to overcome needle phobia and introduction of breathing exercises have been used by patients in other contexts and may be applicable for those patients in home HD.

Central venous catheters are attractive alternatives in home HD because of the ease of use and lower potential for disconnection. Results from a study by Perl et al showed that catheter survival is higher among home nocturnal HD patients compared with in-center HD patients,[6] which may be due, in part, to higher exposure to heparin. The incidence of catheter-related bacteremia was similar between patients undergoing home nocturnal HD and those patients undergoing in-center conventional HD;[26] however, central venous catheters have a higher rate of infectious complications than more permanent vascular access (ie, arteriovenous fistulas and grafts).[27] Similar to arteriovenous access, several safety strategies have been advocated for patients using central venous catheters at home. For example, a number of centers support the use of perforated nonremovable central venous catheter caps (aka, closed-connector devices).

Barriers to Home HD Training

From the patient perspective, learning home HD is often accompanied by a great deal of anxiety.[13] It is reasonable to assume that all patients are confronted to some degree with multiple concerns, including personal lack of confidence, fear of experiencing a catastrophic event while they are on dialysis, fear of burdening family members with care, and apprehension over suboptimal care.[28] It is important to openly discuss and address concerns, and these concerns are almost always surmountable with appropriate support.

Equally important, there are other potential barriers to the implementation of home HD. These barriers include the lack of center, physician, or nursing experience and deficiencies in the actual physical infrastructure for performing and training for home HD. Appropriate workforce development and infrastructure in the home HD hub becomes increasingly important with scaling and expansion of home HD programs, although more modest arrangements are often adequate for start-up or smaller programs (see the modules, "The Home Hemodialysis Hub – Physical Infrastructure and Integrated Governance Structure" and "Workforce Development and Models of Care").

Finally, poor education and planning regarding chronic kidney disease are important modifiable barriers to the adoption of nocturnal and wider home HD.[29] Effective cultivation of patients will improve home dialysis uptake in the predialysis stage, but also, in our experience, improve the receptiveness and engagement of patients during the training process (see the module, "Systems to Cultivate Suitable Patients for Home Dialysis").

Table 7. Key Performance Indicators for Home HD Training

Process Outcomes

- Training time
- Training failure rate
- Training nurse performance
  - » Self-assessment
  - » Patient satisfaction
  - » 360° feedback

Clinical Effectiveness Measures

- Program home HD technique survival
- Patient "near misses" or frequency of intradialytic hypotension
- Patient hospitalization rate
- Patient adherence with treatments, clinical appointment attendance, and blood tests
- Patient adherence with medication, phosphate control, and nutritional and fluid status parameters

Future Studies in Home HD Education

Although home HD training is an important step in encouraging patients to consider undergo dialysis in the home, there is a surprising lack of systematic research in this field. Innovations and research in this area will be pivotal in further promoting a higher acceptance rate of home HD as the renal replacement therapy of choice.

Key Performance Indicators for Home HD Training

As in every clinical process, the outcomes of home HD training should be measured. In our programs, these data have been used in many ways. Documentation of training time and failure rates allow for appropriate planning and funding for growth of the program, and more accurate estimates of training infrastructure requirements in the future. For trainers, individual metrics can be an indicator of their effectiveness and highlight the need for further support or oversight in their roles. For patients, analysis of training data may identify groups of patients with different training requirements, such as the need for more frequent training sessions or simply more of them. In some programs, the analysis of such data has offered insights into the most effective pairings between patients and trainers, and allowed prospective allocation of patients to trainers who may better suit their learning style or cultural or sociodemographic needs. A variety of key performance indicators can be collected, such as those listed in Table 7. At a minimum, 3 process outcomes should be documented along with at least 1 clinical outcome.

References

1. Technology Appraisal No. 48; Guidance on home compared with hospital haemodialysis for patients with end-stage renal failure. London: National Institute for Health and Care Excellence; 2005.
2. Schatell D. MATCH-D: a roadmap to home dialysis therapy. Nephrol News Issues. 2007;21(11):41, 43-44.
3. Moran J, Kraus M. Starting a home hemodialysis program. Semin Dial. 2007;20(1):35-39.
4. Rioux JP, Faratro R, Chan CT. Nocturnal home hemodialysis: implementation, quality assurance and future challenges. Minerva Urol Nefrol. 2010;62(1):103-110.
5. Perl J, Chan CT. Home hemodialysis, daily hemodialysis, and nocturnal hemodialysis: Core curriculum 2009. Am J Kidney Dis. 2009;54:1171-1184.
6. Fortnum D, Ludlow M, Morton RL. Renal unit characteristics and patient education practices that predict a high prevalence of home-based dialysis in Australia. Nephrology (Carlton). 2014;19:587-593.
7. Portolés J, Del Peso G, Fernández-Reyes MJ, Bajo MA, López-Sánchez P. Previous comorbidity and lack of patient free choice of technique predict early mortality in peritoneal dialysis. Perit Dial Int. 2009;29:150-157.
8. Stack AG, Martin DR. Association of patient autonomy with increased transplantation and survival among new dialysis patients in the United States. Am J Kidney Dis. 2005;45:730-742.
9. Nearhos J, Van Eps C, Connor J. Psychological factors associated with successful outcomes in home haemodialysis. Nephrology (Carlton). 2013;18:505-509.
10. Christensen AJ. Patient-by-treatment context interaction in chronic disease: a conceptual framework for the study of patient adherence. Psychosom Med. 2000;63:435-443.
11. Bullington P, Pawola L, Walker R, Valenta A, Briars L, John E. Identification of medication non-adherence factors in adolescent transplant patients: the patient's viewpoint. Pediatr Transplant. 2007;11:914-921.
12. Lacson E Jr, Wang W, DeVries C, et al. Effects of a nationwide predialysis educational program on modality choice, vascular access, and patient outcomes. Am J Kidney Dis. 2011;58:235-242.
13. Wong J, Eakin J, Migram P, Cafazzo JA, Halifax NV, Chan CT. Patients' experiences with learning a complex medical device for the self-administration of nocturnal home hemodialysis. Nephrol Nurs J. 2009;36:27-32.
14. US Renal Data System. USRDS 2013 Annual Data Report: Atlas of Chronic Kidney Disease and End-Stage Renal Disease in the United States. Bethesda, MD: National Institutes of Health, National Institute of Diabetes and Digestive and Kidney Diseases, 2013.
15. Pierratos A, Ouwendyk M, Francoeur R, et al. Nocturnal hemodialysis: three-year experience. J Am Soc Nephrol. 1998; 9:859-868.
16. Kumar VA, Ledezma ML, Rasgon SA. Daily home hemodialysis at a health maintenance organization: three-year experience. Hemodial Int. 2007;11:225-230.
17. Honkanen E, Muroma-Karttunen R, Taponen RM, Grönhagen-Riska C. Starting a home hemodialysis program: single center experiences. Scand J Urol Nephrol. 2002;36:137-144.
18. Lockridge RS Jr, Spencer M, Craft V, et al. Nightly home hemodialysis: five and one-half years of experience in Lynchburg, Virginia. Hemodial Int. 2004;8:61-69.
19. McGregor D, Buttimore A, Robson R, Little P, Morton J, Lynn K, Thirty years of universal home dialysis in Christchurch. N Z Med J. 2000;113:27-29.
20. Pipkin M, Eggers PW, Larive B, et al. Recruitment and training for home hemodialysis: experience and lessons from the Nocturnal Dialysis Trial. Clin J Am Soc Nephrol. 2010;5:1614-1620.

References (cont'd)

21. Connaughton DM, Jamal A, McWilliams J, et al. Home haemodialysis in Ireland. Ir J Med Sci. 2013;182:91-96.

22. The National Renal Office. Epidemiology of ESKD in Adults in Ireland June 2011. ESKD patients on Dialysis. Interim NRO Census. Available from: http://www.hse.ie/eng/about/Who/NRO/census.pdf (accessed date: August 21, 2014).

23. Tanaka H, Sakai R, Kita T, Okamoto K, Mikami M. Overnight home hemodialysis: eight patients and six years of experience in Sakairumi clinics. Contrib Nephrol. 2012;177:133-142.

24. Hudson D, Dunbar-Reid K, Sinclair PM. The incorporation of high fidelity simulation training into hemodialysis nursing education: Part 2—a pictorial guide to modifying a high fidelity simulator for use in simulating hemodialysis. Nephrol Nurs J. 2012;39:119-123.

25. Schachter ME, Tennankore KK, Chan CT. Determinants of training and technique failure in home hemodialysis. Hemodial Int. 2013;17:421-426.

26. Perl J, Lok CE, Chan CT. Central venous catheter outcomes in nocturnal hemodialysis. Kidney Int. 2006;70:1348-1354.

27. Ravani P, Gillespie BW, Quinn RR, et al. Temporal risk profile for infectious and noninfectious complications of hemodialysis access. J Am Soc Nephrol. 2013;24:1668-1677.

28. Cafazzo JA, Leonard K, Easty AC, Rossos PG, Chan CT. Patient-perceived barriers to the adoption of nocturnal home hemodialysis. Clin J Am Soc Nephrol. 2009;4:784-789.

29. Komenda P, Chan C, Pauly RP, et al. The evaluation of a successful home hemodialysis program: establishing a prospective framework for quality. Clin Nephrol. 2009;71:467-474.

7 The Care and Keeping of Vascular Access for Home Hemodialysis Patients

Rose Faratro, RN, BHScN, CNeph(C)[1]

Janine Jeffries, RN[2]

Gihad E Nesrallah, MD, FRCPC, FACP[3]

Jennifer M MacRae, MSc , MD, FRCPC[4]

[1]University Health Network, Toronto, Ontario, Canada; [2]Princess Alexandria Hospital, Brisbane, Australia; [3]Humber River Regional Hospital, Toronto, Ontario, Canada; [4]University of Calgary, Calgary, Alberta, Canada

Implementing Hemodialysis in the Home
A Global Perspective

iSHD
International Society for Hemodialysis

CONTENTS

Abstract

Creating and maintaining a healthy vascular access is a critical factor in successful home hemodialysis (HD). This module aims to serve as a "how-to manual" regarding vascular access issues for both patients and healthcare providers in a home HD program. This module outlines cannulation options for patients with arteriovenous access and describes troubleshooting techniques for potential complications; strategies are suggested to help patients overcome fear of cannulation and address problems associated with difficult cannulation. Technical aspects of central venous catheter care, as well as a guide to troubleshooting catheter complications, are covered in detail. Monitoring for access-related complications of stenosis, infection, and thrombosis is a key part of every home HD program. Key performance and quality indicators are important mechanisms to ensure patient safety in home HD and should be used during routine clinic visits.

Useful Resources*

» La Société Française de l'Abord Vasculaire. History of Buttonhole Technique

» End Stage Renal Disease Network, Cannulation of the AV Fistula

*For hyperlinks see Web version of Manual on ISHD.org

Arteriovenous Fistula

Arteriovenous Fistula Cannulation Options

Cannulation of the arteriovenous fistula (AVF), even when done properly, causes pain and local trauma; repeated cannulation can weaken blood vessel walls and promote wall dilation and the formation of aneurysms.[1,2] Unsuccessful cannulation can result in needle infiltration (swelling that happens when the needle goes through the fistula wall), which in turn causes localized bruising and increases the risk of thrombosis and loss of AVF patency.[3]

Two methods of needling are commonly used: rotating sites/rope ladder (RL) technique, and buttonhole (BH) technique. The standard is RL, wherein the needling site is alternated along the length of the AVF, resulting in minimal scar tissue formation. Many patients are trained on this method of cannulation when beginning home dialysis. While discouraged, some patients prefer particular sites (ie, use the "area wall technique"), which increases the potential for damage to the AVF wall and dilation of the fistula, and can result in the development of an aneurysm.[4-6]

The BH technique, also known as constant site needling, is a cannulation method that uses the same location, angle, and depth repeatedly.[1,2] Sharp needles are used to form a tract of scar tissue for entry into the fistula over time. Once this tract is formed, the patient can begin cannulating using a blunt needle, which is theoretically less traumatizing to the vascular structure and should improve survival of the access.[1]

To date, there are no high-quality clinical trials comparing AVF outcomes with RL vs BH cannulation in home HD patients or other self-needler patients (Table 1). The majority of the evidence supporting the use of the BH technique was generated through observational studies, and the generalizability of the existing observational and clinical trial data to the self-needling patient is unknown.

Table 1. Advantages and Disadvantages of BH Cannulation Technique

Advantages for the Patient	• Reduced needling attempts[1,2] • Fewer hematomas[7] • Reduced number of infiltrations[5,7,8] • Reduced number of aneurysms and aneurysm size[8,9] • Prevents "area" cannulation • Reduced pain (shown in observational studies only)[5,6,10-13] • Beneficial for individuals with needle phobia (opinion only)
Disadvantages for the Patient	• Increased risk of infection[7-14] • Need for meticulous hygiene • Possibility of introducing sharps into tunnel when confronted with difficult needling • If tract moves, BH may require re-siting

Buttonhole Cannulation Technique

In each unit, specialized, highly trained clinic staff are responsible for teaching BH tract creation. Ideally, there should only be 1 cannulator for the BH, and it is best if that cannulator is the patient himself; however, there are cases where a dedicated helper can be taught to cannulate. It is very important that the angle, position of the arm, and tourniquet placement are kept constant with each cannulation in order to create and maintain the BH tract. Previous teachings have suggested that the angle of entry should be 45 degrees for all BH cannulations, but in fact, the angle of entry depends on the depth and the anatomy of the fistula, and, thus, varies with each patient. To provide consistency for the angle of needle insertion, the touch cannulation technique can be taught. This technique refers to the placement of the thumb and forefingers on the needle tubing (and not the wings) while the other fingers rest upon the arm to provide stabilization (for more information and cannulation images, see End Stage Renal Disease Network, Cannulation of the AV Fistula).

Many clinics recommend that 2 separate BH sites (ie, 2 arterial and 2 venous) be created, each 6 to 8 cm apart. Ideally, patients should alternate between these sites and if there is ongoing difficulty with accessing a site or if it becomes infected (see section Increased Risk of Infection with Buttonhole Cannulation), that site should be abandoned.

BH tract creation requires repeated cannulation with a sharp fistula needle, an intravenous (IV) needle, or placement of a polycarbonate peg (eg, BioHole™ Plug, Nipro Corporation, Belgium). With each of these methods (except for the peg, which has no scab formation), the scab on the BH tract is removed before cannulation to allow the access site to be viewed and permit accurate insertion of the needles. The needles are inserted using the exact location, angle, and depth for each HD treatment. Canadian guidelines suggest that topical antimicrobial prophylaxis be applied to the BH site after the dialysis treatment is completed.[15]

The most common way to create a BH tract is with any type of sharp standard HD needle. The BH is initially created after approximately 8 to 12 cannulations using this approach. Once the BH tract is developed, the needles are switched to a dull/ blunt BH needle (eg, Medisystems) or a dull/blunt IV needle with a plastic cannula (eg, Nipro BioHoleTM Cath) to cannulate the BH sites.

Intravenous needles with plastic cannulas (eg, the Supercath™ Clampcath or angiocatheter) have also been used to create BH tracts with repeated needling. As described above, these needles are also inserted into the exact spot, using the same angle and depth for each HD treatment; the scab on the BH is removed before cannulation. Once the BH tract is developed, the blunt version of these needles can be used to cannulate the BH sites. These types of catheters have a large enough cannula to sustain dialysis blood flow, and the plastic (instead of steel) cannula limits the potential for needle infiltration.

Of note, there are descriptions in the literature using these IV needles with plastic cannulas to create a BH by leaving the catheter indwelling for periods of time.[16] Readers should be warned that there are possible complications with these indwelling catheters, namely the chance of infection, needle dislodgement, and cannula breakage with migration into a vessel.[17] The authors have personally treated catheter breakage in patients who have used this technique and we do not recommend this approach.[18]

Polycarbonate pegs are emerging as preferred tools with which to create BHs. The peg is a small, sterile, thumbtack-shaped plug used to maintain the needle tract between cannulations. Scar tissue forms around the peg, which facilitates the development of the BH tract. The use of a polycarbonate peg may lead to improved tract creation, which may in turn improve AVF survival. A randomized trial by Vaux et al[6] used polycarbonate pegs to create BHs, and they found improved AVF survival with BH cannulation at 1 year, whereas with conventional BH tract formation, there was no difference in AVF survival in a comparison with RL needling.[19]

(See "Buttonhole Tract Formation Using Polycarbonate Pegs" in the Appendix) Note that some, but not all, BH protocols include antibiotic prophylaxis.[20, 21]

The BH technique is not recommended for all patients and is contraindicated in patients with arteriovenous grafts (AVGs). In North America and Australasia, the BH technique is considered a relative contraindication for newly created AVFs because the fistula is undergoing dynamic changes that influence the BH tracts; however, this practice is not consistent globally. In Europe, BH cannulation is performed in patients with newly created fistulae.

Indications for and against BH cannulation are summarized in Table 2, and a checklist for assisting clinicians in choosing the best cannulation method for patients can be found in "Criteria for Determining Type of Self-Cannulation" in the Appendix. Choosing a cannulation method is discussed further in the section "Tools to Determine the Best Type of Needling". Patients with limited vision should use prescription lenses or a magnifying glass during the self-cannulation evaluation.

Useful Resources*

- Big D and Me. Dialysis Buttons for your Buttonholes.
- Home Dialysis Central. The Art of Teaching Buttonhole Self-Cannulation.

*For hyperlinks see Web version of Manual on ISHD.org

Table 2. Indications For or Against BH Cannulation Technique

Indications For Its Use	• AVF is short in length or has short usable segments • AVF with tortuous anatomy • AVF with aneurysmal dilatation[6] • AVF is difficult to cannulate. The patient is unable to self-cannulate using the RL technique • AVF is mature • Patient preference. Risk factors discussed and understood by patient • Needle phobia. Patient expresses considerable fear related to self-cannulation
Indications Against Its Use	• AVF is relatively straight • Patient experiences hand tremors. Unsuitable placement of needle on the BH may lead to the creation of multiple tracts within the BH • Patient reports or demonstrates difficulty visualizing the BH site. Poor vision and improper placement of needle on the BH may lead to the creation of multiple tracts within the BH • Patient has bioprosthesis (eg, mechanical heart valve, artificial joint)

Complications of Buttonhole Cannulation

Indentation/Hubbing

Over time BH sites can develop a widening and an indentation at the entry to the skin. This is commonly known as "hubbing". Hubbing occurs when the hub of the needle is buried into the skin, which can result in incomplete scab removal, patient's inability to clean the puncture site, and breakdown of the lining of the tunnel tract.[22] Hubbing can be prevented by leaving space between the hub of the needle and the puncture site.

Trampoline Effect

The trampoline effect describes the motion of a blunt needle meeting resistance and bouncing back toward the cannulator. This occurs because of a thickening of the tunnel tract or poor tract development. When this occurs, the patient's needling technique should be reassessed.

Increased Risk of Infection with Buttonhole Cannulation

Several clinical studies have demonstrated an increased risk of infection with the use of BH cannulation.[5-7, 21-26] The incidence of localized infections is increased with BH and other infectious complications have been reported. These include septic arthritis, bacterial endocarditis, and bacteremia; however, these conditions may not appear until long after the BH technique is initiated.[5, 6, 24-26] While incidence of infection varies between studies (and by patient population and locality), 1 retrospective study reported a rate of bacteremia of 0.073 per 1000 AVF days for BH patients, compared with no bacteremia for RL patients.[26] One systematic review of observational and randomized studies reported an increased risk of AVF-related infections using BH cannulation, with relative risk ranging from 3.15 to 3.34 comparing before and after changes and with RL cannulation, respectively.[27]

Patients should be informed of the increased risk of infection and receive specialized training and frequent evaluations of their cannulation techniques.[15] Strict adherence to aseptic technique in performing cannulations is essential; additional measures of infection prevention are also recommended for BH patients (Table 3).[15, 23, 28, 29] Each clinic should track and regularly review infection rates (see section Key Performance and Quality Indicators)

Table 3. Summary of Measures to Reduce Infection Risk

Adhere strictly to aseptic technique for access skin preparation and BH scab removal Use hand disinfectant prior to decannulation
Perform routine audit of patient cannulation technique on a quarterly basis (recommended) at clinic visits (see the "Arteriovenous Fistula/ Graft Audit Tool" and the "Central Venous Catheter Audit Tool" in the Appendix)
Use face masks on the patient (and staff/ helper if applicable) to lower the theoretical risk of nasal transmission of *Staphylococcus aureus* during cannulation[28]
Discuss and provide topical prophylaxis: Patients considering BH technique require counseling regarding the increased risk of infection and the potential for devastating consequences resulting from infection. Topical prophylaxis is strongly recommended for the prevention of infection[15, 24] • Options for topical agents: » **Polysporin triple ointment:** A formulation of polymyxin B sulfate, bacitracin zinc, and gramicidin used for the treatment of infections caused by bacteria » **Povidone-iodine ointment:** A broad-spectrum antiseptic for the treatment and prevention of infection » **Mupirocin ointment:** Utilized to treat staphylococcal infections or attempt to decrease the incidence of subsequent staphylococcal infections. Note: continued use may result in antimicrobial resistance » **Polyhexamethylene biguanide (PHMB):** A dressing infused with a broad-spectrum antimicrobial for the prevention of infection and promotion of wound healing
Perform routine screening of the nares for *S aureus* and, when present, pursue an eradication program (see the "Mupirocin Protocol" in the Appendix)

Management of BH Infections

The optimal duration and choice of antibiotic therapy to treat BH-related infections has not been directly studied. The following suggestions are based on the authors' opinion. Empiric treatment should begin with a first-generation cephalosporin (eg, cefazolin) or vancomycin, depending on local methicillin-resistant *S aureus* (MRSA) colonization rates. Subsequent choice of antimicrobials should be based on culture and susceptibility results.

- Infection of BH with fever and/or bacteremia: This infection should be treated with appropriate antibiotics for a minimum of 4 weeks. Treatment should be extended to 6 weeks in the case of *S aureus* bacteremia and/or if there is a metastatic complication. If further complications exist, abort use of infected BH site and re-site the BH

- Cellulitis or exit site infection: Local infection without fever and bacteremia should be treated with appropriate antibiotics for a minimum of 2 weeks. Abort use of BH located in the vicinity of cellulitis and re-site the BH. Reevaluate the need to change the dressing type and cleansing agent

- Abscess: Abscess of BH, especially with fever, should be treated with appropriate antibiotics for a minimum of 4 weeks and extended to 6 weeks if bacteremia is present. Treatment may be extended if there is progression of serious metastatic complications. Abort use of infected AVF. The abscess may require surgical intervention[30]

Tools to Determine the Best Type of Needling

For patients with AVF, the RL method of cannulation is the preferred type of needling.[15] In general, RL cannulation is used with an AVF that is of adequate length and superficial depth. In addition, the RL method is favored among patients who have poorer vision or those who have a slight tremor. However, in patients who have an AVF that is of short length, consists of tortuous anatomy, or involves aneurysmal sections, BH cannulation should be considered (see Table 2). Patients with a needle phobia can often overcome this phobia with the BH cannulation technique (see "Fear of Needles" in the Appendix). Due to the increased risk of infections with BH, this technique is not recommended for patients with a history of AVF infections, mechanical heart valves, or other prostheses.

A downloadable tool to assist clinicians in choosing the most appropriate type of self-cannulation can be found in "Criteria for Determining Type of Self-Cannulation" in the Appendix.

Additional Cannulation References*

» End Stage Renal Disease Network, Cannulation of the AV Fistula

» BC Renal. Vascular Access Guideline, Rope Ladder Cannulation of AV Fistulas and Grafts

» Home Dialysis Central. The Art of Teaching Buttonhole Self-Cannulation. Step-by-step PDF booklet with color photos

*For hyperlinks see Web version of Manual on ISHD.org.

Fistula Cannulation Methods

Indications for Use of Standard Sharp Fistula Needles

Standard sharp fistula needles are used if the patient is unable to cannulate using the IV needle with cannula or with the dull/blunt needle at a BH tract. If the sharp fistula needle is used, then the patient is encouraged to cannulate at a new site rather than using the established BH tract. The use of sharp fistula needles for nocturnal dialysis is not preferred due to the potential for needle infiltration during the treatment. However, if sharp fistula needles are used for nocturnal dialysis, it is imperative to ensure that these needles are secured well. See "Taping Methods for Hemodialysis Needle" and "Taping Method of Intravenous Needle with Cannula" protocols in the Appendix. For more information on nocturnal dialysis, see "Prescriptions for Home Hemodialysis".

Indications for Use of IV Needle with Cannula (Examples: Supercath Clampcath Needles, Nipro Biohole Cath)

For nocturnal dialysis, the flexible cannula is used for comfort and to prevent needle infiltration during treatment. The use of this needle system should be considered in:

- Patients who have an allergy to metals
- Restless patients who may be at risk of needle infiltration (ideal use)
- RL technique for the nocturnal HD patient

Protocols on use of IV needle with cannula can be found at:

- "Buttonhole Cannulation for Creation and Maintenance of Tract with Intravenous Needle and Cannula" in the Appendix
- BC Renal, Vascular Access Guideline, Self-Cannulation of Buttonholes on AV Fistulas

Indications for Use of Dull/Blunt Needle

For nocturnal dialysis the dull/blunt needle is used to prevent needle infiltration during treatment. When used with the BH technique, once the BH tract is created, a dull/ blunt needle can be inserted into that tract for the dialysis treatment. Protocols on use of dull/blunt needles can be found at:

- "Buttonhole Cannulation Technique with Dull (Blunt) Bevel" in the Appendix
- BC Renal, Vascular Access Guideline, Self-Cannulation of Buttonholes on AV Fistulas
- BC Renal, Patient Teaching Tool, Self-Needling Your Fistula Using the Buttonhole Method
- BC Renal, Buttonhole Cannulation

Troubleshooting Arteriovenous Fistula Complications

Centers should conduct technique review of self-needling patients every 3 months, with the patient being examined while cannulating in the clinic or during a home visit (see "Arteriovenous Fistula/Graft Audit Tool" in the Appendix). The major focus here is on prevention of infections.

Pain with Needling: Strategies

For patients who experience painful needling, a warm compress should be applied to the access site 5 to 10 minutes before needling. A topical anesthetic (preferred to a subcutaneous injection of lidocaine) should be used to numb the skin surface. Topical lidocaine preparations can be applied to the skin at the desired cannulation sites in a thick layer and then covered with an occlusive dressing or plastic wrap for 60-120 minutes prior to cannulation. Of note, the anesthetic needs to be thoroughly washed off the skin prior to cannulation. It is best to avoid injection of lidocaine into BH sites to minimize the chance for vessel and BH tract movement and potential for vasoconstriction of the blood vessel.

Cannulation Dependency Issues

Some BH patients may become fearful of cannulating using sharp needles at sites other than at the BH site. As a result, these patients can become dependent on the home HD clinic to troubleshoot access issues and reestablish the BH site.

Fear of Needles

Fear of needling can be a barrier to the uptake of home dialysis.[31] Needle fear should not be a contraindication to teaching self-cannulation. In fact, this fear can be overcome if a stepwise approach is followed in which the patient slowly increases his or her comfort level with needles. Patients should start off simply watching the insertion of another patient's needles, followed by watching the insertion of his or her own needles. Becoming familiar with simply holding the needles and holding needle sites after needle removal is also an important step. For more information, please see this website or "Fear of Needles" in the Appendix.

Strategies for Addressing Difficult Cannulation

Patients who experience difficulty with cannulation should be scheduled to return to the home HD unit as soon as possible for a review of their cannulation technique and an access assessment for a possible complication of stenosis or thrombosis (Table 4). Thus, in addition to a physical examination (see, "Physical Examination of the Fistula" approach below), an access flow assessment should be made with a subsequent plan for intervention, if needed.

Regardless of the type of cannulation, patients should be instructed to avoid flipping needles. Flipping a sharp needle can actually damage the vessel, while flipping a blunt needle may be indicative of an underlying access problem.

Some home HD programs will use heparin locks or flushes to ensure patency of the access when patients experience temporary cannulation difficulties (eg, if needling is difficult due to onset of stenosis) or in those who need extra guidance for needling. Locking involves instilling a diluted heparin solution into the cannulas (needles and tubing) of the arteriovenous access and allowing it to dwell for a specified period of time (ie, "locking" the heparin in the lumens); flushing involves passing diluted heparin through the cannula before initiating dialysis. Some programs may substitute citrate 4% for the heparin. Before using this approach, patients should be informed of the potential risk of needle dislodgement and possible sequelae, such as bleeding and infection. More information can be found in the "Heparin Flushing of Cannulas" protocol in the Appendix.

Table 4. Troubleshooting for Buttonhole Cannulation Difficulties
Monitor established sites frequently
Avoid sharp needles in an established BH site. The use of sharp needles in a BH site may lead to excessive scarring
Review AVF for possible underlying access dysfunction and/or re-site BH if patient presents with cannulation difficulties
Reposition the arm, change the angle, and slightly rotate the cannula when resistance is felt during the cannulation of BH
Check for an inflamed or infected BH site. If infection is present, do not cannulate. Cannulation in this instance increases the risk of severe hemorrhage with possible exsanguination
Check for keloid formation at the BH cannulation site
Ensure that the BH needle site aligns with the tract entrance into the AVF. A cannulation failure could occur if the BH needle site does not align properly. A new BH site may need to be created to correct the problem
Check for an enlarged BH needle site that may lead to prolonged bleeding

Appropriate Blood Pump Speeds

The ideal blood pump speed for HD is unknown. However, there are potential deleterious effects of high blood pump speeds on fistula integrity. Needle turbulence is the intense flow that is created by a needle in an arteriovenous access, and has been shown to cause endothelial dysfunction with decreased nitrous oxide formation and loss of endothelial integrity.[32, 33] The effect of higher pump speeds has not been proven, but injury to the endothelial wall from altered flow mechanics of high pump speeds is likely to occur.[34] Expert opinion recommends that lower pump speeds should be used to promote vessel integrity and maintain fistula longevity. More information on pump speeds used for different HD modalities can be found in the "Prescriptions for Home Hemodialysis" module. Regardless of the blood pump speeds utilized, most programs aim to maintain the arterial and venous pressures below -250 and 250 mm Hg, respectively; however, these pressures are not strongly evidence-based. A recent observational study of patients on in-center HD reported an increased risk of access failure with venous pressures outside the range of 100–150 mm Hg.[35]

Physical Examination of the Fistula

The access arm must be examined regularly by the patient. Routine evaluation of the arm using a "look, listen, and feel" approach may help detect access complications and subsequent intervention before the access is lost entirely. For an excellent description of the access physical examination, see Sousa et al.[36]

Monitoring for Complications of Stenosis and Thrombosis

Studies have not been performed to assess the value of access surveillance among home HD patients, but most programs recommend pursuing access flow monitoring when the patient returns for quarterly or biannual clinic visits. In addition, regular physical examination of the access by staff is suggested at these clinic visits.

Home HD patients should be taught how to perform a basic access arm examination regularly using the "look, listen, and feel" approach. Patients should be instructed to assess their access using the Arm Raise Technique. They will pump their hand to make a fist, raise their arm straight in the air, and, while standing in front of a mirror, note if the AVF collapses (normal state) or if the AVF does not collapse, which indicates an outflow obstruction.

It is recommended that patients perform trend analysis by recording the venous and arterial pressures at onset of each run at a blood pump speed of 200 mL/min, and reviewing the changes/trends in these numbers. During dialysis, the maximum arterial pressure should not exceed -250 mm Hg and the maximum venous pressure should not exceed 250 mm Hg. When these pressures are exceeded, the needle should be repositioned and/or the blood pump speed should be decreased. Patients should report to their clinician any changes noted in their routine access arm examination, trend of pressures, or cannulation, and the time of onset of cannulation difficulty.

Recent onset of increased difficulty of needling or prolonged bleeding from the access site after dialysis may be signs of an underlying stenosis and should be investigated. It is important to remember that as the AVF matures, BH tracts may change and new sites may be required, which may lead to difficulties needling. In addition, large fluctuations in body weight or size can alter the BH tracts. Patients and staff should be aware that any new onset of cannulation difficulty can also be due to a hemodynamically significant stenosis or impending thrombosis of the access.

Access flow monitoring is suggested at a frequency of every 4 to 6 months, with the same flow thresholds for intervention as are used with in-center conventional HD patients. The same guidelines have been extrapolated for home HD patients.

Readers should note that there is considerable variability in the frequency of screening AVF/AVG. Some centers assess access flow every 6 months, while others screen more frequently (every

3 months) in cases of AVF with access issues. Other centers only investigate when cannulation difficulties are reported. Screening options include, but are not limited to, formal ultrasound study, Doppler assessment, clinical screening of needling complications, and review of technique quarterly (see "Arteriovenous Fistula/Graft Audit Tool" in the Appendix). Additional information can be found at:

- **Caring for Australians with Renal Impairment (CARI) Guidelines, Chapter 4: Vascular Access Surveillance**
- **Canadian Society of Nephrology, Clinical Practice Guidelines for the Treatment of Patients with Chronic Kidney Disease, Chapter 4: Vascular Access:**

Thrombosis

Often, the first sign of impending thrombosis is what is mistaken for cellulitis, with signs of erythema over the AVF and tenderness to palpation. This is a medical emergency and the patient should be brought in for *immediate physical and ultrasound examination of the AVF*, with arrangements for radiology or surgical thrombolysis made as required. Every effort should be made to salvage the access and avoid catheter placement.

Fistula Hemorrhage

Hemorrhage from fistula has been reported in the in-center HD population,[38, 39] but the incidence of this occurring among home patients is unknown. All patients should be instructed to apply pressure to their site in the event of bleeding and to call for emergency assistance (eg, 911, 991, 999, 112, or 000 as appropriate). For additional information on fistula hemorrhage and patient safety during home HD, please see the module titled, "Ensuring Patient Safety During Home Hemodialysis".

Specific risks for home HD patients include needle dislodgement, or improper threading of the dialyzer, which may lead to significant hemorrhage. Water or enuresis alarms strategically placed under the dialysis machine and dialyzer, as well as under the access arm, help prevent these serious adverse events. Some popular alarms include the following:

- Redsense Venous Needle Dislodgement alarm
  - Training the Trainer
  - Self-Use Instructions
- Zircon Leak Alert™ Electronic Water Detector
- HEMOdialert™ blood leak detector

An aneurysmal fistula that is rapidly enlarging in size could indicate possible rupture and hemorrhage.[40] Thus, aneurismal fistula should be routinely monitored and the diameter of the aneurysms should be noted at each clinical visit. Fistula with necrotic skin as a result of infection can also lead to increased risk of rupture, especially in the case of BH cannulation.

The use of a single needle to minimize bleeding risk has been used in some programs; however, this results in a reduction in clearance and an increase in noise from the double pump system. The routine use of single needle in home HD has fallen out of favor, but it can be a useful technique to provide rest (and avoid a catheter placement) after AVF complications. Programs should have a standardized management plan for patients and caregivers to follow to manage hemorrhage, if it occurs in the home. For more detailed information, please see Home Dialysis Central, The Art of Making Your Fistula or Graft Last or the "Ensuring Patient Safety During Home Hemodialysis" module.

Fistula Infection

AVF infections can manifest as cellulitis, BH exit site infection, or bacteremia. Cellulitis is infrequent in mature AVF without skin lesions, but signs of redness and swelling should be evaluated to rule out thrombophlebitis. With a BH exit site infection, pus and erythema may be present at the needling site. It is important to obtain a swab for culture and sensitivity and 2 sets of blood culture specimens to rule out bacteremia (particularly *S aureus* bacteremia), which is very common with BH sites. See "Increased Risk of Infection with Buttonhole Cannulation" for details.

Two sets of blood culture specimens should be drawn from any HD patient with an unexplained fever. Some units initiate empiric therapy against both gram-positive and gram-negative bacteria, depending on the usual types of infection in that unit. The planned duration of therapy for bacteremia is 4 to 6 weeks, depending on the organism.

Arteriovenous Graft

AVGs do not have the option of BH needling; only the RL and site rotation technique is recommended. Needle options include standard AVF/AVG needles (sharp) or the needle with cannula (angiocatheter) in which a blunt cannula remains in the AVG for dialysis. With the exception of AVG infection (see below), all other sections of the AVF apply to AVG.

AVG Infection

- Often requires surgical intervention, including graft resection
- Treatment requires 6 weeks of antibiotics with double coverage of gram-positive and gram-negative organisms

Central Venous Catheter

Technical Aspects of Catheter Care

Routine placement of catheters in the subclavian vein (central venous catheters [CVCs]) is not recommended because they create a higher risk for central vein stenosis. In general, the internal jugular site is preferred.[41] There are many different catheters available; however, there is no evidence to guide selection of 1 device over another.

Catheter Care Protocols

There are many catheter care protocols available (see "Central Venous Catheter Audit Tool" in the Appendix). In general, donning clean gloves and mask are a requirement when accessing the catheter.[39]

LOCKING

After dialysis, catheters are most commonly locked with citrate 4% and heparin at a concentration of 1000 or 5000 units/mL; however the following should be considered in selecting a lock solution:

- Bleeding risks have been noted with higher heparin concentrations[42] (see "Heparin Locking of Central Venous Catheters" in the Appendix)
- Locking with 30% ethanol/4% trisodium citrate has been demonstrated to prevent the formation of biofilms in catheters in vitro,[43] and weekly 70% ethanol locks have been successfully used for infection prophylaxis (in vivo) in a proof-of-concept study,[44] but ethanol locking is not yet widely used in clinical practice
- Tissue plasminogen activator (TPA) is also used to treat episodes of catheter dysfunction. Please see the following protocols for details:
- "Alteplase Use in Hemodialysis Central Venous Catheters" in the Appendix
- BC Renal. Vascular Access Guideline: Alteplase Use for Occluded Hemodialysis Catheters

DRESSINGS

- Either gauze dressings[41] or nonocclusive transparent dressings can be used at the exit site of catheters[45]
- The lack of a dressing is a potential option for patients with severe skin breakdown or rash at the exit site; however, the evidence for this practice comes from a nondialysis patient population[46]
- Sample guidelines for dressing change and exit site care can be found on the BC Renal website

CLOSED-CONNECTOR DEVICES

A closed-connector device is a device that is designed to decrease the risk of unintentional disconnection examples of which include:

- InterLink (BD)
- Tego Needlefree Hemodialysis Connector (ICU Medical, Inc)
- Swan-Lock (Codan Medical Inc)

As published in the most recent Canadian Society of Nephrology Intensive HD guidelines, a closed-connector device is recommended for patients receiving intensive (home) HD.[15] These closed-connector devices are ideal for home HD patients with a CVC who perform HD without any assistance, as there is less risk for air embolism or chance of inadvertent bleeding. Depending on the device, these closed connectors can be changed under sterile conditions either weekly by the patient at home or monthly by the nurse at the home HD unit. To decrease concerns of air embolism at the time of exchange of a closed-connector device, the patient can be taught to double clamp (ie, use the catheter clamp and another separate clamp on the catheter tubing).

EXIT SITE PROPHYLAXIS

The use of exit site prophylaxis (polysporin, mupirocin/bactroban, medi-honey, povidone-iodone, etc) is very center dependent and not used at every center.[41]

SHOWERING PROTOCOLS

Attached is an example of a protocol for patients from an established home HD program (see the "Showering Protocol" in the Appendix). Remember that the shower and shower head are potential sources of bacteria; therefore, regular cleaning of both is recommended.

Troubleshooting Catheter Complications

Infections

Catheters have a higher rate of infectious complications than arteriovenous accesses, a risk which appears to vary over time according to the length of time the access is in place.[47] Catheter-related infections can be either local (as an exit site or tunnel infection) or systemic (bacteremia).

Exit site infections are defined according to a purulent discharge at the exit site with 2 of the following features:

- Erythema
- Tenderness
- Induration at the exit site
- Sampling of the discharge that results in a culture positive for infection[48]

If left untreated, exit site infections can lead to catheter-related bacteremia. An exit site infection is generally treated with a 2-week regimen of either topical or oral antibiotics.

A tunnel infection should be suspected in a patient who presents with pain or tenderness at the catheter exit site; the tunnel site should be palpated with the intention of expressing a discharge. A tunnel infection is defined as a purulent discharge or aspirate from a tunnel site not contiguous with the exit site and includes 2 of the following features:

- Erythema
- Tenderness
- Induration at a tunnel site
- A culture of serous discharge or aspirate from that site that is positive for infection[48]

Tunnel infections should be treated with a 3-week course of IV antibiotics.

Most HD units use the definition of a probable catheter-related bacteremia, which is 2 or more blood culture specimens that are positive for infection with no evidence for a source other than the catheter. When a patient first presents with a fever and suspected catheter-related bacteremia, start empiric antibiotics that cover both gram-positive and gram-negative organisms. The choice and duration of antibiotics, as well as the decision to remove the catheter, depend on the bacterial organism isolated.[41] An example of a center protocol is included (see "Central Venous Catheter Antibiotic Treatment Protocol" in the Appendix) and detailed treatment guidelines can be found on the CARI website.

Catheter Dysfunction

Catheter dysfunction is a common problem for catheter-dependent patients and results in decreased dialysis efficiency. Definitions of catheter dysfunction vary, but in general they relate to the inability to achieve a certain blood pump speed (from 200 to 300 mL/min) within the venous and arterial pressure limits of 250 and -250 mm Hg, respectively, while dialyzing. Many HD units have developed treatment algorithms for decreased flow, which include checking patient positioning and flushing the lumens with normal saline prior to administering TPA. Home HD units that have adopted these protocols and will either instruct the patient to administer TPA at home or to come back to the unit to have staff administer the thrombolytic. Sample protocols can be found here:

- BC Renal. Alteplase Use for Occluded Hemodialysis Catheters
- "Alteplase Use in Hemodialysis Central Venous Catheters" in the Appendix

Catheter Malfunctions

At times, an HD catheter may develop a crack in the line; generally, these lines will need to be replaced. If the crack develops distal to the "Y" portion, some lines can be repaired. Sample guidelines for determining when a catheter line can be repaired can be found at:

- BC Renal, Vascular Access Guideline: Central Venous Catheter – Repair of Cracked Catheter Adapter, Limb or Clamp

Embolism

There have been reports of air embolism occurring in home HD patients using catheters.[49] Prevention of air embolism by using a closed-connector device, such as those mentioned previously, is recommended.[15] In a survey of Canadian Home HD programs, near misses have been reported in some patients who use connector devices when the device is not applied firmly.

Hemorrhage

Although the closed-connector devices may prevent air emboli, there have been cases of hemorrhage that have occurred in patients because the devices have been used improperly or the membranes in these devices have failed.[15] Wetness detectors can be applied to the catheter for overnight dialysis (see "Ensuring Patient Safety During Home Hemodialysis" module).

Key Performance and Quality Indicators

Key indicators are important operating mechanisms to ensure patient safety in home HD (see "Ensuring Patient Safety During Home Hemodialysis" module). Ensure these key indicators are used and followed during routine clinic visits for home HD patients to minimize complications of infection and to determine access failure:

Performance Measures

1. Use an audit tool quarterly
2. Verify that a form of access screening is occurring (eg, patient reporting the usual venous and arterial pressures at a standardized pump speed)

Quality Indicators

1. What is the infection (local/systemic) rate, according to vascular access type (events per 1000 access days)?
2. What is the rate of access interventions, according to vascular access type (events per 1000 access days)?
3. What is the rate of bleeding (actual or "near misses") from the access site, according to vascular access type (events per 1000 access days)?

Summary

Vascular access is associated with the development of potential complications that can lead to significant morbidity. Thus, the care and keeping of vascular access is a skill that is of utmost importance for home dialysis patients. Teaching patients their cannulation options as well as encouraging them to be vigilant for possible access complications should be a large part of every home dialysis program. Furthermore, routine access screening and review of quality indicators should be instituted on a regular basis to minimize access failure.

References

3. Twardowski Z. Constant site (buttonhole) method of needle insertion for hemodialysis. Dial Transplant. 1995;24:559-560.
4. Twardowski Z, Kubara H. Different sites versus constant sites of needle insertion into arteriovenous fistulas for treatment by repeated dialysis. Dial Transplant. 1979;8:978-980.
5. Lee T, Barker J, Allon M. Needle infiltration of arteriovenous fistulae in hemodialysis: risk factors and consequences. Am J Kidney Dis. 2006;47:1020-1026.
6. Krönung G. Plastic deformation of Cimino fistula by repeated puncture. Dial Transplant. 1984;13:635-638.
7. Verhallen AM, Kooistra MP, van Jaarsveld BC. Cannulating in haemodialysis: rope-ladder or buttonhole technique? Nephrol Dial Transplant. 2007;22:2601-2604.
8. Marticorena RM, Hunter J, Macleod S, et al. The salvage of aneurysmal fistulae utilizing a modified buttonhole cannulation technique and multiple cannulators. Hemodial Int. 2006;10:193-200.
9. MacRae JM, Ahmed SB, Atkar R, Hemmelgarn BR. A randomized trial comparing buttonhole with rope ladder needling in conventional hemodialysis patients. Clin J Am Soc Nephrol. 2012;7:1632-1638.
10. Vaux E, King J, Lloyd S, et al. Effect of buttonhole cannulation with a polycarbonate PEG on in-center hemodialysis fistula outcomes: a randomized controlled trial. Am J Kidney Dis. 2013;62:81-88.
11. Struthers J, Allan A, Peel RK, Lambie SH. Buttonhole needling of arteriovenous fistulae: a randomized controlled trial. ASAIO J. 2010;56:319-322.
12. Ball LK, Treat L, Riffle V, Scherting D, Swift L. A multi-center perspective of the buttonhole technique in the Pacific Northwest. Nephrol Nurs J. 2007;34:234-241.
13. Castro MC, Silva Cde F, Souza JM, et al. Arteriovenous fistula cannulation by buttonhole technique using dull needle. J Bras Nefrol. 2010;32:281-285.
14. Kim MK, Kim HS. Clinical effects of buttonhole cannulation method on hemodialysis patients. Hemodial Int. 2013; 17:294-299.
15. Sukthinthai N, Sittipraneet A, Tummanittayangkoon B, Vasuvattakul S, Chanchairujira T. Buttonhole technique better than area puncture technique on hemostasis and pain associated with needle cannulation. J Med Assoc Thai. 2012;95 Suppl 2:S208-212.
16. Chow J, Rayment G, San Miguel S, Gilbert M. A randomised controlled trial of buttonhole cannulation for the prevention of fistula access complications. J Ren Care. 2011;37:85-93.
17. Nesrallah GE, Mustafa RA, MacRae J, et al. Canadian Society of Nephrology guidelines for the management of patients with ESRD treated with intensive hemodialysis. Am J Kidney Dis. 2013;62:187-198.
18. Marticorena RM, Hunter J, Cook R, et al. A simple method to create buttonhole cannulation tracks in a busy hemodialysis unit. Hemodial Int. 2009;13:316-321.
19. Donnelly SM, Marticorena RM, Hunter J, Goldstein MB. Supercath Safety Clampcath buttonhole creation: complication of catheter breakage. Hemodial Int. 2013;17:450-454.
20. MacRae JM, Tai DJ, Daniw M, Lee J. A simple method to create buttonhole cannulation tracks in a busy hemodialysis unit. Hemodial Int. 2010;14:94-95.
21. MacRae JM, Ahmed SB, Hemmelgarn BR, Alberta Kidney Disease Network. Arteriovenous fistula survival and needling technique: long-term results from a randomized buttonhole trial. Am J Kidney Dis. 2014;63:636-642.
22. Marticorena RM, Hunter J, Macleod S, et al. Use of the BioHole™ device for the creation of tunnel tracks for buttonhole cannulation of fistula for hemodialysis. Hemodial Int. 2011;15:243-249.
23. Toma S, Shinzato T, Fukui H, et al. A timesaving method to create a fixed puncture route for the buttonhole technique. Nephrol Dial Transplant. 2003;18:2118-2121.

References (cont'd)

24. Ball LK, Mott S. How do you prevent indented buttonhole sites? Nephrol Nurs J. 2010;37:427-428, 431.

25. van Loon MM, Goovaerts T, Kessels AG, van der Sande FM, Tordoir JH. Buttonhole needling of haemodialysis arteriovenous fistulae results in less complications and interventions compared to the rope-ladder technique. Nephrol Dial Transplant. 2010;25:225-230.

26. Nesrallah GE, Cuerden M, Wong JH, Pierratos A. Staphylococcus aureus bacteremia and buttonhole cannulation: long-term safety and efficacy of mupirocin prophylaxis. Clin J Am Soc Nephrol. 2010;5:1047-1053.

27. Van Eps CL, Jones M, Ng T, et al. The impact of extended-hours home hemodialysis and buttonhole cannulation technique on hospitalization rates for septic events related to dialysis access. Hemodial Int. 2010;14:451-463.

28. O'Brien FJ, Kok HKT, O'Kane C, et al. Arterio-venous fistula buttonhole cannulation technique: a retrospective analysis of infectious complications. Clin Kidney J. 2012;5:526-529.

29. Muir CA, Kotwal SS, Hawley CM, et al. Buttonhole cannulation and clinical outcomes in home hemodialysis cohort and systematic review. Clin J Am Soc Nephrol. 2013;9:110-119.

30. Ball LK. The buttonhole technique: strategies to reduce infections. Nephrol Nurs J. 2010;37:473-477; quiz 478.

31. Priyesh P, Smith K, Henner D. Effect of implementation of standardized protocol on infection rates in patients utilizing the buttonhole cannulation technique for accessing AV fistulas. Am J Kidney Dis. 2013;61:B77.

32. Tordoir J, Canaud B, Haage P, et al. EBPG on vascular access. Nephrol Dial Transplant. 2007;22 Suppl 2:ii88-117.

33. McLaughlin K, Manns B, Mortis G, Hons R, Taub K. Why patients with ESRD do not select self-care dialysis as a treatment option. Am J Kidney Dis. 2003;41:380-385.

34. Huynh TN, Chacko BK, Teng X, et al. Effects of venous needle turbulence during ex vivo hemodialysis on endothelial morphology and nitric oxide formation. J Biomech. 2007;40:2158-2166.

35. Unnikrishnan S, Huynh TN, Brott BC, et al. Turbulent flow evaluation of the venous needle during hemodialysis. J Biomech Eng. 2005;127:1141-1146.

36. Remuzzi A, Ene-Iordache B. Novel paradigms for dialysis vascular access: upstream hemodynamics and vascular remodeling in dialysis access stenosis. Clin J Am Soc Nephrol. 2013;8:2186-2193.

37. Parisotto MT, Schoder VU, Miriunis C, et al. Cannulation technique influences arteriovenous fistula graft survival. Kidney Int. 2014;86:790-797.

38. Sousa CN, Apóstolo JL, Figueiredo MH, Martins MM, Dias VF. Physical examination: how to examine the arm with arteriovenous fistula. Hemodial Int. 2013;17:300-306.

39. Jindal K, Chan CT, Deziel C, et al. Hemodialysis clinical practice guidelines for the Canadian Society of Nephrology. J Am Soc Nephrol. 2006;17:S1-27.

40. Ellingson KD, Palekar RS, Lucero CA, et al. Vascular access hemorrhages contribute to deaths among hemodialysis patients. Kidney Int. 2012;82:686-692.

41. Gill JR, Storck K, Kelly S. Fatal exsanguination from hemodialysis vascular access sites. Forensic Sci Med Pathol. 2012;8:259-262.

42. Almehmi A, Wang S. Partial aneurysmectomy is effective in managing aneurysm-associated complications of arteriovenous fistulae for hemodialysis: case series and literature review. Semin Dial. 2012;25:357-364.

43. Vanholder R, Canaud B, Fluck R, et al. Catheter-related blood stream infections (CRBSI): a European view. Nephrol Dial Transplant. 2010;25:1753-1756.

44. Yevzlin AS, Sanchez RJ, Hiatt JG, et al. Concentrated heparin lock is associated with major bleeding complications after tunneled hemodialysis catheter placement. Semin Dial. 2007;20:351-354.

References (cont'd)

45. Takla TA, Zelenitsky SA, Vercaigne LM. Effectiveness of 30% ethanol/4% trisodium citrate locking solution in preventing biofilm formation by organisms causing haemodialysis catheter-related infections. J Antimicrob Chemother. 2008;62:1024-1026.

46. Broom JK, Krishnasamy R, Hawley CM, Playford EG, Johnson DW. A randomized controlled trial of Heparin versus EthAnol Lock THerapY for the prevention of Catheter Associated infection in Haemodialysis patients—the HEALTHY-CATH trial. BMC Nephrol. 2012;13:146.

47. Gillies D, O'Riordan L, Carr D, Frost J, Gunning R, O'Brien I. Gauze and tape and transparent polyurethane dressings for central venous catheters. Cochrane Database Syst Rev. 2003:CD003827.

48. Olson K, Rennie RP, Hanson J, et al. Evaluation of a no-dressing intervention for tunneled central venous catheter exit sites. J Infus Nurs. 2004;27:37-44.

49. Ravani P, Gillespie BW, Quinn RR, et al. Temporal risk profile for infectious and noninfectious complications of hemodialysis access. J Am Soc Nephrol. 2013;24:1668-1677.

50. Canada Communicable Disease Report—Supplement. Infection control guidelines: Preventing infections associated with indwelling intravascular access devices. Can Commun Dis Rep. 1997;23(Suppl 8):i-iii, 1-32, i-iv, 1-16.

51. Ouwendyk M, Pierratos A, Francoeur R, Wallace L, Sit W, Vas S. Slow nocturnal home hemodialysis (SNHHD)—one year later. J CANNT. 1996;6:26-28.

Appendix

Vascular Access

Implementing Hemodialysis in the Home
A Global Perspective

iSHD
International Society for Hemodialysis

Table of Contents

Buttonhole Tract Formation Using Polycarbonate Pegs

Procedure

- Remove the hemodialysis needles after dialysis per protocol
- Stop the bleeding
- Insert the peg into the established puncture sites using aseptic technique
- Some centers recommend using topical antibiotic cream at the time of peg insertion, but not all buttonhole protocols include antibiotic prophylaxis
- Cover the pegs with waterproof plaster dressing
- Leave pegs in situ until the next dialysis session
- Remove pegs immediately prior to dialysis session
- Prepare the cannulation sites per unit protocol
- Insert needles into site vacated by the pegs. The BH is created by approximately 8 to 12 cannulations using the peg
- Observe for infection, dislodgement of peg, and bleeding

Criteria for Determining Type of Self-Cannulation

For patients with arteriovenous fistulas (AVF), rope ladder (RL) cannulation technique is the preferred cannulation method for teaching patients self-cannulation. If all indicators are check marked, initiate patient self-cannulation training using RL cannulation technique.

Indications for Rope Ladder Cannulation	Check Items That Apply
AVF is relatively straight	
AVF is newly created and dynamic (developing and changing)	
Patient experiences hand tremors Poor technique may lead to the creation of multiple tracts if buttonhole (BH) cannulation is used	
Patient reports or demonstrates difficulty with vision Poor vision and improper placement of needle on the BH may lead to the creation of multiple tracts if BH cannulation is used	
Patient expresses fear related to self-cannulation, but is nonetheless prepared to attempt self-cannulation	

Total Number of Check Marks:

Indications for Buttonhole Cannulation	Check Items That Apply
AVF is short in length or short usable segments	
AVF has torturous anatomy	
AVF developed aneurysmal dilation	
AVF is mature and no longer dynamic	
AVF is difficult to cannulate The patient is unable to self-cannulate use the RL technique	
Patient displays needle phobia Patient expresses considerable fear related to self-cannulation	

Total Number of Check Marks:

Adapted from Nesrallah G, Mustafa RA, MacRae J, et al. Canadian Society of Nephrology guidelines for the management of patients with ESRD treated with intensive hemodialysis. Am J Kidney Disease. 2013;5:187-198.

Arteriovenus Fistula/Graft Audit Tool

Instructions: **Use a "+" if performed correctly** **Use a "⃠" if not performed correctly**	**Date**	**Date**	**Date**	**Date**
Cannulation: Rope Ladder Technique				
Hand hygiene: wash hands and access with soap and water				
Skin cleansed with antiseptic				
Antiseptic allowed to dry				
Cannulation performed aseptically				
Patient connects aseptically				
Cannulation: Buttonhole Technique				
Hand hygiene: wash hands with soap and water				
Skin and buttonhole sites cleansed with antiseptic				
Scab removed with sterile blunt tip or needle sterile pack				
Needle or pick use 1 time only				
Skin and buttonhole sites cleansed with antiseptic a second time				
Scab removed completely				
No evidence of bleeding after scab removal				
Cannulation performed aseptically				
Patient connects aseptically				

Tool adapted with permission from University Health Network, Toronto, Ontario, Canada.

Arteriovenus Fistula/Graft Audit Tool (cont'd)

Instructions: **Use a "+" if performed correctly** **Use a "⃠" if not performed correctly**	**Date**	**Date**	**Date**	**Date**
Decannulation				
Perform hand hygiene using hand sanitizer				
Antiseptic ointment or cream applied to sites				
Clean gauze or bandage applies to sites				

Comments:

Tool adapted with permission from University Health Network, Toronto, Ontario, Canada.

Central Venous Catheter Audit Tool

Instructions: Use a "+" if performed correctly Use a "⃠" if not performed correctly	Date	Date	Date	Date
Catheter Connection				
Hand hygiene: wash hands with soap and water				
Tego connector changed aseptically every 7 days or as required				
Catheter hub soaked and then scrubbed with antiseptic				
Catheter hub antiseptic allowed to dry				
Tego connector Luer locked aseptically to catheter hub every 7 days or as required				
Tego connector soaked and scrubbed with antiseptic				
Tego connector antiseptic allowed to dry				
Patient connects aseptically				
Catheter Disconnection				
Perform hand hygiene using hand sanitizer				
Patient disconnected aseptically				
Tego connector soaked and scrubbed with antiseptic				
Tego antiseptic allowed to dry				
Catheter locked aseptically				

Tool adapted with permission from University Health Network, Toronto, Ontario, Canada.

Central Venous Catheter Audit Tool (cont'd)

Instructions: Use a "+" if performed correctly Use a "⃠" if not performed correctly	Date	Date	Date	Date
Catheter Exit Site Care				
Hand hygiene: Wash hands with soap and water				
Exit site cleaned with antiseptic				
Antiseptic allowed to dry				
Antimicrobial ointment or cream applied to exit site				
Dressing applied aseptically				
Shower technique				

Comments:

Tool adapted with permission from University Health Network, Toronto, Ontario, Canada.

Mupirocin Protocol: Information for Patients

Muiprocin Nasal Ointment to Eliminate Nasal Carriage of Staphylococcus aureus

Why do I need mupirocin nasal ointment?

Recent nasal swab results have indicated that you are carrying a common type of bacteria called *Staphylococcus aureus* ("staph").

This organism is often found on the skin and in the noses of healthy people where it is generally harmless. In patients who have hemodialysis (HD) access (ie, a catheter, fistula, or graft), this bacteria needs to be treated to prevent any possible spread of infection. An effective treatment to get rid of the bacteria is to apply an antibiotic ointment called mupirocin into both nostrils.

How long will treatment be required?

Treatment for 3 months is required to successfully remove the bacteria. The recommended schedule varies depending on whether you are currently on HD or have not yet started dialysis.

Where can I get the nasal ointment?

You will need to get a prescription for the ointment from your healthcare provider. The ointment can then be purchased at a pharmacy.

Technique for applying mupirocin ointment

- Wash hands well with soap and water or disinfect hands with alcohol gel/rub.
- Open the mupirocin nasal ointment tube.
- Place a small amount of ointment (about the side of a match head) onto a clean cotton swab and massage gently around the inside of the nostril, particularly toward the front of the nostril.
- Do not insert the cotton swab too deeply into the nose—no more than 1 cm inside the nostril.
- Using a new cotton swab, repeat for the other nostril. Using a new cotton swab will prevent contamination of the ointment tube.
- After applying the ointment, press a finger against the nose next to the nostril opening and use a circular motion to spread the ointment inside the nose.
- Wash or disinfect hands after applying the ointment.

Mupirocin Protocol: Information for Patients (cont'd)

Patients on Hemodialysis

Instructions: Apply ointment inside each nostril **2 times per day** for 14 days, and then continue to apply **3 times per week** after dialysis on dialysis days only. Continue course for 3 months in total.

Check each box when you have applied the ointment to remind you when you need to reapply

Stage 1: Apply TWICE daily for 14 days

Day	Date	Morning	Night
1			
2			
3			
4			
5			
6			
7			
8			
9			
10			
11			
12			
13			
14			

Stage 2: After the first 14 days, continue to apply to the inside of each nostril AFTER dialysis on dialysis days ONLY. Continue for a total of 3 months.

Ointment applied after dialysis until the following date: ________________

NOTE: It is extremely important to complete a total of 3 months of treatment. You should have a repeat nasal swab performed at your center after completing the course of therapy to ensure the therapy has been effective.

Mupirocin Protocol: Information for Patients (cont'd)

Patients Not Yet Started on Hemodialysis

Month 1

Day	Date	Morning	Night
1			
2			
3			
4			
5			

Month 2

Day	Date	Morning	Night
1			
2			
3			
4			
5			

Month 3

Day	Date	Morning	Night
1			
2			
3			
4			
5			

Instructions: Apply ointment inside each nostril **2 times per day** for 5 days. Repeat this course of treatment each month for 3 months.

Check each box when you have applied the ointment to remind you when you need to reapply.

NOTE: It is extremely important to complete a total of 3 months of treatment. You should have a repeat nasal swab performed at your center for laboratory testing after completing the course of therapy to ensure the treatment has been effective.

Protocol adapted with permission from Metro South and Ipswich Nephrology and Transplant Services (MINTS), Queensland, Australia.

Fear of Needles

Fear of needles is an important issue to acknowledge and address when the patient is considering home hemodialysis therapy as a treatment modality. Regardless of the cannulation technique that is being considered (rope ladder or buttonhole), instruction on self-cannulation should incorporate strategies for patients coping with fear of cannulation. Presented below are some useful strategies and techniques that can be implemented during training that may help a patient cope when learning to self-cannulate.

Coping strategies to reduce patient distress during self-cannulation

- **Staff behavior:** Patience is a virtue. Staff is encouraged to modify the pace of training based on the patient's skill and level of comfort. Staff can encourage patient involvement by asking the patient to assess the access, preparing the accessories required for cannulation, and observing the cannulation process.
- **Hand holding:** Staff can help patients to slowly engage in self-care by asking them to hold the needle while the nurse cannulates the vessel.
- **Warm compress:** Apply a warm compress to the access site 5 minutes prior to cannulation. This activity has 2 effects. First, the access dilates and becomes engorged, allowing for ease of cannulation. Second, the warmth of the compress is associated with comfort and relaxation.
- **Topical analgesic:** Topical analgesic can be used to reduce the pain associated with needle insertion. Removing the element of pain will allow the patient to focus on self-cannulation.
- **Peer modeling:** Peer support helps connect patients who are diagnosed with chronic conditions such as end stage renal disease. The chronically ill patient is not alone and can find comfort by sharing knowledge and experiences with others who are in similar situations. Peer support can improve patient self-efficacy and attitudes toward self-management.

Useful Resources:

- ESRD Network. Conquering Your Fistula Fear. http://www.esrdnet15.org/QI/FFconquer.pdf
- Home Dialysis Central. Dialysis Needle Fear – Easing the Sting. http://www.homedialysis.org/life-at-home/articles/dialysis-needle-fear
- Peers for Progress. What is Peer Support? http://peersforprogress.org/learn-about-peer-support/what-is-peer-support
- McLaughlin K, Manns B, Mortis G, Hons R, Taub K. Why patients with ESRD do not select self-care dialysis as a treatment option. Am J Kidney Dis. 2003;41:380-385.
- Lawes C, Sawyer L, Amos S, Kandiah M, Pearce L, Symons J. The impact of an education programme for staff working with children undergoing painful procedures. Paediatr Nurs. 2008;20:33-37.

Fear of Needles (cont'd)

- **Imaginal Exposure Therapy:** Imaginal therapy involves the client imagining the situation until acclimatization occurs. Fears should be arranged in a hierarchy from least to most anxiety evolving. The client is encouraged to "be in the scene." The therapist describes the event while the client describes what he or she sees, hears, tastes, smells, and feels. The client is asked to rate the level of anxiety (scale from 0-10, where 10 is extreme) and return immediately to the scene. The session can be recorded and utilized regularly.
- **Hypnotherapy:** Hypnosis can be used to encourage an individual to respond to suggestions and thus alter a habit or attitude for the benefit of health. Hypnotherapy can be used to decrease anxiety and change the patient's reaction and attitude toward needles.
- **Medication:** Medications to alleviate anxiety can be given prior to cannulation. This is a temporary measure and the prescribed medication should be limited to the initial first few cannulation events.

Patient training can become a positive experience when simple strategies are implemented to help the individual cope with fear of needles.

Buttonhole Cannulation Protocol for Creation and Maintenance of Tract with Intravenous Needle and Cannula

(Arteriovenous Fistula Only)

The intravenous (IV) cannula with blunt tip can be used for the maintenance of buttonhole (BH) tracts.

Procedure

1. Wash hands and the arteriovenous fistula (AVF) with soap and warm running water for at least 20 seconds.
2. Dry hands and the AVF with clean towel.
3. Clean the buttonholes (BHs) with a cleansing agent. Note: Some patients find it easier to remove the scab if the BH sites are soaked with cleansing agent or saline saturated gauze. If this is the case, soak for 2 to 5 minutes.
4. Completely remove scab on arterial BH site with 18-gauge blunt needle.
5. Discard 18-gauge blunt needle. **Do not reuse needle.**
6. Completely remove scab on venous BH site with 18-gauge needle.
7. Discard 18-gauge blunt needle. **Do not reuse needle.**
8. Clean AVF with cleaning agent again.
9. Apply tourniquet above the AVF.
10. Remove the IV needle with cannula needle from protector.
11. Align IV needle with cannula at the same angel as previous cannulations, with bevel facing up over the BH site.
12. Insert IV needle with cannula into arterial BH.
13. Blood will backflow into needle hub.
14. Lower the angel of the needle.
15. Continue to advance IV needle with cannula into the AVF approximately 1 cm into blood vessel.

Supplies

1	Clean towel
2	IV needle with cannula (eg, Supercath needles, 17-gauge)
3	18-gauge needles
1	Package 4 × 4 gauze
2	Cleansing swabsticks
1	Dressing to secure needles
2	Forceps
2	10-mL syringes prepared with 6 mL normal saline (0.9%)
1	Tourniquet
1	Alcohol wipe

Buttonhole Cannulation Protocol for Creation and Maintenance of Tract with Intravenous Needle and Cannula (cont'd)

16. With free hand hold the rubber adapter with thumb and forefinger, extend the thumb and pull the inner needle out of the outer needle while the palm of the same hand anchors the inner needle.
17. Continue to advance the outer needle while continuing to withdraw the inner needle until the outer needle is treaded within the vessel completely and the outer needle is completely withdrawn.
18. Release the tourniquet.
19. Secure the needle with dressing.
20. Clamp catheter with forceps.
21. Remove rubber adapter (cap).
22. Luer connect 10 mL syringe prepared with 6 mL normal saline to needle.
23. Remove forceps then aspirate and flush the catheter. Assess flow.
24. Clamp catheter with forceps.
25. Repeat steps 9 through 24. Cannulate venous needle.
26. Continue with dialysis initiation protocol.

Protocol adapted with permission from University Health Network, Toronto, Ontario, Canada, cannulation protocol.

Removal of Intravenous Needle with Cannula

Procedure

1. Retransfuse blood at end of treatment, per protocol.
2. Prepare gauze with a dab of antibacterial cream/ointment.
3. Ensure extracorporeal lines are clamped.
4. Ensure arterial needle is clamped.
5. Ensure venous needle is clamped.
6. Do not disconnect extracorporeal lines from arterial and venous needles.
7. Remove venous needle dressing.
8. Apply gauze with dab of cream/ointment to venous needle buttonhole (BH) site.
9. Apply gentle digital pressure to the venous BH needle site with the free hand.
10. With access hand grip the venous blood circuit tubing between thumb and forefinger and withdraw needle completely while continuing to apply digital pressure with the free hand to BH site.
11. Allow hemostasis to occur.
12. Apply bandage.
13. Remove arterial needle dressing.
14. Repeat steps 8 through 12.
15. Continue with end of treatment protocol.

Supplies

1 Clean towel

3 Package 4 × 4 gauze

2 Bandages

1 Antibacterial cream/ointment

Protocol adapted with permission from University Health Network, Toronto, Ontario, Canada, cannulation protocol.

Buttonhole Cannulation Technique with Dull (Blunt) Bevel

(Arteriovenous Fistula Only)

Procedure

1. Wash hands and the arteriovenous fistula (AVF) with soap and warm running water for at least 20 seconds.
2. Dry hands and the AVF with clean towel.
3. Remove dull/blunt fistula needles from package.
4. Attach 10-mL syringe prepared with normal saline to each needle.
5. Prime the fistula needles.
6. Leave needle line clamps open. Set needles aside.
7. Clean the buttonholes (BHs) with a cleansing agent. (Note: Some patients find it easier to remove the scab if BH sites are soaked with cleansing agent or saline-saturated gauze. If this is the case, soak for 2 to 5 minutes.)
8. Completely remove scab on arterial BH site with 18-gauge blunt needle or BH pick.
9. Discard 18-gauge needle or discard pick. **Do not reuse needle or pick.**
10. Completely remove scab on venous BH site with 18-gauge blunt needle or BH pick.
11. Discard 18-gauge needle or discard pick. **Do not reuse needle or pick.**
12. Clean AVF with cleansing agent again.
13. Apply tourniquet above the AVF.
14. Tighten the tourniquet.
15. Pinch wings of dull/blunt buttonhole needle carefully, remove tip protector.
16. Align BH needle cannula at the same angel as previous cannulations, with bevel facing up, over buttonhole site.

Supplies

1 Clean towel

2 Dull bevel buttonhole needles

3 18-gauge blunt needles

1 Package 4 × 4 gauze

4 Cleansing swabsticks, chlorhexidine 2%/alcohol 70%

2 Normal saline (0.9%) saturated gauze

2 Dressings to secure needles

2 10 mL-syringes prepared with 6 mL normal saline (0.9%)

1 Tourniquet

1 Personal protective equipment (eg, mask)

Buttonhole Cannulation Technique with Dull (Blunt) Bevel (cont'd)

17. Insert needle into established BH site at the same angle as previous cannulations.
18. Advance BH needle along the developed tunnel tract. If mild-to-moderate resistance is met, using gentle pressure, rotate dull/blunt needle back and forth.
19. Allow the dull/blunt needle to seek the vessel entrance, advance dull/blunt needle into the AVF.
20. Release the tourniquet.
21. Check the position of the needle. First, pull back blood into 10-mL syringe, then flush and check the return flow.
22. Clamp needle.
23. Secure the needle with dressing.
24. Repeat steps 14 to 23 to cannulate the second needle.

Protocol adapted with permission from University Health Network, Toronto, Ontario, Canada, cannulation protocol.

Removal of Dull/Blunt Dull (Blunt) Bevel Needles from Arteriovenous Fistula

Procedure

1. Retransfuse blood at end of treatment, per protocol.
2. Prepare gauze with a dab of antibacterial cream/ointment.
3. Ensure extracorporeal lines are clamped.
4. Ensure arterial needle is clamped.
5. Ensure venous needle is clamped.
6. Disconnect extracorporeal lines from arterial and venous needles.
7. Remove venous needle dressing.
8. Apply gauze with dab of cream/ointment to venous needle buttonhole (BH) site.
9. Apply gentle digital pressure to the venous BH needle site with the free hand.
10. With access hand grip the venous needle tubing between thumb and forefinger and withdraw needle completely while continuing to applying digital pressure with the free hand to BH site.
11. Allow hemostasis to occur.
12. Apply bandage.
13. Remove arterial needle dressing.
14. Repeat steps 8 through 12.
15. Continue with end of treatment protocol.

Supplies

1 Clean towel

3 Package 4 × 4 gauze

2 Bandages

1 Antibacterial cream/ointment

Protocol adapted with permission from University Health Network, Toronto, Ontario, Canada, cannulation protocol.

Taping Method for Hemodialysis Needle

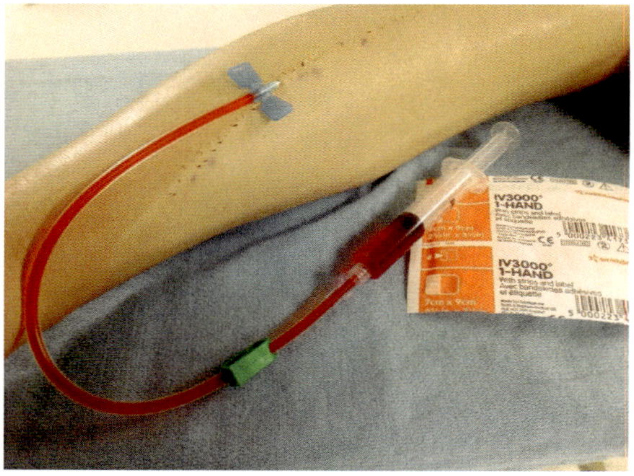

Transparent Dressing

- Transparent dressing is compatible with sensitive skin and adheres well, even when exposed to moisture
- Skin barriers can be used to help prevent irritation
- Apply skin barrier before application of dressing

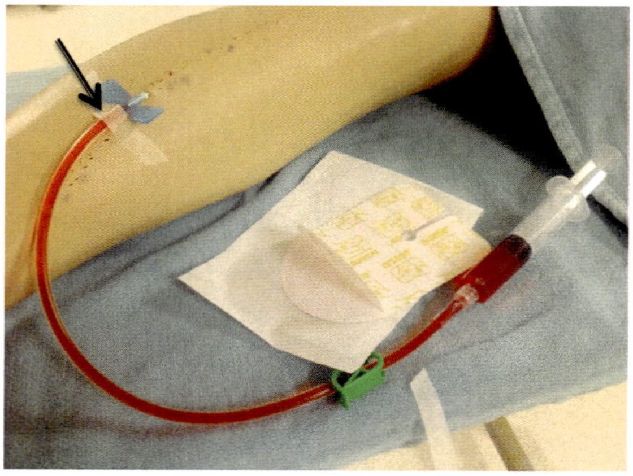

Apply tape strip to secure needle

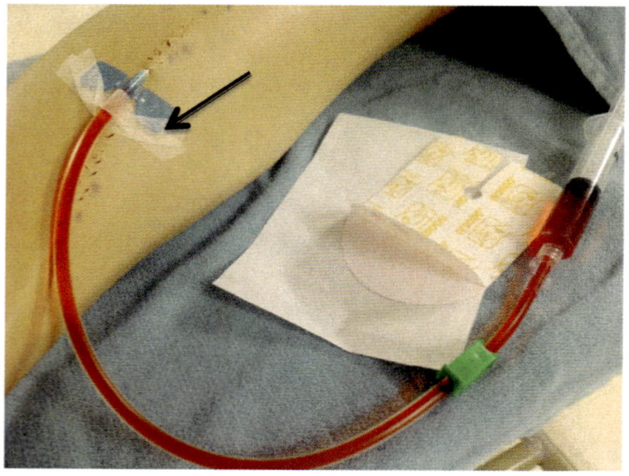

Apply second tape strip under needle and over wings of needle

Rose Faratro, RN, BHScN, CNeph(C)
University Health Network, Toronto, Ontario, Canada

Taping Method for Hemodialysis Needle (cont'd)

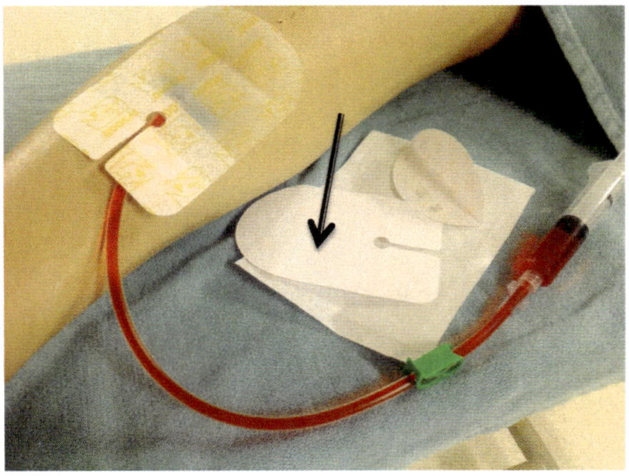

Remove the back lining from the transparent dressing. Apply dressing over needle

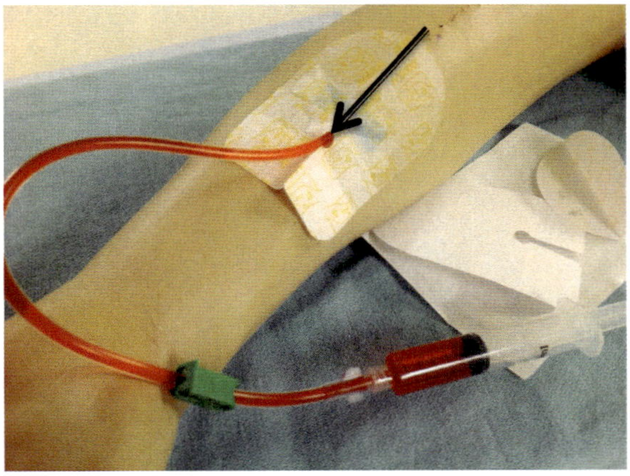

Smooth transparent dressing over the needle and surrounding area. Allow tubing to come through the deep notch of dressing

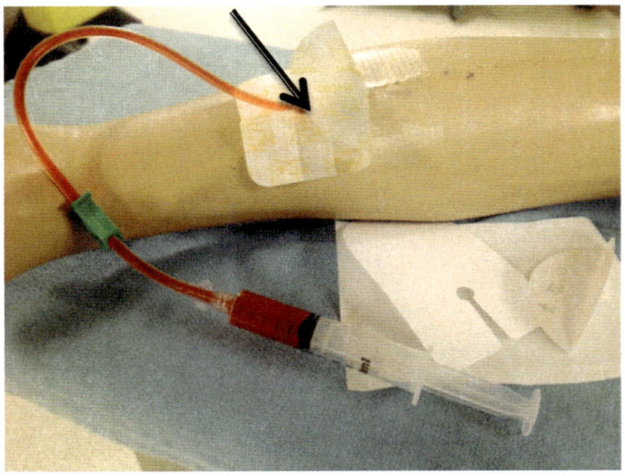

Remove top lining of transparent dressing

Taping Method for Hemodialysis Needle (cont'd)

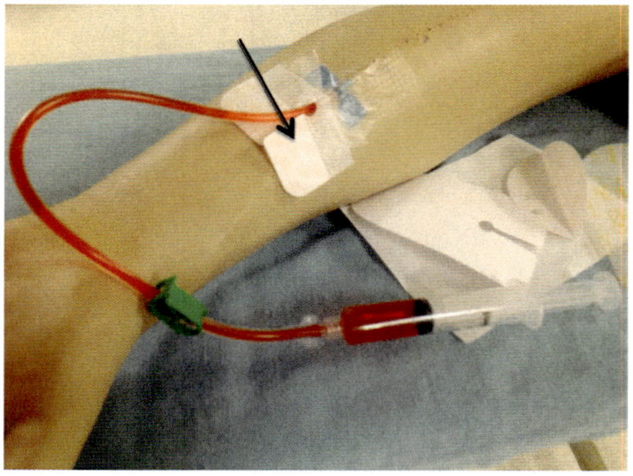

Stabilization fold

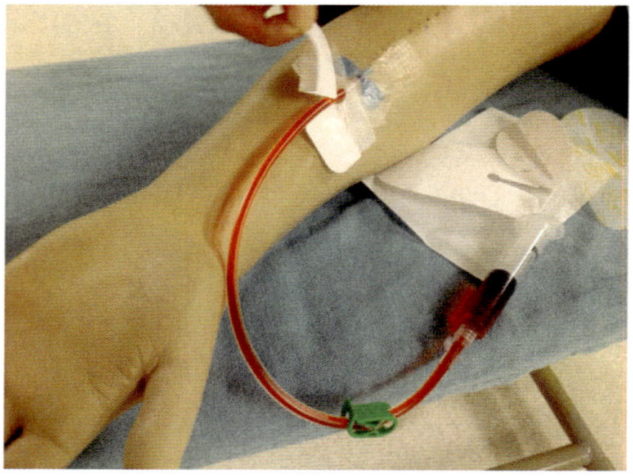

Gently peel off the back lining of the stabilization fold

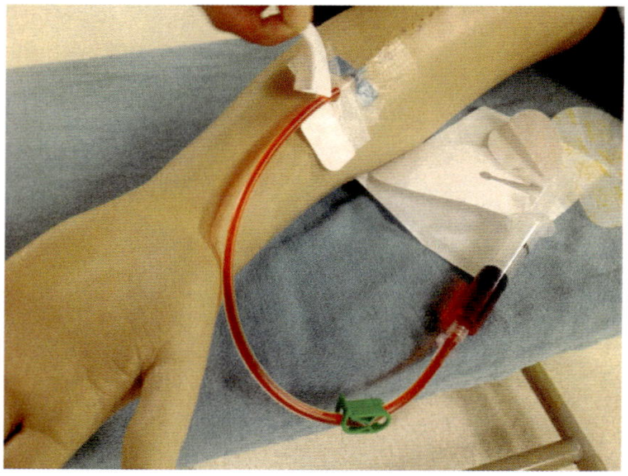

Apply the stabilization fold portion of the dressing and smooth over skin

Taping Method for Hemodialysis Needle (cont'd)

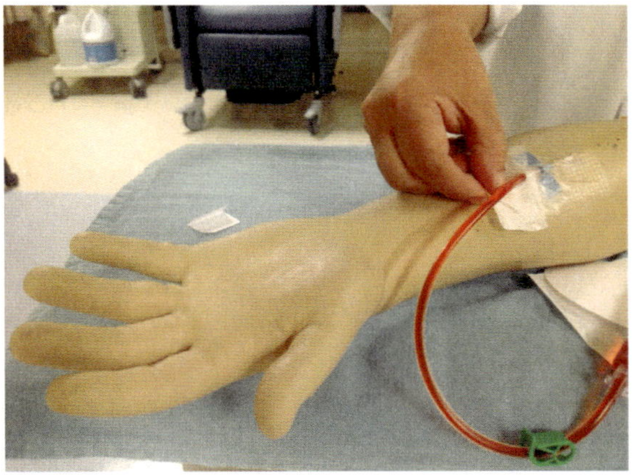

Secure and smooth down second stabilization fold

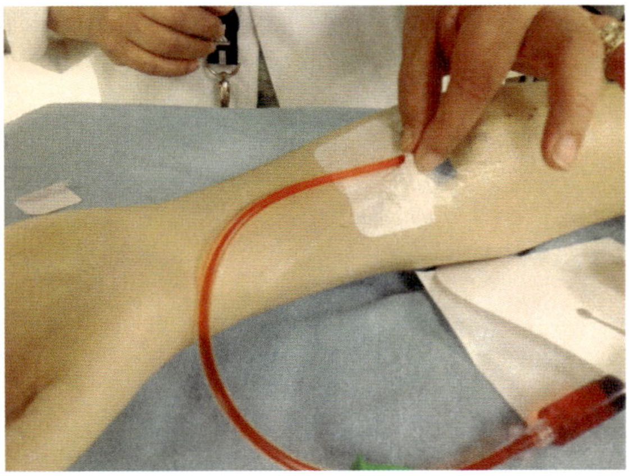

Pinch transparent dressing at the deep notch

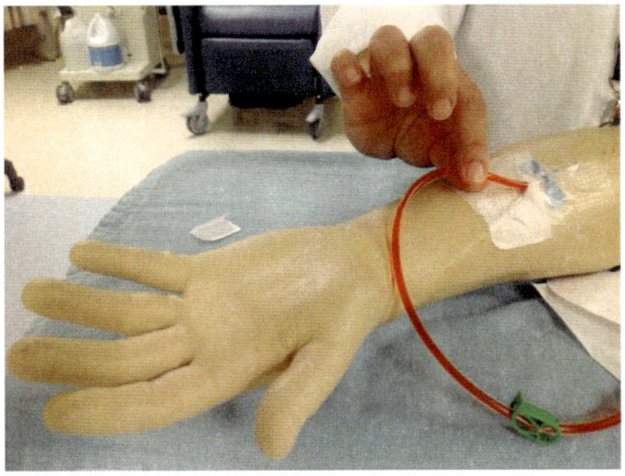

Check stabilization of needle

Taping Method for Intravenous Needle with Cannula

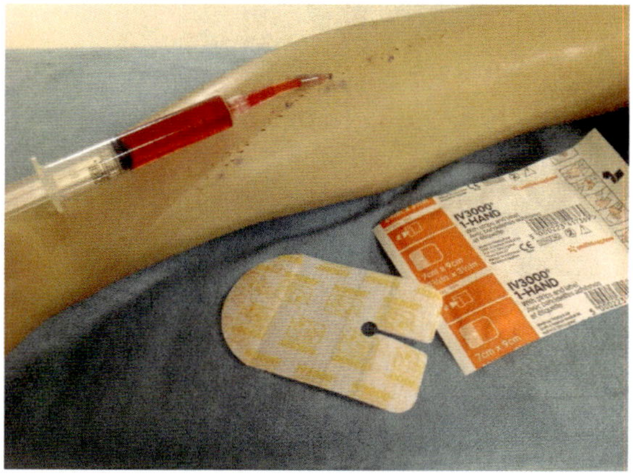

Transparent Dressing

- Transparent dressing is compatible with sensitive skin and adheres well, even when exposed to moisture
- Skin barriers can be used to help prevent irritation
- Apply skin barrier before application of dressing

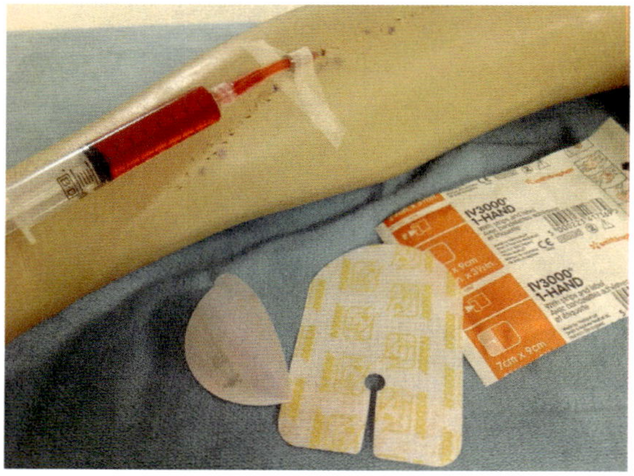

Apply tape strips to secure cannula using the chevron taping method

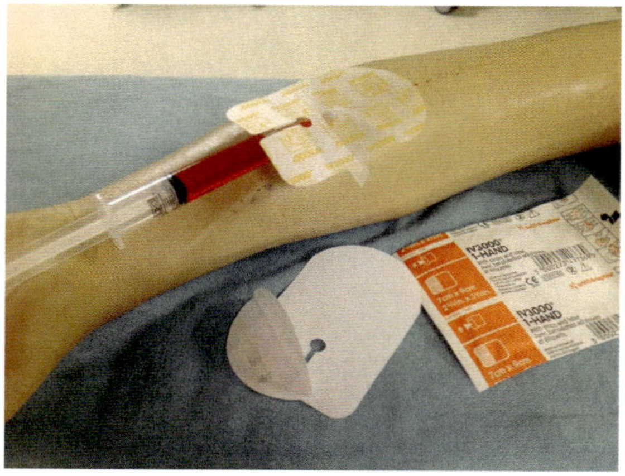

Remove the back lining from the transparent dressing. Apply dressing over cannula

Rose Faratro, RN, BHScN, CNeph(C)
University Health Network, Toronto, Ontario, Canada

Taping Method for Intravenous Needle with Cannula (cont'd)

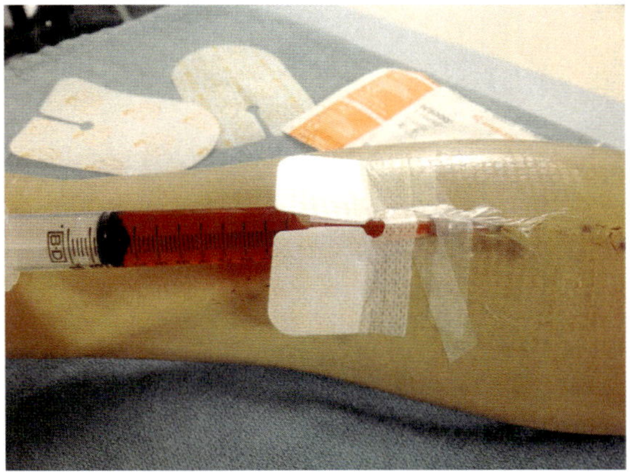

Smooth transparent dressing over cannula and surrounding area

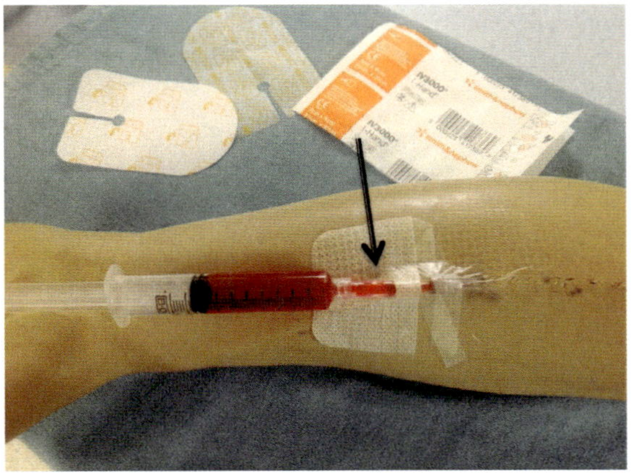

Apply and smooth down stabilization folds

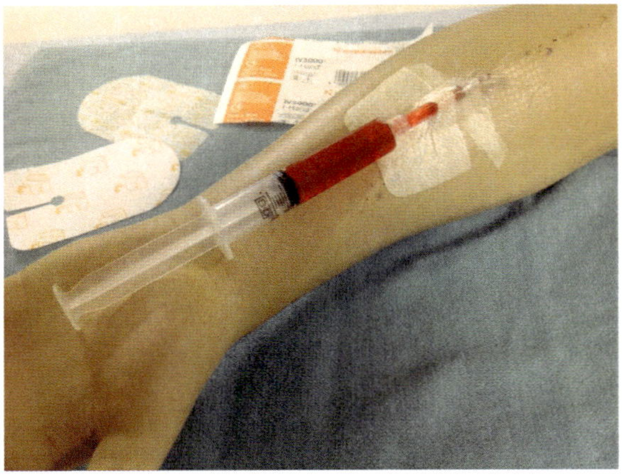

Check stabilization of cannula

Heparin Locking of Central Venous Catheters

Procedure

1. Use alcohol wipe to clean table.
2. Wash hands for 2 minutes. Dry thoroughly.
3. Open supplies and place on table.
4. Wash hands for 30 seconds and apply sterile gloves.
5. Use the 3-mL syringes and needles to draw up the appropriate volume of heparin as indicated on the lumens of each catheter (volume varies).
6. Ensure lines are clamped.
7. Remove caps from lumens. Clean the end of the lumen using the antiseptic wipe or swab. Allow to dry.
8. Connect the heparin-containing syringe to the arterial lumen and instill heparin solution. Replace cap. Repeat for venous lumen.
9. Allow heparin solution to dwell in the lumens until the next dialysis run.
10. Use the antiseptic wipe or swab to clean the ends of the lumens.
11. Aspirate heparin from the lumens using a 3-mL syringe.
12. Use the 10-mL syringes and needle to draw up sodium chloride using separate syringes for each lumen. The total volume in each syringe should be twice that of the lumen. When using Tego connectors, add 0.1 mL to volume.
13. Flush lumens with sodium chloride solution.
14. Perform dialysis, per protocol.
15. Adjust postdialysis heparin bolus to account for heparin used in lock.

Supplies

1 Dialysis dressing pack

1 Personal protective equipment (eg, apron, gloves)

2 10-mL syringe with Luer lock

2 3-mL syringe with Luer lock

2 Sterile Luer lock caps or Tego connectors

2 18-gauge needle

2 10-mL ampules of 0.9% sodium chloride

2 Antiseptic wipe or swab (eg, isopropyl alcohol 70%/ chlorhexidine 2%)

4 6mL heparin sodium, 5000 units per 1 mL (number of ampules determined by volume of catheter, as indicated by lumen)

1 Alcohol disinfecting wipe

Protocol adapted with permission from Metro South and Ipswich Nephrology and Transplant Services (MINTS), Queensland, Australia.

Heparin Flushing of Cannulas

1. Cannulate the access using standard rope ladder or buttonhole protocol.
2. Draw up 1000 units of heparin sodium using a 10-mL syringe and needle.
3. Dilute the heparin in the syringe by drawing up sodium chloride 0.9% to a total volume of 10 mL (concentration now 100 units/mL).
4. Flush each cannula with 5 mL (500 units) of the diluted heparin/sodium chloride solution.
5. Flush cannulas before initiating dialysis using the usual procedure.
6. Reduce the postdialysis heparin bolus by 1 mL (1000 units) to account for the amount used to flush the cannulas.

Note: If patients typically use enoxaparin instead of heparin, advise them to withdraw the heparinized saline from the cannulas (instead of flushing) before using them for HD. Patients should flush the cannulas with sodium chloride 0.9% to ensure proper position before initiating dialysis. Enoxaparin should be administered, as usual.

Protocol adapted with permission from Metro South and Ipswich Nephrology and Transplant Services (MINTS), Queensland, Australia.

Showering Protocol

Procedure

1. Gather all supplies and equipment before entering the shower.
2. Ensure all catheter caps are secure before entering the shower.
3. Remove exit site dressing, dispose of dressing, and inspect the site for signs and symptoms of infection (see below).

- If signs and symptoms of infection are present, DO NOT USE SHOWER TECHNIQUE. Use a covered or modified shower technique. Contact your hemodialysis clinician to notify them of possible infection

4. While in the shower, wash and rinse face, hair, and body using 1 face cloth. The catheter area should be cleaned last.
5. Use the second face cloth and soap to wash the area around the exit site.
6. Rinse thoroughly and exit shower.
7. Dry the catheter area first by gently patting with a dry towel.
8. Dry the rest of the body using a dry towel.
9. Apply a cleansing agent to the area nearest to the catheter and move in a circular pattern away from the catheter.
10. Clean the catheter from the exit site to hub a second time using the cleansing agent.
11. Allow area to dry.
12. If necessary, apply antibiotic ointment to the area.
13. Apply dressing.

Required Supplies

- 2 clean face cloths
- Clean towels
- Mild soap with pump dispenser
- Cleansing agent recommended by the dialysis unit (eg, chlorhexidine, povidone iodine)
- Dressing supplies

Signs of Skin Infection

- Redness
- Swelling
- Unusually warm skin
- Fever
- Fragile skin that bleeds easily
- Pus or other liquid oozing from skin
- Foul odor
- Increased pain or change in pain
- Cracked skin

Protocol adapted with permission from the Home Dialysis Interest Group, Toronto, Canada, document "Shower Technique for Hemodialysis Access".

Central Venous Catheter Antibiotic Treatment Protocol

Purpose

1. To provide evidence-based practice guidelines for the management of suspected systemic central venous catheter (CVC)-related infection in the **hemodialysis (HD) outpatient population**.

   Note: This is a guideline ONLY; there may be times when, based on individual assessments, there is a need to operate outside of this protocol.

2. To provide an accurate and comprehensive record of all vascular access infections via a single point of entry to aid in the development of targeted strategies to reduce vascular related infection rates and optimize patient outcomes.

Personnel Permitted to Perform Procedure

1. Registered nurses (RNs), graduate nurses, and licensed practical nurses (LPNs; in consultation with an RN) who have completed specialized, comprehensive HD training.

2. Patients/designated helpers who have received specialized and comprehensive training by a trained home HD-registered nurse may administer intravenous (IV) antibiotics at home if trained in the procedure and with dosage instructions from the home HD RN (in conjunction with this protocol).

Policy

1. A physician's order is required to initiate the antibiotic protocol

- When a patient presents with suspected CVC bacteremia infection, the attending nephrologist must be notified of any significant clinical findings and diagnostic testing prior to the nurse proceeding with antibiotic treatment (ie, Appendix I: "Phase I — Algorithm for SUSPECTED Systemic Catheter Associated Bacteremia")

- When blood culture specimen results are confirmed to be positive, the attending nephrologist will be notified of the results and the plan to continue with the antibiotic protocol (ie, Appendix II: "Phase II — Antibiotic Protocol for CONFIRMED Catheter Associated Bacteremia")

- Antibiotics should be prescribed in accordance with Appendix III: "Gentamycin, Vancomycin, Cefazolin, Ceftazidime Dosing Charts"

- If the blood culture results are negative, the antibiotic protocol will be discontinued. The attending nephrologist will be notified of the negative results and the clinical status of the patient

Definitions

- Bacteremia: Presence of bacteria in the circulating blood

- Coagulase-negative Staphylococcus (*Staphylococcus epidermidis*): Normal bacterial skin, gut and upper respiratory tract flora. It is a true opportunistic pathogen. Infection is associated with skin penetration from CVC or peritoneal dialysis (PD) catheter insertion; implanted prosthesis (eg, heart valves); and in immunocompromised patients such as those individuals with end-stage renal disease

- *Enterococcus fecalis*: Opportunistic gram-positive bacterium that has become one of the most troublesome pathogens. Lives peacefully in the gut but thrives in wounds. Extremely hardy and can survive for weeks on environmental surfaces

- Gram-negative microorganisms: Examples are *Klebsiella*, *Pseudomonas aeruginosa*, *Escherichia coli* (E coli)

- Metastatic infection: Transmission of infection from an original site to 1 or more sites elsewhere in the body

Central Venous Catheter Antibiotic Treatment Protocol (cont'd)

2. When a patient becomes an inpatient, the attending physician will assume responsibility for management of the infection (ie, will choose to order the antibiotic protocol or provide individualized prescriptive care).
3. The access nurse and/or designate unit-specific access expert will be notified of all suspected and/or confirmed infections.
4. Strict aseptic technique must be used when performing CVC-related interventions.
5. In the event of suspected catheter-related infection, patient assessment will include the following general clinical manifestations of bacteremia (see Appendix I, "Phase I — Algorithm for SUSPECTED Catheter Associated Bacteremia").

   Note: Patients who have artificial heart valves or those who are taking steroids or immunosuppressant medications are more prone to develop systemic infection.

- Fever ≥ 38°C and/or chills and rigors
- Hypothermia
- Confusion or altered level of mental state
- Hyperglycemia
- Nausea and/or vomiting
- Complaint of general and unusual feeling of unwellness
- Signs and symptoms of any of the following:
    - Respiratory infection (eg, cough, colored phlegm or sputum production, hemoptysis, shortness of breath, crackles and/or wheezes on auscultation, oxygen desaturation on room air, increased need for oxygen replacement)
    - Gastrointestinal infection (eg, diarrhea, abdominal cramps, loss of appetite, abdominal distention and/or tenderness)
    - Genitourinary infection (eg, hematuria, pyuria or dysuria in patients with some residual function, pain in lower back, hips or thighs)
    - Integumentary or access site infection (eg, redness, tenderness, serous or purulent exudates, pallor or bruising, cool or warm to touch, edema)
    - Metastatic infection (eg, red, tender, and/or swollen joints; new or worsening cardiac murmur, congestive heart failure)
- Elevated white blood cell (WBC) count

Definition (cont'd)

- Sepsis: Severe and potentially fatal illness caused by overwhelming infection of the bloodstream by toxin producing bacteria
- *Staphylococcus aureus*: Gram-positive microorganism that commonly colonizes the human skin and nasal mucosa. Can enter into the blood stream through breakage of the skin or may be ingested in contaminated food particles. Once in the body, it can produce poisons and toxins causing severe illness
- MSSA: Methicillin-sensitive *S aureus*
- MRSA: Methicillin-resistive *S aureus*
- *Streptococcus viridans*: Hemolytic streptococcus that is usually the main culprit for endocardial infection

Central Venous Catheter Antibiotic Treatment Protocol (cont'd)

6. An RN or an LPN (in consultation with a RN), without a physician's order, may obtain the following laboratory specimens:

- Blood culture specimens: 2 sets of 2 (4 total) or 1 set of 3 (local laboratory dependent)
- Complete blood cell count
- Swab(s) for culture and sensitivity from sites where exudate is present
- Sputum and/or urine for culture and sensitivity if indicated
- Predialysis antibiotic levels if the patient is already being treated for suspected or confirmed infection
    - If the CVC is locked with an antibiotic solution, draw antibiotic levels per PT/INR method (start dialysis, wait 5 minutes, and then draw level). Consult physician if unable to withdraw antibiotic lock solution from the CVC
    - If the predialysis antibiotic levels are not available before the patient completes the dialysis session, the next antibiotic dose can be given during the next session unless the levels are below target. In this case, it is advisable to bring the patient back for dosing. If the patient refuses or there is uncertainty (ie, close to target), check with the nephrologist

7. Unless otherwise ordered, the patient's standard lock solution will continue to be used. Note: There may be some situations where the physician requests use of vancomycin/heparin OR ceftazidime/heparin lock solution (to replace the patient's standard lock solution).
8. Antibiotics will be adjusted based on the following predialysis antibiotic levels:

- Vancomycin greater than 19 mg/L: Hold vancomycin
- Gentamicin less than 1.5 mg/L or greater than 3 mg/L: refer to Appendix III. "Gentamycin, Vancomycin, Cefazolin, Ceftazidime Dosing Charts"

Note for home HD patients: Alternatively, vancomycin 25 mg/kg load followed by 500 mg every HD session to a maximum of 4 sessions/week, may be given without pursuing vancomycin levels.

Procedure for Antibiotic Lock Preparation

(refer to Appendix II — "Phase II Antibiotic Protocol for CONFIRMED CVC Associated Bacteremia According to Bacterial Organism")

1. Prepare **vancomycin and heparin** lock solution, if ordered, for CVC Locks:
   Note: Vancomycin lock solution **should be prepared immediately prior to administration** as it is good for 72 hours only (this will ensure potency is maintained within the catheter lumen until the next run). Also note that prevancomycin levels may be influenced by the vancomycin/heparin lock solution and unusual results should be brought to the attention of the physician.

   a. Gather equipment/supplies
      - Vancomycin **500-mg** vial
      - Sterile water for reconstitution
      - Heparin **10,000-units/mL** vials
      - Sodium Chloride 0.9% 50 mL minibag
      - Needles, 18 gauge × 5
      - Syringes, 3 mL × 3; 10 mL × 4
      - Medication labels, if required

   b. Prepare vancomycin 2.8 mg/mL
      - Add 10 mL sterile water for injection to a 500-mg vial of vancomycin powder to make a 50-mg/mL solution
      - Shake to dissolve
      - Withdraw and discard 4 mL from a 50-mL minibag of sodium chloride 0.9% (this is the standard average overfill in a minibag)
      - Inject 3 mL (150 mg) of vancomycin into the minibag and apply medication label
      - Final concentration: 150 mg in 53 mL = 2.8 mg/mL vancomycin

Points of Emphasis

- Patients must be educated on the signs of CVC access infection and the need to seek immediate medical attention in urgent or emergent situations (eg, septicemia)
- Antibiotic doses may be verified by 2 nurses (1 must be a RN) or 1 nurse and 1 pharmacist at the discretion of the RN

Procedure for Antibiotic Lock Preparation (cont'd)

c. Prepare heparin lock solution
- Into a 3-mL syringe, draw 0.3 mL (3000 units) from a 10,000-units/mL vial of heparin
- Using the same syringe, withdraw 2.7 mL (7.5mg) of vancomycin from the above minibag
- Repeat above 2 steps, using a second 3-mL syringe
- Flush both lumens with 10-mL sodium chloride 0.9%
- Instill vancomycin/heparin lock solution equal to the volume of CVC lumens
- Apply medication labels to the lumens

d. Final products (reflected on medication label)
- Vancomycin 7.5 mg/3 mL= 2.5 mg/mL
- Heparin 3000 units/3 mL=1000 units/mL

2. If **ceftazidime/heparin** lock is ordered
For inpatients: Order from pharmacy
For outpatients: Mix as follows (prepare immediately prior to administration)

a. Gather equipment/supplies
- Ceftazidime **1-g** vial
- Heparin **10,000-units/mL** vials
- Sterile water for injection 10 mL
- Sodium chloride 0.9% 50-mL minibag
- Needles, 18 gauge × 5
- Syringes, 10 mL × 4; 3 mL × 3; 1 mL × 1
- Syringe-to-syringe transfer device × 2
- Medication labels

b. Reconstitute cettazidime
- Inject 4.4 mL sterile water for injection to 1-g vial of ceftazidime
- Shake well to reconstitute
- Yields a 200-mg/mL solution

Bibliography

Allon M. Dialysis catheter related bacteremia: Treatment and prophylaxis. Am J Kidney Dis. 2004;44:779-791.

Allon, M. Saving infected catheters, why and how? Blood Purif. 2005;23:23-28.

Ariano RE, Fine A, Sitar DS, Rexrode S, Zelenitsky SA. Adequacy of vancomycin dosing regimen in patients receiving high flux hemodialysis. Am J Kidney Dis. 2005;146:681-687.

Chiou et al. Antibiotic lock technique reduces the incidence of temporary catheter related infections. Clin Nephrol. 2006;65:419-422.

CSN Hemodialysis Clinical Practice Guidelines. J Am Soc Nephrol. 2006; 17:S1-27.

Falk A, Prabhuram N, Parthasarathy S. Conversion of temporary hemodialysis catheters to permanent hemodialysis catheters. Semin Dial. 2005;18:425-430.

Jaber BL. Bacterial infections in hemodialysis patients: Pathogenesis and prevention. Kidney Int. 2005;67:2508-2519.

Mokrzycki MH, Zhang M, Cohen H, Rosenberg S. Tunnelled hemodialysis catheter bacteremia: risk factors for bacteremia: recurrence infections complications and mortality. Nephrol Dial Transplant. 2006;21:1024-1031.

Poole CV, Carlton D, Bimbo L, Allon M. Treatment of catheter related bacteremia with an antibiotic lock protocol: effect of bacterial pathogen. Nephrol Dial Transplant. 2004;19:1237-1244.

Tanriover B, Carlton D, Saddekni S. Bacteremia associated with tunneled dialysis catheters: comparison of two treatment strategies. Kidney Int. 2000;57:2151-2155.

Vercaigne LM, Ariano RE, Zacharian JM. Bayesian pharmacokinetics of gentamycin in a hemodialysis population. Clin Pharmacokinet. 2004;43:205-210.

Procedure for Antibiotic Lock Preparation (cont'd)

c. Prepare lock solution
   - Draw up 0.25 mL (50 mg) ceftazidime
   - Draw up 2.5 mL (25,000 units) heparin using the 10,000-units/mL solution
   - Using a syringe-to-syringe transfer device, transfer the contents of both syringes to a 10-mL syringe
     - Fill this final syringe to 10 mL using sodium chloride 0.9%
     - Mix well
     - Using syringe-to-syringe transfer device, fill 2, 3-mL syringes with ceftazidime/heparin lock solution
     - Flush both lumens with 10 mL sodium chloride 0.9%
     - Instill ceftazidime/heparin lock solution equal to the volume of CVC lumens
     - Apply medication labels to lumens
   - Final product (reflected on medication label):
     - Cettazidime 5 mg/mL + heparin 2500 units/mL lock solution

Bibliography (cont'd)

Zipporah K, et al. Management of hemodialysis catheter related bacteremia with an adjunctive lock solution. Kidney Int. 2002;61:1136-1142.

Protocol adapted with permission from Southern Alberta (Canada) Renal Program, Alberta, Canada.

Appendix I. Phase I - Algorithm for Suspected Systemic CVC-Associated Bacteremia

Patient with HD CVC

↓

Presents unwell

(symptomatic or asymptomatic)
For example, fever ≥ 38°C, chills, rigors, hypothermia, confusion or altered mental state, hyperglycemia, nausea and/or vomiting, complains of general or unusual/vague feeling of unwellness

↓

Perform clinical assessment

(refer to Policy Statement 6)
Signs and symptoms of respiratory, gastrointestinal, genitourinary, integumentary, or metastatic infection, elevated WBC

↓

Obtain lab specimens

(refer to Policy Statement 7)
Blood cultures; CBC; swab(s) for culture and sensitivity from sites where exudates are present; sputum and/or urine for culture and sensitivity, if indicated; pre-dialysis antibiotic levels if patient is already being treated

↓

Check for allergies

To vancomycin, cefazolin, gentamicin, and ceftazidine

↓

If allergies exist to any antibiotics

- Check with pharmacy to determine if applicable to any of the protocol recommended drugs
- Defer to the physician for individualized care
- Do NOT proceed with the Antibiotic Protocol

If no allergies and pending cultures,

obtain physician order to initiate the Antibiotic Protocol

→

Initiate Antibiotic Protocol

- If patient presents clinically unwell (ie, symptomatic) obtain physician order to administer vancomycin + cefazolin + gentamicin*, consider immediate CVC removal (unless another source of infection has been identified), and admit patient to hospital
- If patient appears clinically well (ie, complains of general or unusual/vague feeling of unwellness but otherwise asymptomatic), administer vancomycin + gentamicin*, leave CVC in place, and treat as an outpatient until cultures return
- If patient is gentamicin intolerant, substitute with ceftazidime*

Predialysis Antibiotic Levels

Vancomycin target = 15 - 19 mg/L

- For home HD patients, refer to Policy Statement 9
- Vancomycin level will be reduced by 30% after dialysis

Gentamicin target = 1.5 - 3.0 mg/L

- Patients should be questioned regularly about hearing problems and/or dizziness (signs of ototoxicity)

- If blood culture results are known to be positive, with no other obvious source of infection, the attending nephrologist will be notified of the results and the plan to continue with the Antibiotic Protocol physician (proceed to Appendix II: Phase II for antibiotic choice and duration of therapy)
- If positive swab but negative blood cultures, check with physician for exit site treatment
- If positive sputum, would and/or urine, check with physician for next steps
- If all diagnostic tests are negative, notify physician and, unless the patient is clinically symptomatic, discontinue antibiotic therapy

*Dosing per Appendix III

Appendix II. Phase II – Antibiotic Protocol for Confirmed CVC-Associated Bacteremia According to Bacterial Organism

Treatment for Organism-Specific CVC-Associated Bacteremia

Note: Significant if ≥ 2 culture bottles positive for organism listed below

Coagulase-Negative ***Staphylococcus*** (antibiotics x 3 weeks)

- If clinical assessment is negative, leave catheter in place, give IV vancomycin* x 3 weeks total; use standard lock solution unless vancomycin/heparin lock solution ordered
- If clinical assessment positive, obtain physician order to remove the CVC

Note: Significant if ≥ 1 culture bottle positive for organism listed below

Staphylococcus aureus (antibiotics x 4 to 6 weeks)

- Given the high risk of metastatic complications it is ideal practice to remove the CVC and replace at a new site even if clinical assessment is negative (guidewire exchange should not be done)
- If MSSA positive, give cefazolin* x 4 weeks
- If MRSA positive, give vancomycin*
- If clinical assessment positive, admit patient to hospital and physician will assume responsibility for prescribing antibiotics (cloxacillin 2 g IV q 4 - 6 h x 4 weeks is recommended)
- If metastatic complications, treatment duration is 6 weeks

Note: Significant if ≥ 1 culture bottle positive for organism listed below

Entercoccus fecalis (antibiotics x 3 weeks)

- Plan for CVC removal and hospital admission; physician will assume responsibility for prescribing antibiotics (ampicillin 2 g IV post HD x 3 weeks is recommended)
- If CVC is left in place, physician will assume responsibility for prescribing antibiotics (vancomycin/ampicillin + gentamicin is recommended)
- Follow sensitivity to ampicillin; if resistant, change to vancomycin

Clinical Assessment

If any of the following are positive, the ideal practice is to remove the catheter and insert a new catheter at a new site:

- Patient is clinically unwell (eg, general malaise, hypotensive, septic, altered mental state, chills, sweating)
- Persistent fever ≥ 38°C
- Recent CVC bacteremia (with same CVC)
- Signs and symptoms of exit site infection or metastatic infection
- History of prosthetic heart valve

If the catheter is left in place, the physician may order one of the following antibiotic locks (refer to Procedural statements 1 and 2 for mixing):

Vancomycin/heparin lock

- Vancomycin 7.5 mg/3 mL = 2.5 mg/mL
- Heparin 3000 units/3mL = 1000 units/mL

Ceftazidime/heparin lock

- Ceftazidime 5 mg/mL
- Heparin 2500 units/mL

Draw follow-up blood cultures 2 weeks after the last dose of antibiotics

*Dosing per Appendix III

Appendix II. Phase II – Antibiotic Protocol for Confirmed CVC-Associated Bacteremia According to Bacterial Organism (cont'd)

Treatment for Organism-Specific CVC-Associated Bacteremia

Enterococcus fecium (antibiotics x 3 weeks)

- Plan for CVC removal and hospital admission; physician will assume responsibility for prescribing antibiotics (may order Antibiotic Protocol)
- Combination therapy: ampicillin 2 g q24h (post HD on HD days) x 3 weeks and gentamicin recommended
- Follow sensitivity to ampicillin; if resistant, change to vancomycin
- Look for abdominal source or endocarditis

Streptococcus viridans (antibiotics x 3 weeks)

- Guidewire exchange OK if clinical assessment negative
- Give cefazolin

Gram-negative organism (antibiotics x 3 weeks)

- Remove CVC (guidewire exchange OK) if clinical assessment positive
- If clinical assessment negative, leave CVC in and give ceftazidime or gentamicin
  x 3 weeks (according to sensitivities) and ceftazidime lock if ordered

Pseudomonas aeruginosa (antibiotics x 4 weeks)

- Irrespective of clinical assessment, removal of catheter is recommended
- If catheter is not removed, use dual antibiotics (ceftazidime + gentamicin x 4 weeks) pending verification of cultures
- If multidrug resistant, consult the infectious disease team

Draw follow-up blood cultures 2 weeks after the last dose of antibiotics

*Dosing per Appendix III

Appendix III. Gentamycin, Vancomycin, Cefazolin, Ceftazidime Dosing Charts

Gentamicin LOADING Dose		
Patient Weight, kg	Gentamicin Dose, mg (1.5 mg/kg rounded to the nearest 10th)	Gentamicin Dilution Amount Required, mL (gentamicin 40 mg/mL vial)
40-43	60	1.5
44-50	70	1.75
51-56	80	2.0
57-63	90	2.25
64-70	100	2.5
71-76	110	2.75
77-83	120	3.0
84-90	130	3.25
91-96	140	3.5
97-103	150	3.75
104-109	160	4.0
110-116	170	4.25
117-123	180	4.5
124-129	190	4.75
> 130	200 (maximum recommended dose)	5.0

Notes

- Draw predialysis gentamicin level on next session after gentamicin loading dose
- If level is therapeutic (1.5 - 3.0 mg/L) or greater than 3.0 mg/L, proceed with maintenance dose
- If level is < 1.5 mg/L, proceed with a maintenance dose that is increased by 25%

Appendix III. Gentamycin, Vancomycin, Cefazolin, Ceftazidime Dosing Charts (cont'd)

Gentamicin MAINTENANCE Dose		
Patient Weight, kg	Gentamicin Dose, mg (1.5 mg/kg rounded to the nearest 10th)	Gentamicin Dilution Amount Required, mL (gentamicin 40 mg/mL vial)
40-44	40	1.0
45-54	50	1.25
55-64	60	1.5
65-74	70	1.75
75-84	80	2.0
85-94	90	2.25
95-104	100	2.5
105-114	110	2.75
115-124	120	3.0
> 134	130 (maximum recommended dose)	3.25

Notes

- Draw predialysis gentamicin level at least twice weekly and the next dialysis session after a dose change or nontherapeutic level
- If level is < 1.5 mg/L, increase dose by 25%
- If level is > 3.0 mg/L, hold next dose, then decrease dose by 25% once level has returned to therapeutic range (1.5 - 3.0 mg/L)
- Question patient at each session about hearing problems or dizziness (signs of ototoxicity)

Appendix III. Gentamycin, Vancomycin, Cefazolin, Ceftazidime Dosing Charts (cont'd)

Ceftazidime Dose
2 grams IV every dialysis session up to a maximum of 4 doses per week

Vancomycin Dose		
Patient Weight, kg	Vancomycin Dose, mg (20 mg/kg rounded to the nearest 250mg)	Vancomycin Reconstitution Amount Required, mL (vancomycin 1000mg/20mL sterile water)
31-43	750	15
44-56	1000	20
57-68	1250	25
69-81	1500	30
82-93	1750	35
> 94	2000 (maximum recommended dose)	40

Cefazolin Dose		
Patient Weight, kg	Cefazolin Dose, mg (20 mg/kg rounded to the nearest 500mg)	Cefazolin Dilution Amount Required, vials (cefazolin 1000mg/10mL sterile water))
≤ 60	1500	1.5
> 60	2000 (maximum recommended dose)	2

Notes

- Draw vancomycin levels before each dialysis session
- If level is > 19 mg/L, hold next vancomycin dose

Alteplase Use in Hemodialysis Central Venous Catheters

Purpose

To use a fibrinolytic agent to restore and maintain patency of occluded hemodialysis (HD) central venous catheters (CVCs). This may involve 1 or both lumens of the CVC.

Policy

1. This procedure may be done on tunneled or nontunnelled CVCs, but only with a physician's order.
2. Strict aseptic technique is to be used when performing this procedure.
3. The reconstituted product must be carefully inspected for particulate matter and not administered if it is present. To minimize risk, a 5-µm filter needle must be used to withdraw the reconstituted product from the vial prior to patient administration.
4. Before alteplase use, the CVC should be thoroughly evaluated to determine other causes of occlusion and/or inability to sustain required flows.
5. Indications of CVC malfunction include:

- Difficulty aspirating and/or infusing
- Inability to maintain a sustained blood flow rate (QB) > 250 mL/min for 2 consecutive HD sessions
- Inability to initiate a QB > 200 mL/min for 1 HD session
- Arterial pressure of ≤ -250 mm Hg and/or venous pressures of ≥ 250 mm Hg
- Line reversal to achieve QB > 250 mL/min

6. All efforts should be made to limit a maximum of 2 doses of alteplase within a 2-week time period and/or a maximum allotment of 4 mg per dialysis session. If this has occurred, the patient's primary nephrologist should be notified and CVC viability should be assessed.

- Note: Alteplase should not be ordered for CVCs that have been placed within 1 week, as problems related to occlusion of CVCs during this period are likely a result of mechanical problem; therefore, line exchange should be considered

7. All patients whose lumens are routinely locked with alteplase (indication for this is rare)

- Will receive 1 mg per lumen of alteplase lock solution
- Will be assessed by the vascular access team and primary nephrologist for other potential alternatives

Points of Emphasis

1. Alteplase contains no antibacterial preservatives and should be reconstituted immediately before use. Reconstituted solution may be used within 24 hours after reconstitution if stored in the refrigerator
2. Relative contraindications to alteplase include:

- Recent (within 2 months) central nervous system surgery or severe trauma
- Known active internal bleeding

3. Lyophilized (not reconstituted) alteplase should be stored at refrigerated temperature
4. No other medications should be added to solutions containing alteplase

Alteplase Use in Hemodialysis Central Venous Catheters (cont'd)

Procedure

1. Evaluate and troubleshoot the patency of the catheter as instructed in the Appendix "Alteplase Algorithm".
2. If indicated, obtain physician's order for alteplase administration, verifying the method of administration.

- 30-minute dwell (for lumen occlusion)
- Intravenous infusion (for sluggish flow)
- Lock

3. Obtain alteplase and reconstitute as follows:
   a. Reconstitute the 2-mg vial of alteplase with 2.2 mL sterile water for injection (result is 1 mg/mL alteplase)
   b. Inject the sterile water into the 2-mg alteplase vial, directing the diluent stream into the powder. Slight foaming may occur; allow the vial to stand undisturbed until large bubbles have dissipated
   c. Mix by gently swirling the vial until the contents are completely dissolved. DO NOT SHAKE
   d. Inspect the product for foreign matter and discoloration. The reconstituted 2 mg alteplase preparation should appear as a colorless to pale yellow transparent solution
4. Explain the procedure to the patient. Obtain baseline vital sign measurements and document them in the patient chart.
5. Instill the alteplase solution as follows:

Equipment

- On/off supplies
- 3-mL syringes
- 10-mL prefilled normal saline (0.9%) syringes
- Blunt fill needles
- Gauze (4 × 4)
- Two 5-μm filter needles
- Alteplase 2-mg vial
- Sterile water for injection
- Labels for syringes

Alteplase Use in Hemodialysis Central Venous Catheters (cont'd)

30-minute dwell

a. Note: If resistance is felt at any time, use a gentle push/pull motion to instill the lumen. Never use excessive force

b. Using a 5-μm filter needle, withdraw 1 mL reconstituted alteplase (1 mg) into 2 separate 3-mL syringes. Apply alteplase labels to the syringes

c. Using 2 additional 3-mL syringes, withdraw normal saline solution equal to the remaining volume of each lumen plus 0.9 mL (used to advance alteplase)

d. Instill 1-mL alteplase solution (1 mg) into each lumen

e. Instill normal saline equal to the volume of each lumen, then advance alteplase by 0.3 mL (0.6 mL will be left in each syringe)

f. Clamp lumens, leaving syringes attached. Wait 10 minutes

g. Advance alteplase by 0.3 mL using saline solution (0.3 mL will be left in each syringe)

h. Clamp lumens and leave syringes attached. Wait 10 minutes

i. Advance alteplase using the last 0.3 mL of saline. Clamp lumen. Wait 10 minutes

j. Use prefilled 10-mL normal saline syringes to briskly flush and aspirate each lumen to assess function

k. If unable to flush or withdraw alteplase, attempt to reposition the patient and ensure the catheter is not kinked. Attempt again to flush with 10 mL normal saline

Bibliography

Allon M. Current management of vascular access. Clin J Am Soc Nephrol. 2007;2:786-800.

BC Renal Agency. Vascular Access Guideline. Alteplase use for occluded hemodialysis catheters. Updated March 4, 2011. Available at: www.bcrenalagency.ca/sites/default/files/documents/files/Use-of-Alteplase-FINAL-March-4-2011.pdf. Accessed June 9, 2014.

Beathard GA. Catheter thrombosis. Semin Dial. 2001;14:441-445.

Cathflo® Activase® (alteplase) [package insert]. South San Francisco, CA: Genentech, Inc; 2005.

Daugirdas JT, Blake PG, Ing TS. Handbook of Dialysis, Volume 236. 4th ed. Philadelphia, PA: Lippincott Williams and Wilkins; 2007.

Deitcher SR, Fesen MR, Kiproff PM, et al. Safety and efficacy of alteplase for restoring function of occluded central venous catheters: results of the cardiovascular thrombolytic to open occluded lines trial. J Clin Oncol. 2002;20:317-324.

Dinwiddie LC. Managing catheter dysfunction for better patient outcomes. Nephrol Nurs J. 2006;31:653-660, 671.

Jindal K, Chan CT, Deziel C, et al. Hemodialysis clinical practice guidelines for the Canadian Society of Nephrology. J Am Soc Nephrol. 2006;17(Suppl 1):S4-27.

National Kidney Foundation. KDOQI Clinical Practice Guidelines for Vascular Access, Update 2006. Available at: http://www2.kidney.org/professionals/KDOQI/guideline_upHD_PD_VA/. Accessed June 06, 2014.

Alteplase Use in Hemodialysis Central Venous Catheters (cont'd)

Intravenous infusion

a. Use a 5-µm needle to withdraw 2 mL reconstituted alteplase (2 mg) into a 3-mL syringe

b. Add 2 mg alteplase to a 50-mL minibag of 0.9% normal saline solution

c. Attach minibag to the infusion pump, and then to the venous chamber of the blood line

d. Infuse alteplase over 1 hour (rate of 50 mL/h) as follows:

- With the CVC lumens in the "reverse" position for the first 30 minutes
- With the CVC lumens in the "normal" position for the last 30 minutes. If unable to infuse in the "normal" position, administer the last 30 minutes in the "reverse" position

Alteplase lock

a. Use a 5-µm needle to withdraw 1 mL reconstituted alteplase (1 mg) into 2 separate 3-mL syringes

b. Using 2 additional 3-mL syringes, withdraw normal saline equal to the remaining volume of the lumen plus 0.2 mL each (used to advance alteplase)

c. Instill alteplase 1 mL (1 mg) into each lumen

d. Instill normal saline equal to the remaining volume of each lumen, then advance alteplase by 0.2 mL

e. Clamp lumen, apply injection clamps, and apply alteplase labels to the lumens

f. Allow alteplase to dwell in the lumens until the next HD treatment

6. If catheter is patent, commence dialysis and administer heparin as prescribed.
7. If catheter is patent and the heparin lock solution has been flushed through the catheter, commence dialysis but do not administer heparin bolus as prescribed.
8. If the alteplase procedure (30-minute dwell or infusion) was performed at the end of dialysis or on a nondialysis day, flush the lumens with 10 mL 0.9% saline and lock with anticoagulant.

Bibliography (cont'd)

Ponec D, Irwin D, Haire WD, et al. Recombinant tissue plasminogen activator (alteplase) for restoration of flow in occluded central venous access devices: a double-blind placebo-controlled trial–the Cardiovascular Thrombolytic to Open Occluded Lines (COOL) efficacy trial. J Vasc Interv Radiol. 2001;12:951-955.

Protocol adapted with permission from Southern Alberta Renal Program, Alberta, Canada.

Appendix

Alteplase Algorithm

CVC Troubleshooting Performed with No Success

Lumens occluded

- ☐ Inability to aspirate and flush lumens

CVC lumens sluggish

- ☐ Inability to maintain a blood flow >250 mL/min, and/or
- ☐ High venous and low arterial pressure, and/or
- ☐ CVC lumen can be flushed but not aspirated

- ☐ Patient has received ≥ 2 doses of alteplase in a 2-week time period
- ☐ Patient has already received maximum allotment of 4mg alteplase during this treatment
- ☐ CVC was placed < 1 week ago

Yes to any

- ☐ Call physician for possible line exchange and inform vascular access team

No to all

- ☐ Lumen remains occluded

Call physician for alteplase **30 minute dwell**

Instill alteplase 1mg into lumen (procedural statement 5a)

- ☐ Blood flow < 200 mL/min, or
- ☐ Inability to maintain blood flow > 250 mL/min for 2 consecutive HD sessions

Call physician for alteplase **infusion**

Initiate alteplase infusion 2mg/50 mL (procedural statement 5b)

Resume dialysis and slowly attempt to maximize pump speed

If unsuccessful, flush lumens using a brisk motion

Note: when flushing the CVC, watch the point where the catheter is attached to the hub. If ballooning occurs at this point of the catheter, stop the flush. Ballooning indicates too much pressure is being exerted and may cause catheter rupture.

If catheter is occluded, <u>do not flush</u>
Determine which lumen aspirates/flushes easiest and select this lumen to flush

- ☐ Briskly flush the lumen with 5-10 prefilled syringes, sequentially and without aspirating between flushes
- ☐ Attempt to aspirate, giving 2-3 brisk flushes/aspirations/flushes with the blood that has been aspirated

Resume dialysis and slowly attempt to maximize pump speed

Target weight loss may need to be adjusted to reflect the normal saline flush amount

If unsuccessful, notify vascular access experts and/or the physician for consultation and consideration of line exchange

Note: If unsuccessful, alteplase may be repeated once (maximum 4 mg/day)

8 Home Hemodialysis: Infrastructure, Water, and Machines in the Home

John W M Agar, MBBS, FRACP, FRCP[1]

Anthony Perkins, RN[1]

James G Heaf, MD, DMSc[2]

[1]Renal Unit, University Hospital, Barwon Health, Geelong, Victoria, Australia; [2]Herlev Hospital, Copenhagen University Hospital, Herlev Ringvej, Denmark

Implementing Hemodialysis in the Home
A Global Perspective

ISHD
International Society for Hemodialysis

CONTENTS

Abstract

We describe the infrastructure that is necessary for hemodialysis (HD) in the home, focusing on physical requirements, the organization of plumbing and water, and the key features that should guide the selection of machines that are suitable for home use.

Introduction

Hemodialysis (HD) in the home requires specific physical infrastructure, careful organization of plumbing and water, and thoughtful selection of machines that meet the requirements of the patient and his or her environment.

Infrastructure

Technical Requirements Necessary for a Dwelling to be Adapted for Home Hemodialysis

There are few dwellings that cannot be adapted for home HD; however, minimum technical requirements must be met. A checklist of infrastructural considerations for home HD can be found in Appendix 1.

Legal and Financial Requirements

There should be no legal restrictions (either central or local government) concerning the use of the dwelling for home HD. There are multiple different financial responsibilities in home HD, and these should be transparent among stakeholders, and formalized through binding agreements (Table 1).

Building Prerequisites

A sound structure is necessary, which should not be affected by dampness, mold, or excessive environmental pollution.

Electricity Supply

The dwelling must have an appropriate electricity supply to accommodate HD. The supply should be compatible with all equipment, as recommended by the manufacturer, and compliant with local regulations (eg, separate circuit requirements, grounding, trip protection). A stable electricity supply is required, usually via the main power source to the dwelling. Supplemental renewable power supplies, such as solar or wind, can also be considered. If it is likely that there will be frequent power failures, the best option is uninterrupted power supply battery backup, which will bridge the power failure until emergency rinse-back or disconnect procedures can be completed. Some HD machines have built-in battery capacity, and most provide a manual wind-back function. Another

Table 1. Potential Legal Concerns to Address when Starting Home HD

Issue	Stakeholders
Binding agreements between major stakeholders to establish financial responsibilities (unless mandated by law)	• Patient • Provider (hospital and/or dialysis center) • Dialysis machine supplier • Local government authority • Landlord • Tax authorities (some expenses may be deductible)
Compliance with regulations concerning use of land and dwelling, water supply, plumbing, electricity supply, and fluid and solid waste disposal	• Provider (hospital and/or dialysis center) • Government authorities • Landlord
Compliance with regulations concerning medical responsibility for treatment in the home, and delegation of medical responsibility to the patient	• Provider (hospital and/or dialysis center) • Government authorities

option is a stand-by generator installed at the dwelling with associated control equipment, although this is more costly and complicated. For more information on power outages, see the following:

- Home Dialysis Central, "Disaster Planning for PD and Home HD" (for patients)
- "NxStage Home Hemodialysis Patient, Planning Guidebook for Non-Medical Emergencies"
- Disaster planning discussion in "The Home Hemodialysis Hub: Physical Infrastructure and Integrated Governance Structure" module

Water Supply

The dwelling must have sufficient water supply for HD. In most cases, the feed water for dialysis is sourced from a municipal water supply; occasionally, it is sourced from an alternative supply (eg, tank, bore, or well). Water consumption varies from 500 mL/min to 1500 mL/min, depending on flow rate of dialysate and the percentage of water rejected during the reverse osmosis (RO) process.

In most cases, RO machines require a certain level of water pressure to function. Inadequate water pressure can occur for several reasons. Occasionally, the pressure from water mains is inherently unsatisfactory. In other cases, the HD site may be located above ground floor in a high-rise building, thereby reducing supply pressure. Occasionally, there is transient decrease in pressure when other water-consuming equipment in the house is used (flushing a toilet, running a dishwasher, etc). In these situations, the easiest solution is to install a booster pump on the feed water line. This is seldom necessary for ground floor dwelling installations (~5% of installations), but not uncommon for installations in high-rise buildings. Another option is to install a header tank at the dwelling, although this is more costly and complicated. If transient decreases in water pressure are unavoidable and troublesome, consideration can be given to a "flow-fed" rather than "pressure-fed" RO unit; flow-fed RO units have, in effect, a built-in miniaturized header tank, which allows for about approximately 60 seconds of reduced supply before inadequate pressure results in RO malfunction.

Water temperatures across the globe are variable and it may be necessary to cool or heat the feed water. Water temperature issues can make RO units inefficient and sometimes inoperative, so it is important to address water temperature problems when planning for home HD. Where the feed water is too cold, it can be heated by mixing hot and cold water with a thermostatic mixing valve. Where it is too hot, it can be cooled through the use of a heat exchanger.

Plumbing Requirements

Reject water from the RO unit is usually disposed of via the dwelling's storm-water drainage system, although reject water can be redirected back to the RO unit for further generation of permeate in areas where there are severe water shortages. Rather than disposing of reject water, strong consideration should be given to its collection and domestic reuse. Reject water is usually potable, but slightly salty, which limits it for some uses. Notwithstanding, there is abundant experience of reject water reuse as high-grade "gray water" for gardening and horticulture, watering of livestock and agriculture, showering, laundry, general cleaning, toilet flushing, etc.[1] For more information, see The Geelong Experiment, available here.

The dwelling will need to have options for environmentally sound disposal of dialysate effluent, which is usually managed through sewerage systems or septic tanks. The use of septic tanks for drainage of dialysate effluent is, to some degree, a matter of local customary practice and experience. Large volumes of effluent may result in a requirement for emptying of the tank at an unsustainable frequency. Of note, septic tanks are not usually used to collect RO reject water, which will dilute the natural microorganisms in the tank that are required to break down sewerage. Theoretically, such dilution can also occur if the volume of dialysate effluent is very large, as might be the case for a patient on nocturnal or daily HD. Another consideration is the disinfection method used for the dialysis machine. If chemicals are used (eg, bleach), the dialysate effluent will be bactericidal and may drastically reduce the microorganism count in the septic tank. These variations in circumstances lead to corresponding variations in practice. For example, as a generalization, dialysate effluent is not usually drained to the septic tank in Australia, whereas it is in New Zealand.

The disposal of waste into municipal storm water or sewerage systems usually requires a tundish (Figure 1), which is a standard plumbing fitting that provides a point of physical separation ("air break") between a machine and/or patient and municipal drains. This prevents the accidental back-siphoning of drain waste into dialysis machinery, which can occur with cyclical changes in pressure in directly connected drain lines.

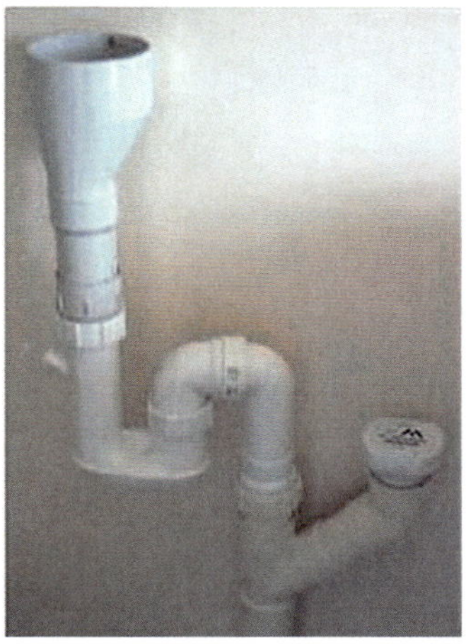

Figure 1. Tundish (photo courtesy of John Agar).

In most locations, a device to prevent back-flow from the intake of the RO unit into the municipal potable water supply is required. This device is called a back-flow preventer and it functions as a one-way valve on the feed water line. Back-flow preventers are installed to eliminate the potential risk of back-pressure forcing contaminants (eg, bleach) from the dialysate circuit into potable water piping. The device is not merely a check valve, but a complex and expensive technical assembly involving test cocks and shut-off valves. The back-flow preventer requires careful installation and regular calibration. For dialysis facilities, these devices are mandatory. For home HD, the consequences of back-flow are somewhat mitigated by the more prevalent use of heat disinfection rather than chemical disinfection. Some countries do not require installation of a back-flow preventer, although it is still the default practice and recommended in a guideline established by the International Organization for Standardization (ISO) 23500:2014.[2]

Plumbing requirements are complex, and the plumber used for installations should be familiar with dialysis systems. The plumbing should be nontoxic with an internally smooth surfaces (with no grooves or sharp corners) and no dead space. In addition, unattractive and circuitous plumbing is unacceptable, and the layout should as aesthetically pleasing and as efficient as possible.

Plumbing services are usually provided to patients in 2 main ways: via an independent commercial provider whose services have been contracted by the patient, or plumbing professionals who have been contracted through the patient's dialysis provider. In both cases, it is important to ensure reliable, expert service from the vendor. Table 2 contains a checklist of plumbing questions that should be considered before beginning home HD.

Solid Waste Disposal

HD produces large amounts of waste, primarily plastic products, and those that have had blood contact (dialyzer, lines, etc) are considered biohazardous. The dwelling is usually required to have an extra waste bin exclusively for dialysis-generated wastes, which should be secured but accessible for pick-up and disposal. All sharps waste should be collected in dedicated containers; disposal arrangements and costs are usually the responsibility of the caring home HD program. For other solid waste, options will vary depending on local regulations. For some, dialysis solid waste can be double bagged and thrown in the regular household garbage. For others, local authorities require extra payment for medical waste disposal. Home HD programs should understand local regulations around storage and disposal of medical (and particularly biohazardous) waste and the recycling of plastics.

Communication

The dwelling must have options for adequate communication, and at a minimum should have access to a fixed or cellular telephone network, and ideally connection to the Internet as well.

Table 2. Necessary Plumbing Questions Checklist

Questions	Done/Not Done
Is the chosen site accessible to plumbing? • Site assessment • By whom?	 ☐ ☐
What are the requirements for dialysate effluent and reverse osmosis reject water drainage? • Sewer • Septic tank	 ☐ ☐
What external/internal connections are required? • List of required connections (eg, tundish, back-flow preventer)	 ☐
Is the installation on the ground floor or on a higher floor? • Ground • Second floor or higher	 ☐ ☐
If elevated (second floor or above), consider water pressure and the requirement for: • Pump system • Header tank • Additional plumbing complexity and cost	 ☐ ☐ ☐

Infrastructure in Community House vs Home Hemodialysis

Two options may be available to patients desiring to undergo independent HD. HD can be performed in either an unstaffed community-based setting ("community house" HD) or in a residential dwelling (home HD). A community house setting is not as common, so it will be discussed only briefly here.

Community house HD is performed in a home-like setting that is adapted from a previous residential dwelling or dialysis facility.[3-6] The community house is shared by a group of patients who come and go as they choose and are responsible for their own HD, just as they would if they were performing home HD. Each patient has a space with a machine bay and other dialysis equipment and consumables. A key requirement for successful operation of community house HD is the ability to create a home-like, noninstitutional atmosphere with flexible scheduling that is comparable to home HD. For those patients who dialyze 5 or more times per week at a community HD location, it is best that they have their own dedicated machine and space, while those who dialyze 3 times per week or perform alternate-day HD can usually share a machine. The home HD program is responsible for the infrastructure of the HD system and maintenance of the equipment in the community house. Patients using the community house for HD have their own secure access, as do maintenance and professional staff from the caring dialysis center.

The technical details of HD are common to both the community house and home HD, although community house HD requires consideration of the following issues related to infrastructure and processes within the house:

- Demarcation of operational tasks. There should be clear agreement by all participating patients that define responsibility for specific tasks. This process is usually implemented through "community house rules" and "patient contracts"; these responsibilities include:
  - » Cleaning of the house: Performed by either participating patients themselves or by a contracted cleaning staff
  - » Care of machinery: Patients should leave machines in a suitable condition for the next user. The caring center is responsible for technical machine maintenance
  - » Patient rostering: Performed by internal agreement among patients
  - » Communication arrangements for both routine and emergency situations:
    - – At a minimum, a landline telephone is required
    - – Explicit and agreed to arrangements should exist so that patients know who, how, when, and where to call in the case of clinical, technical, or emergency problems, or when there are concerns about the building or the machines
- Financial and legal responsibilities: Home HD programs will need to give consideration to the payment and/or provision of the following services for an affiliated community house:
  - » Insurance of the building and contents
  - » Building rent and taxes
  - » Building maintenance
  - » Property security
  - » Supply and payment of electricity, water, and other utilities

Although content can often be applied to community house HD, the remainder of this module is concerned with HD performed in the patient's personal residence.

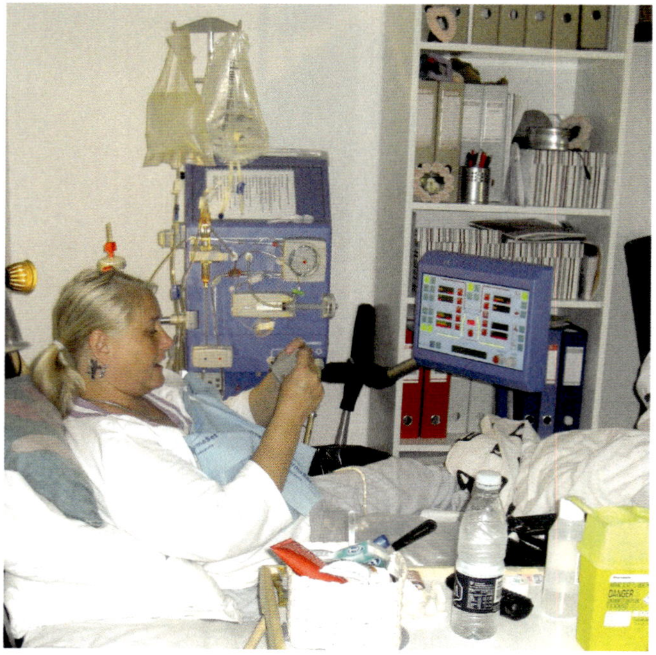

Figure 2. The dialysis room. The dialysis room should feel like "home" (photo courtesy of James Heaf).

The Dialysis Room

The room chosen for HD should be functional and conducive to safe and convenient home HD (Figure 2). The room should also be comfortable and allow for the room's other social requirements (eg, family activities). Safety should also be a prominent consideration in all decisions around infrastructure and machinery choice and placement. The room should have or offer the following:

- Adequate lighting (ie, 900 lumens)
- A low humidity and comfortable temperature
- No overt safety risks or hygiene hazards (eg, no open fireplace, drafts, frequent through traffic, clutter), with restricted access to small children and pets during HD
- Surfaces and furnishings that are easy to clean. Curtains and carpets are generally undesirable and, if possible, should be replaced with wet-wipe surfaces (plastic/synthetic blinds, tiles, linoleum, hard flooring)
- In-room telephone access
- Easy access to washbasins, which ideally should have hands-free elbow taps or an automatic sensor system for turning water on and off

Safety

Safety should be a prominent consideration in decisions regarding infrastructure and choice of HD machines for the home.

Exsanguination

Exsanguination is a rare complication of home HD and has the potential to be life-threatening. Full discussion of prevention and management of this and other complications is provided in the "Ensuring Patient Safety During Home Hemodialysis" module, although the following points are relevant to a discussion of infrastructure and machinery for home HD:

- All dialysis machines should be equipped with monitors for exact measurement of venous and arterial pressure, which should be set to appropriately narrow alarm bands. Importantly, there are limitations of pressure-based safety systems to detect line separation. The core methods to guard against that hazard involve adherence to standard operating procedures on securing and taping of needles, closed connector devices for tubing connections, and wetness detectors to detect blood and dialysate leaks (see "The Care and Keeping of Vascular Access for Home Hemodialysis Patients" module)
- Real-time monitoring of home HD treatments has been provided by some centers in the past, but is not generally recommended[7]
- An automatic alarm ("panic button/alarm") to contact the local paramedic unit may be an appropriate option available for some patients

Intradialytic Hypotension

Intradialytic hypotension (IDH) is a common complication which, in extreme situations, can lead to loss of consciousness and serious consequences. In the home setting, the absence of onsite staff makes IDH a potentially more sustained and therefore threatening event. To help prevent and mitigate IDH, each dialysis treatment should be arranged to permit rapid administration of therapy (eg, intravenous [IV] fluid administration and reduction in blood flow and ultrafiltration rate). Also, patient seating should permit rapid adjustment to a supine position.

Intravenous Drugs

Treating clinicians are responsible for prescribing IV therapy in the home. Secure (and sometime refrigerated) storage is required for such medications. Some drugs have the potential to cause anaphylaxis; therefore, patients should have their first administration of these drugs performed in the dialysis center to ensure that no problems will occur with the prescription.

The following drugs are typically *not* problematic:

- Erythropoietin-stimulating agents
- Vitamin D analogues
- Albumin

Machinery Breakdowns

The most common malfunctions leading to machine shutdown include power failure and interruptions in water supply. If a shutdown does occur, a patient should terminate his or her dialysis session and as soon as possible contact the dialysis center for service.

Configuration of the HD Space

The location and configuration of the home HD space will be determined by the size of machinery and the available space in the home. In some home HD programs, a choice of different HD machines with different size specifications is available. In most programs, choice is limited. The size of the available dialysis machine will often dictate where the home HD space will be located within the home.

Water Treatment Units

Water treatment units do not require a large amount of space. In choosing and situating these types of units, the following are important considerations:

- Noise and vibration
- Adequate servicing access
- Leakage protection with wet-resistant flooring
- Adequate drainage access

For systems using home dialysate batch generation, the size of the dialysate bath should also be included in the space calculation. At present, the only available batch dialysate home HD machine has a unit that contains 60 L of dialysate (see section on "Low-flow Systems").

Storage

Patients need a cupboard or a closet for storing dialysis equipment (scales, tubing, needles, plaster, filters, etc), with additional space for their dialysis machines, should they choose to store it as well (Figure 3). Depending on the logistics of the dialysis program and the type of dialysis being performed, a single cupboard or closet may not be adequate for supply storage and this should be carefully assessed.

Placement and Location of Dialysis Machinery and Peripherals

Choosing the appropriate location for the dialysis machine within the residence is a key issue. Substantial dwelling alterations are sometimes required to accommodate machinery. Before home modifications are made, there should be a clear agreement between parties (preferably based on a unit policy) about who is financially responsible for making the required alterations.

There are several factors and requirements that may be relevant to machine placement. Some questions patients may wish to consider include the following:

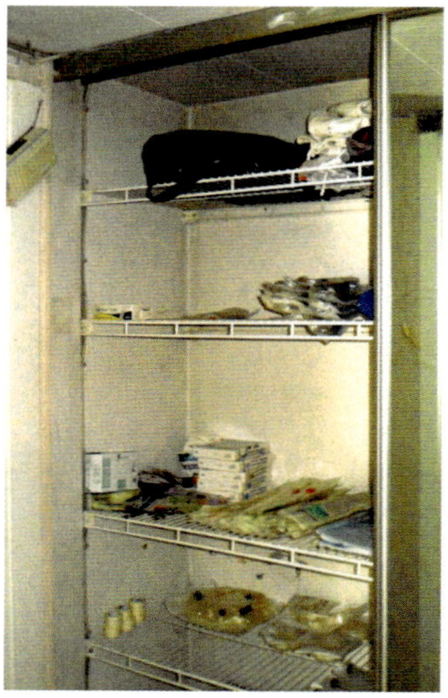

Figure 3. Home HD storage (photo courtesy of James Heaf).

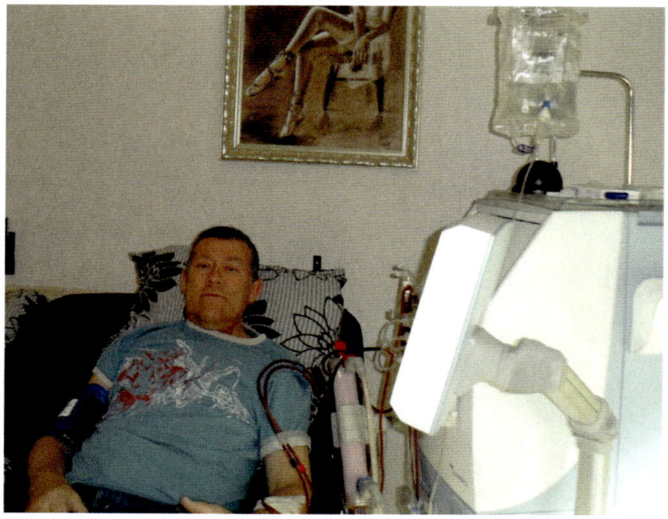

Figure 4. Placement of the home HD machine. This patient initially chose the living room, but changed his mind because the armrest on his sofa was too wide (photo courtesy of James Heaf).

- Where is the best place to perform dialysis?
  - » The bedroom is the only option for patients who choose nocturnal HD. Despite this, some patients choose to sleep in reclining chairs due to fear of moving too much while asleep and disconnecting needles (Figure 4)
  - » Patients who choose HD during daytime hours can perform dialysis in the bedroom or another dedicated space within the home
  - » Many patients find HD equipment unattractive and clinically sterile looking, and will therefore prefer to keep their HD equipment out of view
  - » The HD machine should be placed close to the patient and oriented to permit ease of adjustment. Some machines have mobile control panels that provide more flexibility
  - » The HD machine needs to be close to a water supply and drains, and the room must be able to accommodate extra plumbing, if required
- What if I want to perform dialysis privately or in the same room with family members present?
  - » If the patient prefers more social dialysis, the living area is best; however, machine placement is an issue, and there should be consensus within the family on placement
  - » If a patient prefers private dialysis, the machine should be placed in the bedroom or a spare room
- What do I want to do while performing dialysis?
  - » For example, watch television, perform work, talk on the phone, use a computer
  - » Patients with flexible access to telephone and Internet (eg, Wi-Fi) will have an increased choice of placement

No matter where a patient chooses to perform dialysis, access to a landline or cellular telephone is mandatory.

Multiple Placements

Patients who have the larger, more static HD machines may be limited in terms of options for machine placement. However, this is not necessarily true for those patients who use mobile batch dialysis equipment (eg, NxStage). Because these units are considered portable, they can be more easily moved from one location to another, as long as the appropriate outlets and peripheral equipment are in place in the dialysis area. Patients using the portable equipment are able to dialyze in various rooms throughout a house. In addition, patients with the more portable units are able to dialyze at a second dwelling (eg, a weekend cottage or vacation home) or in a travel caravan (recreational vehicle). It is very important to note that each location requires a separate plumbing, drainage, and electrical installation, which can result in added setup costs. It is also important to remember that water supplies that are not used frequently may lead to water stasis, which, in turn, could result in potential water contamination. This fact must be taken into consideration when planning for dialysis at weekend cottages or vacation homes. Each manufacturer will have special protocols required for water flushing and water connection if a water treatment system has not been used recently.

Convenience

Lighting

In addition to room lighting, a reading light is desirable. A back-lit magnifier can be considered for needle insertion, if appropriate.

Seat/Bed

For nocturnal HD, there are few requirements for the bed used. If the patient wishes to use the bed for HD during the day, a bed with an independent head adjustment can be considered.

Seating requirements for dialysis are more rigorous. A dedicated dialysis chair should be provided. It should be comfortable, easy to clean (ie, vinyl or leather, rather than fabric), and have arm rests and an adjustable back rest. The patient must be able to assume a supine position quickly and without effort if symptomatic hypotension occurs. If possible, consider letting the patient choose his or her own chair.

Noise

Dialysis is generally a quiet process; however, excessive noise can be a problem and a major disincentive to home HD. Noise is a particular issue for patients performing nocturnal HD and for their partners who share the bedroom in the dwelling.

The RO unit usually generates most of the noise that does occur. If the noise is bothersome, one easy solution is to install the RO unit in an adjacent and separate room, and run plumbing through the intervening wall. Alternatively, a purpose-built, insulated cover box for the RO system is an option if it must be located in the same room as the patient and machine. HD machinery with squeaky pumps or other moving parts may also be sources of excess noise. It is important to ensure that all moving parts on the machine are as silent as possible.

Hygiene

A clean environment is necessary to prevent infectious complications associated with home HD. Two problems need to be addressed:

- Home structure and configuration
- Patient and family adherence to standard hygiene procedures

Staff need to be satisfied that both of these elements are satisfactory before home dialysis is allowed.

Patient and Family Requirements

The following applies primarily to the patient, but family members living in the same dwelling should be advised to follow the same hygienic rules, particularly if they help with the dialysis process.

- The home and the dialysis room should be kept clean and dry. Vacuum cleaning and cleaning of all surfaces should be performed regularly. Textiles and upholstered furniture that remain in the room should be deep-cleaned frequently
- Dirty clothing during dialysis should be avoided by both patient and care partner
- The patient and care partner should always practice good hand hygiene when performing any dialysis-related procedures. The value of both soap and chlorhexidine or alcohol washing should be emphasized
- Small children and pets pose a safety and hygiene risk for dialysis. In general, pets should not be present during dialysis. Until it can be established through supervised visits that a pet will not chew, pull, or bat at the dialysis lines, it is recommend

to keep pets out of the dialysis room. Even if a pet proves well behaved enough to be present during treatment, it is best to keep it out of the room during cannulation

Environment

The environmental impact of a home HD program should be assessed. A particular area of concern is electricity and water consumption.[8] Strong consideration ought to be given to:

- Reject water reuse[9]
- "Green" energy, such as solar, wind, etc[10]

Responsibility

Ultimately, the home HD program or provider is held accountable for clinical outcomes within the service; however, the provision and undertaking of home HD involves a division and sometimes sharing of responsibilities between the patient and program. It is vital that patients and their care partners understand the responsibilities that are assigned to them, as opposed to those responsibilities that fall under the purview of the home HD program. There should be no ambiguity, and agreement between the 2 parties should be formally documented through either patient contracts, or embedded in unit policies and procedures. These documents should be written in simple, easy-to-understand, nontechnical language so that they are accessible and useful to patients.

Responsibilities should be clear from the time of the initial home feasibility study and site evaluation. Patients and their care partners should understand whether they have a choice of machine and other equipment, and whether they are responsible for any of the costs or processes involved with building renovations and/or installation. There should be clear understanding and agreement around use and ownership of dialysis machinery, communication and monitoring equipment, and home storage modifications and infrastructure.

In most instances, the program is responsible for home HD equipment costs, although some costs may fall to the patient, depending on the country in question and, occasionally, personal factors. The following factors will affect equipment and financial responsibilities:

- Local, regional, national subsidy schemes
- Public or private insurance arrangements
- Patient preference for a system that is not offered, and whether the patient has the means to pay for or contribute to home care

Communication and monitoring equipment can include home landline or cellular telephone and information technology systems and hardware (eg, email, fax, modem, Wi-Fi). These may be the responsibility of the patient, home HD program, or both. If this equipment is provided, there should be clear understanding of ownership and agreement on appropriate use. Often, shelving and storage facilities are part of the installation for home HD, and the patient and program should be clear about who "owns" these modifications, who is responsible for their maintenance and repair, how maintenance and repairs should be handled, and who is responsible for removing and/or restoring these home modifications to predialysis status should the patient move or no longer require home HD.

There are numerous responsibilities related to HD machine support and troubleshooting, and maintenance of the supply chain. Patient contracts or unit policies and procedures should clearly define which responsibilities accrue to the patient, the home HD program, and the manufacturer. In general, the costs of HD machine support and troubleshooting will not be borne by the patient; however, the patient and his or her care partner have responsibility for the timely communication of equipment issues, general care and cleaning of the machine's external surfaces, and performance of some routine maintenance procedures. It is vital to establish what is expected from whom, how, and when.

- Who is responsible for communication of equipment issues, and to whom?
- What is the contractual responsibility of the manufacturer with the program/provider?
  - » Equipment updates
  - » Timely advice regarding equipment issues
- Who is responsible for maintenance of supply chain for consumables and stock control in the home?

Water

Water can contain many different natural and artificial contaminants that can be harmful to humans. The intake of water for a healthy individual is estimated at approximately 2 L per day (14 L/week). An HD patient is exposed to around 360 to 580 L of water per week (depending on dialysate flow rates, dialysis duration, and dialysis frequency), and this water is separated from blood only by a thin, semipermeable membrane. Ensuring that water used in the HD process is of excellent quality is important to reduce the risk of patient exposure to harmful contaminants.

Home HD patients will often be exposed to more water than those patients undergoing conventional dialysis, because they typically dialyze longer and more frequently. As a result, home HD patients depend even more on having excellent water quality. The importance of water quality in HD, regardless of modality, therefore, requires a number of essential water-treatment processes to ensure patient protection by the removal of all contaminants. Because water is an integral part of the HD process and requires frequent review, maintenance, and surveillance, a number of guidelines have been developed to ensure that the water used in the HD process meets best practice standards. ISO guidelines for hemodialysis water quality and treatment can be purchased here. Relevant guidelines include the following:

- ISO 11663:2014, "Quality of dialysis fluid for haemodialysis and related therapies". Available here.
- ISO 13958:2014, "Concentrates for haemodialysis and related therapies". Available here.
- ISO 13959:2014, "Water for haemodialysis and related therapies". Available here.
- ISO 23500:2014, "Guidance for the preparation and quality management of fluids for haemodialysis and related therapies". Available here.
- ISO 26722:2014, "Water treatment equipment for haemodialysis applications and related therapies". Available here.

Feed Water

Apart from municipal water, feed water can be sourced from a variety of different places, such as rivers, streams, dams, bores, and wells. Some systems like the NxStage (see the section on "Low-flow Systems") have the option of using batch dialysate provided by the manufacturer. In this case, the responsibility for water quality lies with the manufacturer. In all other cases, batch or single-pass dialysate preparation requires water that is subjected to properly designed and maintained water treatment systems, such that it meets appropriate chemical and microbiological standards for purity (Figure 5).

Feed water should meet ISO 13959:2014 ("Water for haemodialysis and related therapies") for maximum allowable levels for certain elements that may be toxic in hemodialysis and those that are normally included in dialysate.[11] ***A full chemical analysis should be performed on any water that is being considered for use in HD.*** This analysis should then be compared with ISO 13959:2014 to ensure safety.

Water Purification Processes

A cascade of processes is required in HD to ensure that water is at a level of purity that is acceptable for use. While not all processes are necessary in all cases, water of lower purity may require additional purification for use in HD (Figure 6). The following equipment and filters may be required to ensure higher water purity:

Water Softeners

- Common purification devices that are used in locations where the local water supply has a high mineral content ("hard water")
- They are a form of deionizer that exchanges calcium and magnesium ions for sodium ions
- Although calcium and magnesium ions are effectively removed by RO, use of a water softener along with the RO unit will protect the RO membranes from calcification by calcium and magnesium salts, thereby reducing system maintenance costs

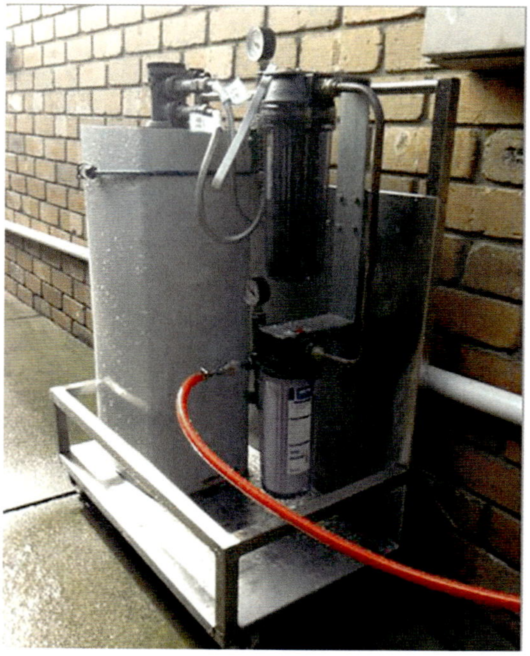
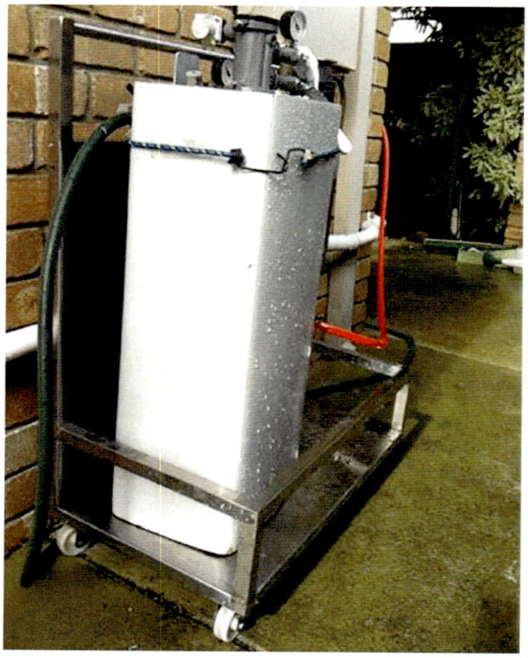
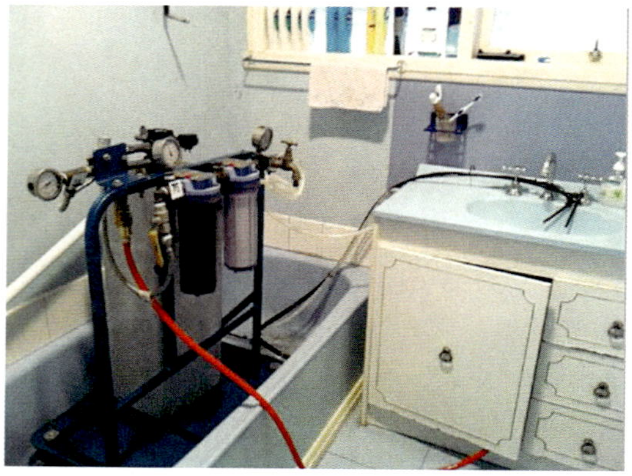

Figure 5. Examples of temporary water configurations. Home HD should not be excluded from those who have rental agreements that prevent permanent installation of fittings and equipment (photos courtesy of Anthony Perkins).

- Water softener tanks have a finite capacity and must be regenerated. Monitoring RO conductivity will indicate when softener tanks should be regenerated
- Water softeners used for HD processes must include a lock-out system to prevent brine from entering the softener's product water stream
- Some jurisdictions do not permit water softeners because of the discharge of salt during regeneration

Activated Carbon

- Activated carbon is the standard method used to remove monochloramine (commonly referred to as chloramine) from water
- Chloramine is toxic. All water treatment systems should include carbon beds, unless it is clear that the water supply is disinfected by a means other than chlorination, such as ozone
- Carbon also provides nonspecific removal of organic contaminants from water
- Carbon beds cannot be regenerated and have a finite capacity for chloramine absorption

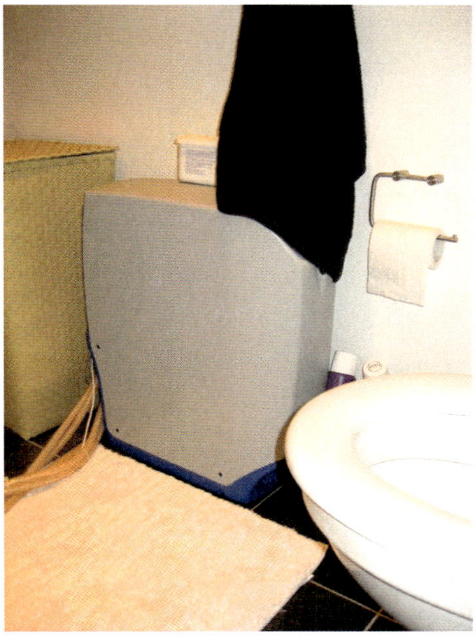

Figure 6. Water purification unit (photo courtesy of James Heaf).

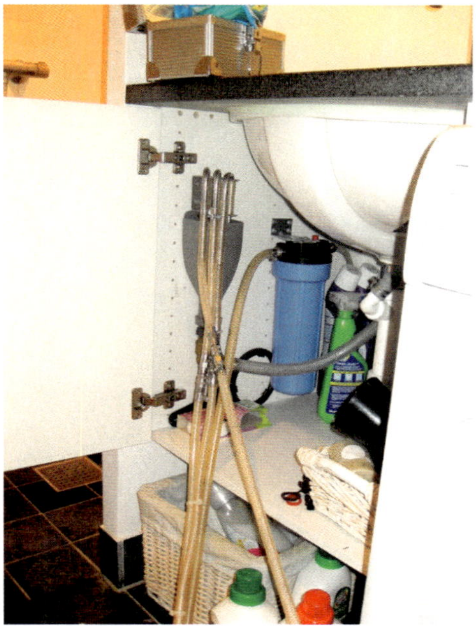

Figure 7. Water filter (photo courtesy of James Heaf).

- To prevent inadvertent exposure of patients to chloramine as the capacity of the carbon is exhausted, 2 carbon beds are installed in series
- Block carbon filters can offer an alternative to conventional granular activated carbon beds when space is limited

Particle Filters

- Particle filters remove coarse particulate matter from the water, and can also remove finer particles from washed out carbon beds (Figure 7). This also helps protect the RO membrane from clogging and fouling

Ultraviolet Irradiation

Ultraviolet (UV) irradiation is a common water purification process for facility-based systems, but is less commonly used in current home-based systems. This method involves a low-pressure mercury vapor lamp enclosed in a quartz sleeve that emits a germicidal 254-nm wavelength and provides a dose of radiant energy of 30 mW • sec/cm^2 to kill bacteria.[11] UV irradiation penetrates bacteria, which alters their DNA such that they are neutralized or unable to replicate. It has also been suggested that UV could be used for dechlorination, as it has been successfully implemented for this purpose in the food and pharmaceutical industry.[12]

- Of note, some bacteria are or can become resistant to UV irradiation, and the presence of biofilm will reduce its effectiveness
- UV irradiation does not destroy endotoxin, and the levels of endotoxin may even increase as a result of the release of bacterial fragments. Therefore, UV irradiation should be followed, at some point, by ultrafiltration
- The UV irradiation device should be sized for the maximum anticipated flow rate according to the manufacturer's instructions
- Regular maintenance of the UV irradiation device includes continuous monitoring of radiant energy output that activates

an audible and visual alarm, routine cleaning of the quartz sleeve, and replacing the lamp at least annually or sooner if recommended by the manufacturer

Reverse Osmosis

- RO is a common, but not mandatory, process used to produce water of quality suitable for HD. RO uses a high transmembrane water pressure gradient to force water across a membrane to create permeate, the product water
- Small and portable RO machines are customary for home installations, where space is at a premium. These machines require a routine maintenance and disinfection program
- Heat disinfection is the best method to prevent the formation of biofilm and keep microorganisms within allowable limits

Deionizers

A secondary purification step after RO may be required where RO alone is not sufficient to provide water of the required quality. A deionizer is a device that can be added to aid in the water purification process.

- Deionizers can produce water of very high purity. They are effective in removing ionic contaminants; however, they do not remove microbiological contaminants. In fact, they provide a good environment for bacterial proliferation and often worsen the microbiological quality of water passing through them
- It is necessary to incorporate bacterial control equipment after the application of a deionizer

Ultrafilters in the Dialysate Pathway

- Work by using adsorption of endotoxin; they have a finite capacity
- These filters are the last line of defense against endotoxin and the potential contamination of the HD machine fluid pathway
- Ultrafilters need regular replacement per manufacturer specifications

Water Quality

ISO has developed easily adaptable guidelines pertinent to HD water quality. Adherence to these guidelines will help in setting up an appropriate water program for home HD.

- Guidelines
  - » ISO 13959:2014, "Water for haemodialysis and related therapies"
  - » ISO 26722:2014, "Water treatment equipment for haemodialysis applications and related therapies"
  - » ISO 23500:2014, "Guidance for the preparation and quality management of fluids for haemodialysis and related therapies"
- Frequency of sampling and testing
  - » Many guidelines recommend monthly testing and sampling of dialysate for microbiological contamination; however, the frequency of testing should be dependent on the quality of feed water. Feed water of poorer quality (eg, from rivers, streams, dams, bores, and wells [public and private]) may need more frequent testing to ensure the best quality of dialysate is produced
  - » Biochemical analysis should also be performed frequently. In most cases, analysis may only need to be performed annually, but in areas where there is poor water quality, or areas where there is a higher usage of chemicals in agriculture, industry, or the environment, more frequent testing will be necessary to ensure a suitable water supply used for dialysis
- Bacteria
  - » The maximum allowable levels are at 100 cfu/mL[11]
  - » Low-nutrient agar (R2A) at room temperature (22°C [71°F]) is the best medium for culturing bacteria
- Endotoxins
  - » The maximum allowable levels are at 0.25 EU/mL[11]

» Endotoxin levels can be tested using the Limulus amebocyte lysate (LAL) test, which can be performed by either the quantitative turbidimetric assay (most sensitive and expensive) or the qualitative gel-clot assay (less sensitive but also less costly). The most common method used in dialysis quality assurance programs is the latter

- Biofilm

    » Bacteria are extremely difficult to remove from a water distribution system once they have had an opportunity to colonize, especially if they form a mature biofilm on the interior surfaces of the water distribution system. To minimize biofilm formation, all water distribution systems should be disinfected on a regular basis using a schedule designed to limit bacterial proliferation, rather than to eliminate bacteria once proliferation has occurred. Regular heat disinfection of the water distribution system is recommended to prevent the formation of biofilm

    - Prevention is better than cure
    - Disinfection with hypochlorous acid/hypochlorite or bleach has been shown to be inadequate for disinfection of fluid pathways to remove biofilm[13]
    - Frequent heat disinfection

- Maintenance

    » Regular maintenance and cleaning processes should be scheduled to prevent contamination of the water pathways within the equipment. Heat disinfections can help prevent the formation of biofilm, but hard-to-reach areas within water equipment needs to be manually cleaned. In some cases, harsh chemicals, such as peracetic acid, need to be used

    » Annual replacement of inflow hoses between the RO unit, HD machine, and dialysate hoses can help prevent the formation of biofilm problem areas

- Relationships

    » Building relationships with microbiology experts goes a long way in setting up appropriate water quality surveillance programs. Good relationships with municipal water providers should also be established

Pure vs Ultrapure

Clinical trial and observational evidence suggest that ultrapure water or dialysate may have beneficial clinical outcomes, particularly in relation to inflammation and the reduction of inflammatory markers in patients exposed to high-quality/ ultrapure water.[14-22] To achieve ultrapure water, stringent considerations need to be adhered to, including:

- Design of the water distribution system to avoid areas of stagnation
- Attention to the preparation of concentrates
- Frequent disinfection of the treated water distribution system and dialysis machines
- Regular surveillance and microbiological analysis of water

Machines

Which Machine Is Most Appropriate?

The choice of machine is commonly the single greatest per-patient capital outlay for home HD. It is also the most problematic to discuss without commercial bias, as this is the chief domain of commercial competition between dialysis equipment providers. Many of the currently available systems have been designed for facility-based dialysis and are over-engineered and unnecessarily complex for home HD. The easier and more intuitive the machine is to operate, the better it will be for a home HD program. However, 1 fact is paramount: *any currently available HD machine is capable of providing home HD. No particular machine is, or should be considered to be, a requisite for good, sustained and effective home hemodialysis.* Thus, the answer to the question "which machine?", the response is "any machine", as long as it meets the patient's specific needs and requirements.

All machines have strengths and weaknesses, whether they are used in facilities or in the home. Key considerations are differences in size, and also differences in the way that dialysate is delivered. Some machines require water treatment systems to generate on-line or batched dialysate, and others come with prepackaged dialysate in bags.

As with the dialysis machines themselves, each of the generative options for creating suitable dialysate has strengths and weaknesses. These include: purity of water, ease of manufacture, availability, handling, and cost. The choice of machine and the fluid delivery pathway will depend on a range of individual factors that will vary between countries, services (and sometimes, within a service), and patients.

Single-pass Systems

Single-pass systems (SPS) have been the HD standard around the world for over 50 years. SPS are well understood and widely used systems, where dialysate is produced within the machine. This production is performed by proportionally mixing a purified water source with a pair of acid and base concentrates, the buffer component of which is now commonly bicarbonate. The reconstituted dialysate is tested for conductivity, which is a check system to ensure correct proportioning, and then is heated, deaerated, and pressurized. The dialysate is then directed as a single-pass, high-flow, pure or ultrapure fluid to the dialyzer for transmembrane contact with the patient's blood. Common examples of SPS for home HD include, but are not limited to, systems manufactured by Baxter, Braun, Fresenius, Gambro, Jihua, Nikkiso, and Nipro.

SPS machines have a number of advantages:

- Physician and nursing dialysis staff everywhere are familiar with operating characteristics of SPS. This also applies to unit technical staff who are familiar with the strip-down and replacement practices required for machine maintenance
- Although SPS machines are complex, most current systems have on-screen instructions for nurses (and, in the situation of home HD, the patients) to follow
- On-screen instructions are commonly matched by a number of fail-safe warning systems to alert the user to any missteps made during the set up process
- SPS systems allow for multiple variations in dialyzer and dialysis fluid parameters, for example, dialyzer surface area, and the sodium concentration of the dialysate
- A wide range of commercially available dialysis fluid concentrates permits individualization of fluid component electrolytes, in particular, potassium and calcium, allowing customization of the dialysis prescription
- The high dialysis fluid-to-blood-flow ratio of SPS machines allows higher clearance rates, particularly for small molecular solutes

SPS systems also have a number of disadvantages:

- SPS machines are often large and heavy. This limits—indeed, effectively prevents—portability and, in addition, introduces a range of occupational health and safety (OH&S) issues. This is particularly pertinent to home HD, where current SPS machines are of such bulk that OH&S rules usually prevent a single technician alone being sent to maintain (and especially move) the system
- Importantly, the maintenance requirements for SPS machines are extensive. The systems are "wet" systems—this means that a fluid circuit exists within the machine. O-rings wear or leak; electrical circuits are exposed to the risk of moisture; and internal dialysis fluid pathways must be sterilized, de-scaled, and decalcified to properly maintain the system
- As equipment failures and maintenance requirements introduce additional cost, most HD services will be well aware that machine maintenance and servicing comprise a significant component, both in time and money, of the provision of their services

Low-flow Systems

The only currently available example of a low-flow system (L-FS) is the NxStage system. This system is currently the most frequently used within the United States, although it is not as widely available or used as frequently outside the United States.

An L-FS machine depends on a quite different clearance concept when compared to SPS systems. In some ways it is more akin to peritoneal dialysis (PD), where dwell time allows a greater equilibration between blood and dialysate across a semipermeable membrane. SPS systems use a dialysate flow to blood flow (Qd:Qb) ratio of 2:1, but the low-flow dialysate rate used by L-FS reverses this ratio, so Qd:Qb is between 1:2 and 1:3. As a result, an L-FS operates at a different site on the diffusion curve, allowing far greater transmembrane dialysis fluid equilibration with blood than occurs in the more rapid pass profile of an SPS. A good peer-reviewed discussion of the principles of L-FS dialysis is given by Kohn et al.[23] Home HD prescriptions using L-FS are discussed in the "Prescriptions for Home Hemodialysis" module. There are 2 current options for the NxStage L-FS:

1. Using dialysis fluid that is bagged in a clear 5-L plastic bag (similar to that provided to patients for PD) and which provides a travel-suitable option
2. Using an on-line dialysis fluid generator (PureFlow™, NxStage Medical, Inc., Lawrence, MA) that provides 60-L batched dialysis fluid that is manufactured on-line by an additional on-line, ultrapure fluid generator. The PureFlow™ is not intended to be a travel-suitable dialysate source, but is intended for a permanent or semipermanent installation.

The NxStage L-FS system has several advantages. All blood and dialysis fluid, dialysate, and wet flow systems are disposable and attached to the external surfaces of the machine such that the machine has no internal wet contact areas, which makes the machine safe from corrosion and its electronic circuitry is protected. The machine weighs 32 kg (71 lb) and is therefore potentially portable. This weight lies within single technician and O&HS handling parameters, which makes servicing simpler and relatively inexpensive. Finally, it uses a preformed plastic cartridge that incorporates all lines, the dialyzer, and fluid pathway ports. The patient need only insert the cartridge into the machine, after which all pathways are opened and engaged automatically.

The NxStage machine also has disadvantages. At 32 kg, the machine still demands significant organization and commitment from patients in terms of planning travel logistics. In addition, patients must travel with or ensure that adequate quantities of dialysate will be available throughout their trip. In addition, only 1 dialyzer option is available in the preformed cartridge, which limits individualization of prescription. Finally, the maximum volume of dialysate that can be used during a single treatment is 60 L. This may be inadequate for some patients with high generation of uremic toxins, without substantial increases in treatment frequency to essentially daily dialysis.

Other Systems

Among many, 4 other home HD systems are in advanced stages of development; however, they are not yet commercially available. These include the Fresenius Portable Artificial Kidney (PAK) (United States), the Baxter Vivia system (United States), the Quanta SC+ System (United Kingdom), and the Physidia home HD/HDF system (France).

- The Fresenius PAK is a sorbent-based system for reprocessing and regenerating dialysis fluid online and during dialysis
  - » Sorbent systems, once commercially competitive in the 1970s and 1980s as the REDY dialysis system, fell from popularity in the 1990s
  - » Many newer dialysis systems in development seeking portability and/or wearability will depend on sorbent dialysis principles
  - » More information on sorbent principles is given by Agar[24]
- The Baxter Vivia machine is an SPS with integrated water treatment that allows multiple uses of its dialyzer and blood sets

- The Quanta SC+ is a small SPS machine that is RO-dependent, but designed to be portable
- The Physidia system will have the capacity to provide either HD or hemodiafiltration (HDF) treatment options, which is in line with the growing European preference for HDF
  - » As HDF is a process that combines diffusive and convective principles and necessitates the reinfusion of 20 to 30 L of water back into the patient, the water that is produced on-line must be ultrapure
  - » While the requirement for ultrapure water has placed potential practical and financial limitations on HDF in the home, HDF has been used successfully for home dialysis in the United Kingdom, Australia, New Zealand, and in Europe

The Concept of Portability

The NxStage system is a portable system and, indeed, many patients travel with it; however, traveling with any current dialysis system available is not easy, nor is it for the uncommitted. The machine remains heavy and cumbersome for travel, and requires 25 to 30 L of bagged dialysate per treatment. While bagged dialysis fluid can be delivered to most regions and sites, multisite delivery for during travel is difficult and costly. Newer dialysis systems based on recirculating sorbent regeneration of dialysis fluid (currently in development) will potentially reduce the total water requirements for dialysis fluid generation to ≥ 6 L of tap water, and may make genuinely portable HD machines a reality in the future.

In some places, "portable" HD is available in the form of fitted mobile vans for hire. In particular, for more than 30 years, New Zealand has offered vacation vans for subsidized public hire that are fitted with dialysis machines and RO systems, which are supported by various New Zealand dialysis services (see this website). However, because the machines that have been fitted and built into the vans may not be familiar to all patients—a patient trained on 1 system may be unable to manage a different, unfamiliar machine or RO system—care must be taken when arranging a van for hire to ensure that the equipment fitted in the van is suitable for the patient-vacationer. Patient-vacationers will also need to ensure that a stable power supply will always be available at their selected destination. Effluent drainage is, by and large, tank-captured for later disposal at a suitable drainage site.

What Machine Features Are the Most Important for Successful Home Dialysis?

The choice of machine should be tailored to meet the individual requirements of the patient and his or her home circumstances, and the capacity of the home HD program to provide support and maintenance.

A key issue determining choice is that of space. Ideally, the home HD machine should take up as little space as possible (Figure 8).

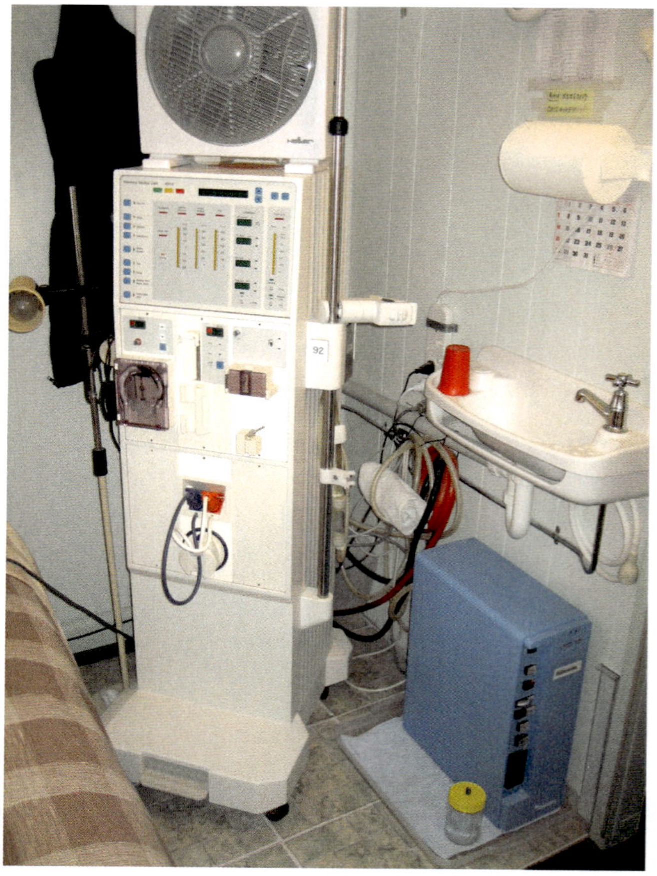

Figure 8. Practical and accessible home HD room (photo courtesy of John Agar).

In general, large machines do not provide sufficient technological superiority to justify their use, but price will ultimately be a deciding factor. Most HD machines have NOT been designed for home installation. In many bedrooms, such as in Europe and Asia, bed-to-wall space is narrow and limits the installation of large-based systems. In this regard, the current best options are those machines with narrower width/depth footprints.

Purchasers should be aware of 2 methods of assessing size:

- Gross size = maximum breadth × maximum length × maximum height. Determining size requirements is probably the most important factor, because many patients place their machines in a cupboard or closet when not in use
- Net size, or how many cubic centimeters the machine will fill. Smaller units will have an aesthetic advantage. Often, the problem for home dialysis machines is not the size requirements, but the necessity of having a broad base on the machine to prevent accidents

A second key issue determining machine choice is that of ergonomics. The features of the machine should be chosen such that the system is well suited to the intended dialysis site. Ultimately, the most significant challenge in home dialysis is one that must be directed toward the manufacturers, namely, to create a dialysis system that meets the needs of potential home HD patients. The ideal home HD machine should be:

- Compact enough to meet space requirements
- Reliable
- Quiet
- Accessible
- Easy to learn and use
- Simple for patients with limited dexterity to use
- Simple and quick to set up and take down
- Easy to clean
- Able to be hidden when not in use
- Affordable

Currently, no available machine fits all these criteria, so the choice of machine should be such that it meets as many as possible.

Environmental Considerations

Environmental issues are important to consider in any home HD program for several reasons:

- Utility costs are generally borne by the dialysis service in facility-based care, but are transferred to the patient in most home HD models
    - » While some countries offer variable water and power subsidies to patients, this is not applicable to all. As an example, the subsidies offered by the Australian government are available at the Kidney Health Australia website.
    - » As a result, water and power usage can be a paramount financial consideration for many patients who wish to pursue home HD where subsidies either do not exist or fall short of the amount required to cover water and power costs
    - » Waste disposal—both at practical levels of volume and type and, potentially, from a cost perspective as well—may also present significant environmental and cost problems for the patient
    - » Governments are placing an increasing emphasis on carbon generation and carbon footprints—a growing concern for health systems worldwide—and the carbon footprint of dialysis is particularly large. The carbon footprints of several dialysis systems in relation to the duration and frequency of prescriptions and associated wastes have been calculated by Connor et al.[25]
    - » Machine systems and prescriptions can generate a 4-fold increase in the carbon footprint, which becomes a potential area of concern for patients wishing to undergo home HD. Carbon issues are fast becoming government policy platforms that affect subsidies, and this in turn can impact directly on the program costs for patients

With these issues in mind, machines that are water and/or power efficient, and systems that minimize waste generation, can be important considerations for the home HD patient and his or her support network.

References

1. Agar JW. Personal viewpoint: hemodialysis-water, power, and waste disposal: rethinking our environmental responsibilities. Hemodial Int. 2012;16:6-10.
2. International Organization for Standardization. ISO 23500:2014. Guidance for the preparation and quality management of fluids for haemodialysis and related therapies. 2014. Available at: http://www.iso.org/iso/catalogue_detail.htm?csnumber=61863. Accessed January 22, 2015.
3. Marshall MR, van der Schrieck N, Lilley D, et al. Independent community house hemodialysis as a novel dialysis setting: an observational cohort study. Am J Kidney Dis. 2013;61:598-607.
4. Marley JV, Dent HK, Wearne M, et al. Haemodialysis outcomes of Aboriginal and Torres Strait Islander patients of remote Kimberley region origin. Med J Aust. 2010;193:516-520.
5. Villarba A, Warr K. Home haemodialysis in remote Australia. Nephrology (Carlton). 2004;9(Suppl 4):S13-S137.
6. Kneipp E, Murray R, Warr K, Fitzclarence C, Wearne M, Maguire G. Bring me home: renal dialysis in the Kimberley. Nephrology (Carlton). 2004;9(Suppl 4):S121-S125.
7. Marshall MR, Pauly RP, Peirratos A. Delivering home hemodialysis: is there still a role for real-time treatment monitoring? Semin Dial. 2014;28:176-179.
8. Agar JW, Simmonds RE, Knight R, Somerville CA. Using water wisely: New, affordable, and essential water conservation practices for facility and home hemodialysis. Hemodial Int. 2009;13:32-37.
9. Perkins A, Simmonds RE, Boddington J, Hungerford R, Agar JW. Green nephrology in Australia: recirculating reject water. J Ren Nurs. 2010;2:281-283.
10. Agar JW, Perkins A, Tjipto A. Solar-assisted hemodialysis. Clin J Am Soc Nephrol. 2012;7:310-314.
11. International Organization for Standardization. ISO 13959:2014. Water for haemodialysis and related therapies. 2014. Available at: http://www.iso.org/iso/home/store/catalogue_ics/catalogue_detail_ics.htm?csnumber=61862. Accessed April 18, 2014.
12. James R. Dechlorination by ultraviolet radiation: a suitable alternative to activated carbon in dialysis water systems? J Ren Care. 2009;35:205-210.
13. Suman E, Varghese B, Joseph N, Nisha K, Kotian MS. The bacterial biofilms in dialysis water systems and the effect of the sub inhibitory concentrations of chlorine on them. J Clin Diagn Res. 2013;7:849-852.
14. Susantitaphong P, Riella C, Jaber BL. Effect of ultrapure dialysate on markers of inflammation, oxidative stress, nutrition and anemia parameters: a meta-analysis. Nephrol Dial Transplant. 2013;28:438-446.
15. Schiffl H, Lang SM, Stratakis D, Fischer R. Effects of ultrapure dialysis fluid on nutritional status and inflammatory parameters. Nephrol Dial Transplant. 2001;16:1863-1869.
16. Schiffl H, Lang SM. Effects of dialysis purity on uremic dyslipidemia. Ther Apher Dial. 2009;14:5-11.
17. Sitter T, Bergner A, Schiffl H. Dialysate related cytokine induction and response to recombinant human erythropoietin in haemodialysis patients. Nephrol Dial Transplant. 2000;15:1207-1211.
18. Hsu PY, Lin CL, Yu CC, et al. Ultrapure dialysate improves iron utilization and erythropoietin response in chronic hemodialysis patients - a prospective cross-over study. J Nephrol. 2004;17:693-700.
19. Honda H, Suzuki H, Hosaka N, et al. Ultrapure dialysate influences serum myeloperoxidase levels and lipid metabolism. Blood Purif. 2009;28:29-39.
20. Rahmati MA, Homel P, Hoenich NA, Levin R, Kaysen GA, Levin NW. The role of improved water quality on inflammatory

References (cont'd)

markers in patients undergoing regular dialysis. Int J Artif Organs. 2004;27:723-727.

21. Arizono K, Nomura K, Motoyama T, et al. Use of ultrapure dialysate in reduction of chronic inflammation during hemodialysis. Blood Purif. 2004;22(Suppl 2):26-29.

22. Furuya R, Kumagai H, Takahashi M, Sano K, Hishida A. Ultrapure dialysate reduces plasma levels of beta2-microglobulin and pentosidine in hemodialysis patients. Blood Purif. 2005;23:311-316.

23. Kohn OF, Coe FL, Ing TS. Solute kinetics with short-daily home hemodialysis using slow dialysate flow rate. Hemodial Int. 2010;14:39-46.

24. Agar JW. Review: understanding sorbent dialysis systems. Nephrology (Carlton). 2010;15:406-411.

25. Connor A, Lillywhite R, Cooke MW. The carbon footprint of home and in-center maintenance of hemodialysis in the United Kingdom. Hemodial Int. 2011;15:39-51.

Appendix

Home Hemodialysis: Infrastructure, Water, and Machines in the Home

Implementing Hemodialysis in the Home
A Global Perspective

iSHD
International Society for Hemodialysis

Home Infrastructure Checklist

Considerations

Machine Considerations

Width, depth, and height

- ❑ Does the installation area (eg, bedside to wall space) fit the chosen machine?

Servicing and cleaning

- ❑ How accessible is the machine to servicing and cleaning?
- ❑ How available is the water treatment plant to servicing and cleaning access?
- ❑ Does the weight of machine hinder easy movement?
    - ❑ Do local occupational health and safety (OH&S) standards allow for 1 or require 2 servicing personnel to service the chosen system?

Machine ergonomics

- ❑ Patient needs and ability will determine machine interface
    - ❑ Are the controls built into the machine and "machine-determined"?
    - ❑ Are the controls separate (ie, tablet device) and "patient-determined"?
- ❑ If "machine-determined", are controls, screens, alarms, etc, all within reach of patient's chosen dialysis position (eg, recumbent, sitting) and do they allow access at a full range of patient positions (eg, lying or seated patient height)?
    - ❑ OH&S issues
    - ❑ Clinical safety issues

Need or desire for variability and operating characteristics

- ❑ Dialyzer variability
    - ❑ Some current systems provide a cassette-based, drop-in consumable pack with no choice of dialyzer
- ❑ Blood flow variability
- ❑ Dialysis fluid flow variability
- ❑ Single vs double needle options

Home Infrastructure Checklist (cont'd)

User friendliness

- ❑ Console design and complexity
- ❑ Console height and/or variability
- ❑ Console dimmer switch

Patient lifestyle

- ❑ Is there a requirement or preference for travel and/or machine portability?

Dwelling and Room Considerations

Chair-situated dialysis vs bed-situated home HD

- ❑ Is there sufficient space?
- ❑ Comfortable?
- ❑ Adequate lighting?
- ❑ Ability to recline?
- ❑ Is the set up care partner friendly?

Storage

- ❑ Is there sufficient storage for dialysis consumables?
- ❑ Does the machine need to be out of the way or out of sight when not in use?
    - ❑ Is it easy to relocate the machine after it has been moved out of sight?
    - ❑ Is there a secure (and, if needed, refrigerated) storage area for medications?
- ❑ Aesthetics

Communication options

- ❑ Is there access to a land line or cellular telephone network?

Home Infrastructure Checklist (cont'd)

Hygiene and cleanliness considerations

- ❑ Can the room be regularly and completely cleaned?
- ❑ Is there easy access to solid waste disposal (eg, medical waste, recycle)?
- ❑ Is there easy washbasin access, which ideally should have hands-free elbow taps or an automatic on-off sensor system?

Utilities

- ❑ Can the room be appropriately equipped with electricity and plumbing?
- ❑ Are backup systems available in the event of an outage?

Plumbing Considerations

- ❑ Wet-resistant flooring
- ❑ Installation of back-flow preventer
- ❑ Consideration of water pressure issues and the requirement for a feed water pump or header tank
- ❑ Installation of reverse osmosis (RO) system with or without housing
- ❑ Determine if there is a potential for the reuse of RO reject water; drain if no reuse planned
- ❑ Installation of drainage points for reject water and effluent
    - ❑ Is disposal into a septic tank?
    - ❑ Will installation require a tundish?

Home Infrastructure Checklist (cont'd)

Other Considerations

- ❑ A reliable and accurate set of scales for pre- and postdialysis weight recording
- ❑ Optional access to a centrifuge for laboratory work
  - ❑ Home patients are capable of—and can be taught to—collect and spin down their own pre- and postdialysis blood samples. To facilitate this, access to a light-weight, easy-to-operate blood sample centrifuge can be offered
- ❑ Social requirements
  - ❑ Are the needs of family and care partners met?
  - ❑ Are there appropriate provisions for home entertainment and Wi-Fi/Internet?

Maintenance Considerations

- ❑ In-house maintenance programs
  - ❑ On-site or off-site?
  - ❑ By whom?
  - ❑ How often?
- ❑ Dialysis company maintenance
  - ❑ On-site or off-site?
  - ❑ By whom?
  - ❑ How often?

9 Prescriptions for Home Hemodialysis

Robert Lockridge, MD[1]
Tom Cornelis, MD[2]
Carolyn van Eps, MBBS, PhD, FRACP[3]

[1]Lynchburg Nephrology Physicians, Lynchburg, Virginia, USA;
[2]Department of Internal Medicine, Division of Nephrology, Maastricht University Medical Center, Maastricht, Netherlands;
[3]Princess Alexandra Hospital, Brisbane, Australia, NSW

Implementing Hemodialysis in the Home
A Global Perspective

ISHD
International Society for Hemodialysis

CONTENTS

Abstract

Prescribing a regimen that provides "optimal dialysis" to patients who wish to dialyze at home is of major importance, yet there is substantial variation in how home hemodialysis (HD) is prescribed. Geographic location, patient health status and clinical goals, and patient lifestyle and preferences all influence the selection of a prescription for a particular patient—there is no single prescription that provides optimal therapy for all patients, and careful weighing of potential benefit and burden is required for long-term success. This module describes how home HD prescribing patterns have changed over time and provides examples of commonly used home HD prescriptions. In addition, associated clinical outcomes and adequacy parameters as well as criteria for identifying which patients may benefit most from these diverse prescriptions are also presented.

Introduction

Throughout the world, there is significant variation in the percentage of prevalent dialysis patients performing hemodialysis (HD) in their homes (Figure 1).[1] Not only is there a difference in the percentages of home HD patients between countries, but there is also a difference in the number of patients doing home HD within each country.

Similarly, there is considerable variation in how home HD treatment is prescribed. Most home HD patients throughout the world use traditional machines designed for in-center or self-care HD. In the United States, the large majority of home HD patients are treated with short daily HD using a non-traditional, low-flow dialysate rate machine.[2]

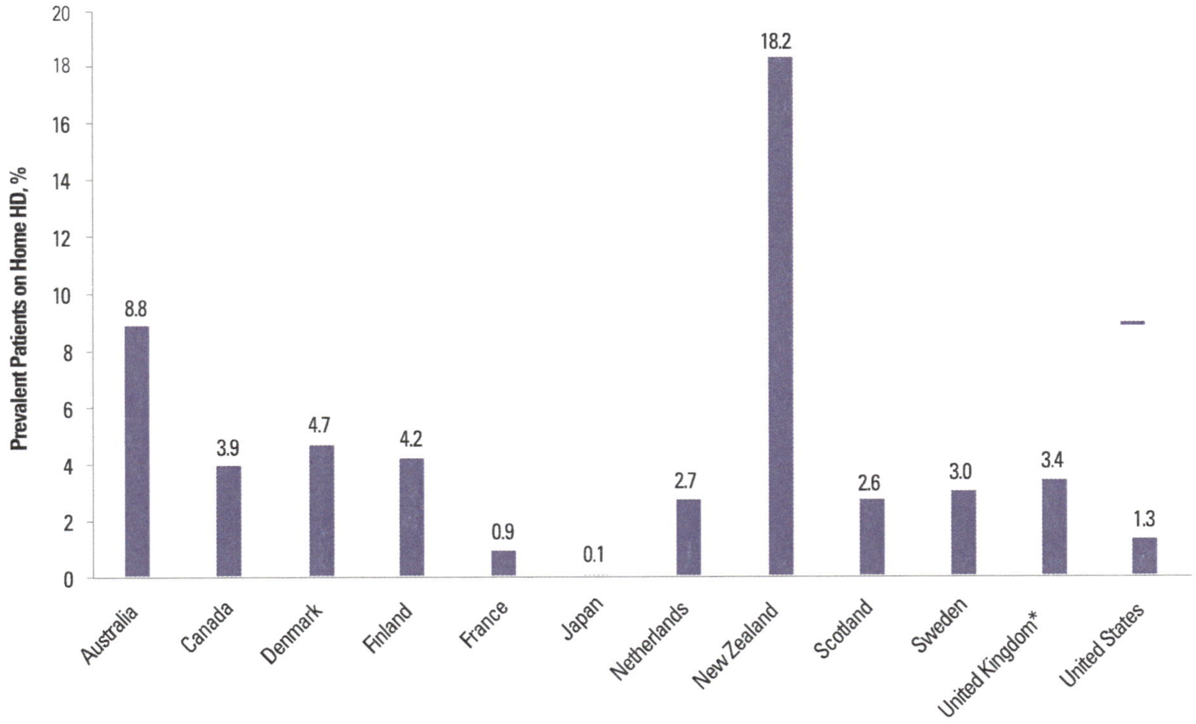

Figure 1. Proportion of prevalent dialysis patients on home hemodialysis

*United Kingdom includes England, Wales, and Northern Ireland. Scotland data reported separately.

Table 1. Fundamental Principles of Home HD Prescription
Minimum adequate HD can be defined as urea reduction ratio > 65% and a single-pool Kt/V of 1.2 per treatment for 3 times per week HD[4]
Increased total hours of HD per week is associated with improved survival[5-12]
Avoidance of high interdialytic weight gains (> 3–4 kg) and chronic fluid overload is associated with improved survival[12-14]
Avoidance of a long 3-day interdialytic break is associated with improved survival[15, 16]

HD = hemodialysis.

In the early years of dialysis therapy, practitioners recognized that clinical well-being formed an important part of the assessment of dialysis adequacy. Modern thinking has again embraced this concept. Instead of providing adequate dialysis, we should strive for "optimal dialysis", defined in terms of excellence in quality of life, control of symptoms, and normalization of risk factors, including blood pressure, cardiac structure and function, mineral balance, nutrition, hormonal status, and survival.[3] If we, as clinicians, define optimal dialysis in these terms, it is unlikely that any single dialysis prescription will be optimal for all patients, but rather that we should strive to offer a range of HD prescriptions for patients that best address their individual needs.

There are 4 fundamental principles of home HD prescriptions that have emerged from international studies (Table 1).[4–16] The benefits of these principles must be weighed with the goals of the patient, as well as the burden to the patient and patient care partner.

This module will describe the most commonly used home HD prescriptions, focusing on outcome data and descriptions of patients who may benefit from the particular prescriptions.

Rationale for Home HD Prescriptions

Throughout the world, HD is currently most commonly prescribed as 3 sessions per week (Mondays, Wednesdays, and Fridays or Tuesdays, Thursdays, and Saturdays), with each session lasting 3 to 5 hours.[16,17] This regimen has emerged as the most popular as a result of multiple logistic and patient factors. In the very early years of dialysis, treatment was prescribed as 2 to 3 sessions weekly, 8 hours per session. Over time, HD session durations have shortened to 3 to 5 hours, primarily on the basis that with the improving technologies, small-molecule clearance appeared to be adequate using this dialysis dose,[18] and it was logistically and financially easier to deliver therapy to the growing patient population. Regular dialysis every second or third day adequately controls accumulations of minerals (eg, potassium) and water that are known to have negative short-term effects, while also offering reasonable control of more long-term concerns, such as uremic symptoms and general well-being, for the majority of patients. It is possible for patients to sit attached to the dialysis machine for these 3- to 5-hour durations while still allowing some time for other activities that enhance quality of life. Dialyzing on the same days each week makes it easier for patients to schedule work and other important life commitments around dialysis. This scheduling is also easy for dialysis units and allows up to 6 shifts to be accommodated each week while avoiding excessive overnight and weekend overtime pay rates, as well as the associated life disruption for patients and staff.

Patients always desire the lowest possible dialysis treatment durations and frequency to avoid unnecessary intrusion of chronic disease on their lives.[19,20] From the late 1970s, HD treatment grew in numbers; technical advances in dialysis equipment allowed more efficient clearance of a broader range of toxins and potentially shorter treatment sessions, and financial constraints created an interest in defining clinical efficacy in a mathematical way (ie, identifying the lowest dialysis dose that would produce satisfactory clinical outcomes).[18,21] This resulted in the birth of the concept Kt/V as a measure of dialysis adequacy, where K is clearance of a molecule, t is the time on dialysis, and V is the volume of distribution for the molecule.[4] Clearance on dialysis of any substance can be defined in terms of Kt/V. Urea was one of the first identified and best understood uremic toxins and its quantification was easy and readily available. Therefore, Kt/V urea became the central focus of efforts to define a minimal dialysis requirement.[19]

In the modern era, there is a divergence of opinion and practice between clinicians from different countries in terms of the use of urea kinetic modeling for home HD patients. In the United States, urea kinetic modeling is deeply embedded in customary practices and clinician belief systems, and this extends to home HD. In fact, there are regulatory and reimbursement requirements that demand regular reporting and monitoring of Kt/V urea for all dialysis patients, including those on home HD. This situation is unique and contrasts with the policies in most other countries. In Australia and New Zealand, for instance, only about half of home HD patients have either a urea reduction ratio or Kt/V urea measured, and it is usually only calculated for those patients undergoing thrice-weekly schedules.[17] Many clinicians believe there are insufficient data to correlate Kt/V with clinical outcomes in home HD patients because frequency of dialysis and session length are markedly different from facility HD norms. Notwithstanding, Kt/V urea is a fundamental determinant of home HD prescription in some countries such as the United States, and it is important that the clinicians from those countries understand the underlying principles of Kt/V urea as applied to home HD.

The minimum adequate HD dose for patients being treated with standard thrice-weekly HD regimens has been defined as a single-pool Kt/V urea of 1.2 per dialysis session.[4] This target is primarily based on the results of 2 sentinel multicenter randomized controlled trials. The National Dialysis Cooperative Study examined outcomes in 151 patients undergoing HD for 3 sessions weekly.[22] Patients were randomized to either short (2.5 to 3.5 hours) or long (4.5 to 5.0 hours) session duration and within these groups, to either high-efficiency (time averaged blood concentration of urea [TAC urea] 50 mg/dL) or low-efficiency (TAC urea 100 mg/dL) dialysis. Participants in the high TAC urea groups experienced more hospitalizations ($P < .001$) and withdrawals from dialysis ($P < .001$). In both the high and low TAC urea groups, those patients dialyzed for the shorter therapy duration experienced more hospitalizations than did those patients undergoing long therapy duration (P = 0.06).[22] Subsequent analyses of these data in a mechanistic study by Gotch and Sargent[23] and of the final data set by Keshaviah[24] found that Kt/V urea < 0.8 was associated with increased patient failure rates,[23] and that there were similar failure rates for patients with single-pool Kt/V values of 0.9 to 1.5.[21,24]

In the HEMO Study, 1846 patients were randomized to either standard (Kt/V goal of 1.05) or high-dose HD (Kt/V goal of 1.45), and to either low- or high-flux dialysis membranes.[25] The mean single-pool Kt/V urea was 1.32±.09 for the standard dose and 1.71±.11 for the high-dose group; however, no improvement in survival was observed with either intervention, although in subgroup analysis, there were some associations of mortality benefit in female participants.[25]

It should be noted that Kt/V has only been established as a surrogate marker of dialysis outcomes for short-hours, thrice-weekly dialysis regimens. Although there have been studies examining the effect of quotidian HD regimens on urea reduction estimated by various equations, its role for predicting patient outcomes in long-hour regimens has not been determined.[4,26] However, The National Kidney Foundation's Kidney Disease Outcomes Quality Initiative (KDOQI) has suggested a standardized weekly Kt/V of 2.0 for more frequent and longer HD treatments as well as for continuous ambulatory peritoneal dialysis (CAPD) and continuous cycling peritoneal dialysis (CCPD) as a minimal adequacy standard.[4]

The ultimate objective of any prescription is to provide the best long-term clinical outcomes possible for any given patient. This contrasts with the early days of HD, where dialysis was exclusively used short-term for treatment of acute kidney injury and subsequently, as a bridge to kidney transplantation for those who did not recover kidney function.[18] Over time, HD has evolved into a long-term therapy for patients with end-stage renal disease (ESRD) who for whatever reason cannot receive a kidney transplant. Lengthy transplant waiting lists in some regions also means that many patients require maintenance dialysis for substantial periods before a suitable organ becomes available. These changes have demanded a refocus of our attention to improving longer-term survival for dialysis-dependent patients with ESRD. The choice to dialyze at home relieves patients from many of the logistic influences on dialysis frequency and duration that have shaped our in-center HD regimens. Further, previous studies have shown that quality of life is higher in patients who are provided with a choice of dialysis modality,[27] and it is therefore possible that providing home HD patients with the autonomy of alternating between different HD modalities may further increase quality of life. The best renal replacement therapy will always be kidney transplantation; however, only a minority of ESRD patients will receive one. For the rest, the flexibility of home HD prescriptions—which can be modified based on preferred frequency, duration, personal schedule, and on clinical needs—can provide patients with improved clinical and quality-of-life outcomes while they are on dialysis, which are the closest outcomes to those achieved with transplant, had these patients been fortunate enough to receive one.

Traditional Standard-Hours Home HD Using Standard Dialysate Flow Machines

Outcome Data

Standard-hours home HD 3.0 to 3.5 times per week is a suitable prescription for use in the home (Table 2). For those dialysis units that are new to offering patients home HD, it can be easiest to begin providing this familiar regimen while unit personnel gain experience supervising HD at home.

Survival of patients with HD-dependent ESRD managed with the conventional thrice-weekly regimen is markedly lower than that of the age-matched general population.[17] Overall mortality rates for ESRD patients managed with standard chronic HD regimens in developed countries range from 5% to 27%, and the mortality in these patients is primarily related to cardiovascular disease, infection, and voluntary withdrawal from treatment.[17,28,29]

Table 2. Traditional Standard-Hours Home HD Prescription Using Standard Dialysate Flow Machines

Frequency	3.0-3.5 sessions per week
Session Duration	3.5-5.0 hours
Blood Flow Rate	300-400 mL/min
Dialysate Flow Rate	500-800 mL/min
Membrane	1.4-2.5 m^2 high flux
Dialysate Sodium	138 mmol/L (range, 134-140 mmol/L)
Dialysate Potassium	2 mmol/L (range, 2-3 mmol/L)
Dialysate Calcium	1.25 mmol/L (range, 1.0-1.5 mmol/L) 2.5 mEq/L (range, 2.0-2.5 mEq/L)
Dialysate Bicarbonate	34 mmol/L (range, 32-36 mmol/L)
Anticoagulation	• Standard heparin bolus (50 U/kg) • Low-molecular-weight heparin is also effective, but is used less commonly due to cost. Dose is typically administered as a bolus; it may be fixed or weight-based, depending on the patient and local policies
Assessment of Adequacy	Kt/V urea > 1.2 per session URR > 65% per session
Special Considerations	Excellent regimen for dialysis units that are new to home HD to use while experience is gained

HD = hemodialysis; URR = urea reduction ratio.

In addition to reduced quantity of life, ESRD patients also experience reduced quality of life as a consequence of symptoms of uremia that include fatigue, weakness, reduced sensation, impaired cognitive functions, dizziness, disturbed sleep, restless leg syndrome, neuropathy, anorexia, nausea, altered taste and smell, itching, cramps, sexual dysfunction, infertility, and depression and anxiety.[30] Currently available dialysis therapies place a great burden on patients and their families as they require a substantial time commitment, adherence to intrusive dietary restrictions, and the use of multiple medications. In addition to the effects of uremia, the HD procedure itself has been associated with symptoms including fatigue, headache, nausea, restlessness, cramps, hypotension, and cognitive dysfunction. This has been termed the dialysis disequilibrium syndrome.[29]

The ability to teach patients to perform their own HD at home has been associated with improved survival and quality-of-life outcomes during traditional home HD.[31,32] Therefore it is still a worthwhile exercise to teach patients to dialyze at home even if they are only willing to use a standard HD prescription.

Patients Who May Benefit From this Prescription

We would recommend standard-hours dialysis for patients where minimizing time committed to HD therapy is of paramount importance, such as patients with palliative treatment goals or patients who, despite appropriate counseling about the benefits of increased frequency and extended-hours HD regimens, insist on performing a standard-hours HD regimen. Patients should be advised to avoid the standard prescription as it relates to the 3-day interdialytic break, as this long interdialytic interval is associated with increased cardiovascular events and mortality.[15,16]

There may also be a role for standard-hours regimens for patients who are newly commencing HD and who still have considerable residual renal function. These patients can usually achieve excellent control of fluid, serum parameters, and symptoms with fewer dialysis treatment hours for the first months, and dialysis dose can be gradually titrated upwards. This approach can assist patients in developing good habits with diet and fluid restrictions that will be compatible with excellent control of blood chemistry and fluid balance on an optimized dialysis regimen once residual renal function is lost. It can also be advantageous for patients starting dialysis at home to schedule their sessions during office hours, when maximum staff assistance is available; standard-hours regimens are particularly amenable to this. However, some patients may have difficulties adjusting to gradually increasing dialysis hours and may be better placed commencing a more intensive HD routine at the outset.

Alternate-Night Nocturnal Home HD Using Standard Dialysate Flow Machines

Outcome Data

There are no randomized, controlled data supporting the use of home alternate-night nocturnal HD (NHD) for the management of ESRD; however, there are data from observational and non-randomized, controlled studies that suggest benefits over conventional HD regimens. An example prescription is presented in Table 3.

Extended-hours HD, 3 sessions weekly has been practiced in-center in Tassin, France, for many years with reportedly excellent survival rates, control of hypertension, and higher clearance parameters.[18,33]

The Turkish Long Dialysis Study Group compared patients managed with a thrice-weekly (8 hours per session) in-center NHD regimen (n = 247) with matched control patients managed with a 4-hours-per-session conventional HD regimen (CHD; n = 247) in a prospective, controlled study over 12 months.[34] Use of an NHD regimen was associated with a 72% risk reduction for overall mortality ($P < 0.01$), a lower hospitalization rate, improved nutritional status, and improvement in echocardiographic

Table 3. Alternate-Night Nocturnal Home HD Prescription Using Standard Dialysate Flow Machines

Frequency	3.5 sessions per week
Session Duration	6-10 hours
Blood Flow Rate	250-350 mL/min
Dialysate Flow Rate	300-500 mL/min
Membrane	1.4-2.1 m^2 high flux
Dialysate Sodium	138 mmol/L (range, 135-138 mmol/L)
Dialysate Potassium	2 mmol/L (range, 2-3 mmol/L)
Dialysate Calcium	1.5 mmol/L (range, 1.5-1.75 mmol/L) 3 mEq/L (range, 2.5-3 mEq/L)
Dialysate Bicarbonate	32 mmol/L (range, 28-35 mmol/L)
Anticoagulation	• Minimum to prevent dialysis circuit thrombosis • Usually an extra 1000 U of unfractionated heparin bolus will be required above the standard regimen requirement. Thereafter, unfractionated heparin infusion at the same hourly rate used for standard HD regimens can be used and adjusted upwards if evidence of clotting is observed in the circuit • If fractionated heparin is used, an infusion following the initial bolus may be required to prevent clotting in patients prescribed longer session hours • Low-molecular-weight heparin is also effective, but is used less commonly due to cost. Dose is typically administered as a bolus; it may be fixed or weight-based, depending on the patient and local policies
Assessment of Adequacy	• Meets internationally accepted guidelines for electrolyte control and fluid balance • No or minimal requirement for antihypertensive medications and phosphate binders • Excellent reported quality of life
Special Considerations	• Arguably, this is the easiest of the extended-hours HD regimens to maintain long term • Very little increase in consumable requirement that of above standard-hours HD (associated little increase in cost or stock storage requirements) • May reduce dialysis access complications compared with daily HD regimens • Addition of phosphate to the dialysate is rarely required. Addition of phosphate to the acid component of the dialysate in the form of Fleet® 5-40 mL may be required if serum phosphate predialysis is < 1 mmol/L and post-dialysis is lower than the recommended normal reference range when phosphate binders have been ceased and dietary phosphate intake is encouraged • Greater loss of water-soluble vitamins. Routine replacement of vitamins C, B group, and folic acid is recommended • Requires reliable monitoring for blood leak (eg, blood leak sensor and alarm system and/or remote monitoring) • Requires a large receptacle to hold 2 bottles of acid component of dialysis and a large size bicarbonate bag to ensure there are enough dialysate components to complete the treatment

HD = hemodialysis

parameters (eg, chamber diameters, left ventricular hypertrophy) compared with CHD. NHD was associated with a significant reduction in serum phosphate level and accompanied by a reduction in phosphate binder use; similarly, hemoglobin levels increased and the use of erythropoietin was reduced. While there was no significant difference in blood pressure between groups, use of antihypertensive therapies was reduced with the NHD regimen ($P = .02$). Cognitive functions were improved with NHD but not CHD, and quality-of-life scores remained stable with NHD but deteriorated in the CHD group.[34]

Fresenius Medical Care in the United States compared 746 patients converted to 3 sessions weekly in-center NHD with 2062 matched control patients followed over a 2-year period.[8] This study reported a survival advantage of 25% with NHD ($P = .004$). While the interdialytic weight gain was higher with NHD, phosphate control was significantly improved and ultrafiltration rates were decreased owing to the longer session duration.[8]

A regimen of 3 to 4 NHD sessions weekly is the most commonly prescribed extended-hours HD regimen for HD patients in Australia.[35] Jun et al.[36] examined all-cause mortality, technique failure, and access complication rates in 286 Australian ESRD patients managed with extended-hours HD (> 24 hours per week). The majority of patients performed alternate-day, extended-hours HD. The overall survival rates (98%, 92%, and 83%) and technique survival rates (90%, 77%, and 68%) at 1, 3, and 5 years, respectively, were excellent. Increased frequency of HD was associated with an increased likelihood of developing an access event; however, access-related adverse event–free survival rates were 80%, 68%, and 61% at 1, 3, and 5 years, respectively.[36]

Reports from Brisbane, Australia, on patients who converted from home CHD (3 to 5 sessions weekly, 3 to 6 hours per session) to alternate-night home NHD (6 to 10 hours per session, 3 to 5 sessions weekly) describe improvements in blood pressure control with reduced antihypertensive requirement[37]; lower serum phosphate, calcium-phosphate product, and parathyroid hormone levels with reduced requirement for phosphate binding medications[37-39]; reduced vascular and ectopic calcification[38]; lower prolactin and higher testosterone levels in male patients[40]; reduced erythropoietin requirement[39,40]; improvements in general health and overall health ratings, physical function, physical role, and energy and fatigue scores on the kidney disease quality of life (KDQOL) assessment tool[39,40]; longer distance covered during the 6-minute walk test[39]; and improved small and middle molecule clearances.[39] The risk of dialysis access infectious complications appeared to be increased, particularly when the buttonhole cannulation technique was used in conjunction with extended-hours HD.[40] In contrast to the cardiovascular benefits reported in previous studies, no improvements in cardiovascular structure and function or hospitalization rates were observed following conversion to alternate-night NHD in this study.[37,41] Notably, the majority of patients in these studies dialyzed 3.5 to 4.0 sessions weekly and avoided a 3-day-long interdialytic break both at baseline and follow-up. The allowance of an interdialytic break of > 2 days on a regular basis should be discouraged as this longer dialysis-free interval has been associated with increased cardiovascular events and mortality.[16]

Interdialytic weight gains remain higher with alternate-day, extended-hours HD regimens compared with daily HD regimens. High interdialytic weight gains may be an indicator of improved nutritional status, but also remain a source of ongoing cardiovascular stress that may counteract the effects of improved control of other uremic toxins.[14-16] Interdialytic weight gains greater than approximately 3 to 4 kg and ultrafiltration rates higher than 10 to 13 mL/kg/h have been associated with increased mortality in adult long-term HD patients. This is the result of extracellular fluid expansion, which promotes hypertension and congestive cardiac failure, and high ultrafiltration rates, which promote cardiovascular instability and organ ischemia during dialysis sessions.[14-16]

Patients Who May Benefit from this Prescription

Alternate-night NHD is best suited to patients who desire their waking hours to be largely free of dialysis and are able to sleep while undergoing dialysis treatment, and those who do not have reason to frequently get up at night and do not wish or are unable to sustain a daily HD regimen.

The 2-day break may lead to large, problematic interdialytic weight gains. Thus, alternate-night NHD is ideal for patients who struggle to maintain reasonable interdialytic weight gains or who have significant cardiac dysfunction.

Arguably, this prescription is the easiest of the extended-hours HD regimens to maintain long term. There is very little increase in consumable requirements for this treatment above standard-hours HD, so the increase in cost and storage requirements is minimal. This prescription may be associated with fewer vascular access-related complications compared with daily HD regimens.

Traditional Short Daily Home HD Using Standard Dialysate Flow Machines

Outcome Data

The short daily HD regimen (Table 4) is supported by results from many cohort and non-randomized studies that have suggested survival, cardiovascular, and quality-of-life benefits.[42-44] Short daily HD is also the regimen with the most robust randomized, controlled evidence for associated meaningful health benefits when compared with standard HD regimens. The Frequent Hemodialysis Network (FHN) conducted a randomized, controlled trial in which 125 patients managed with 6 sessions weekly, 1.5 to 2.75 hours per session, were compared with 120 patients managed with 3 sessions weekly, 2.5 to 4.0 hours per session HD, over 12-months.[45-47] The short daily HD regimen was associated with significantly better outcomes, including composite outcome of death or change in left ventricular mass, composite outcome of death and physical health composite score, decreased left ventricular mass, and improved hypertension and serum phosphate control. There was no difference between the 2 groups in cognitive performance, depression scores, albumin, erythropoietin sensitivity, the composite measure of death and hospitalization rates, serum calcium, parathyroid hormone, or rate of loss of residual renal function. Short daily HD was associated with an increased need for vascular access interventions in this group compared with the interventions experienced in the standard HD frequency group.[45-47] It should be noted that the FHN trial included a relatively small number of highly selected participants and the mortality outcomes were composite measures, so results of this trial may not apply to all patients or patient populations.

Patients Who May Benefit from this Prescription

Any patient who is willing and able to sustain dialyzing on a daily basis may benefit from a short daily regimen. Patients who are unable to tolerate increased hours per session, particularly when sleeping during dialysis or when sitting for long periods is not possible, may benefit the most. Short daily schedules may be the preferred option that fits best around some patients' other daily commitments such as employment or education, particularly if these patients do not tolerate or are not willing to perform nocturnal HD regimens.

Although fluid gains between treatments are usually reduced, high ultrafiltration rates may remain a problem with substantially shortened session durations. Also, daily HD regimens consume increased amounts of disposable supplies per week compared with thrice-weekly HD, which generates increased cost and a need for increased storage space in the home. Patients with cannulation phobias or vascular access that is difficult to cannulate or those prone to complications may be less suited to daily HD regimens (see "The Care and Keeping of Vascular Access in Home Hemodialysis Patients" module).

Table 4. Traditional Short Daily Home HD Prescription Using Standard Dialysate Flow Machines	
Frequency	5-6 sessions per week
Session Duration	2.5-3.5 hours
Blood Flow Rate	350-450 mL/min
Dialysate Flow Rate	350-600 mL/min
Membrane	1.4-2.1 m^2 high flux
Dialysate Sodium	138 mmol/L
Dialysate Potassium	2 mmol/L
Dialysate Calcium	1.25 mmol/L (range, 2.5 mEq/L)
Dialysate Bicarbonate	32-36 mmol/L
Anticoagulation	• Standard heparin bolus (50 U/kg) • Low-molecular-weight heparin is also effective, but is used less commonly due to cost. Dose is typically administered as a bolus; it may be fixed or weight-based, depending on the patient and local policies
Assessment of Adequacy	• Achieve a single pool Kt/V of 1.2 per treatment and/or a standardized weekly Kt/V of 3.0 • Maximize fluid control resulting in less blood pressure medications with optimal blood pressure control • Liberalize dietary intake • Provide > 12 hours of RRT per week
Special Considerations	To receive adequate therapy, patients must perform at least 5-6 treatments per week, which results in increased supplies, increased storage requirements, and increased cost for the provider. Fluid gain between treatments is less; however, with shorter treatment time, the amount of fluid required to remove per hour may exceed a safe ultrafiltration rate

HD = hemodialysis; RRT = renal replacement therapy.

Traditional Nocturnal Home HD Using Standard Dialysate Flow Machines

Outcome Data

There are two randomized, controlled trials that examine patient outcomes with traditional daily NHD regimens (Table 5) compared with standard-hours HD regimens. Culleton et al.[48] conducted a randomized, controlled trial comparing outcomes in 27 patients receiving daily NHD with 25 patients receiving CHD over a 6-month period. Daily NHD was associated with improved left ventricular mass measured by cardiac magnetic resonance imaging, effect of kidney disease and burden of kidney disease domains of the KDQOL Scale, blood pressure with associated reduction in antihypertensive use, and serum phosphate with reduction in phosphate binder requirement. There was no benefit detected in overall quality of life or anemia management parameters.[48] The FHN Group[49] conducted a randomized, controlled trial comparing outcomes in 45 patients managed with daily NHD with 42 patients managed with CHD regimens. Daily NHD was not associated with improvement in the study's primary composite outcomes: death or change in left ventricular mass, and death or physical health composite score. Nocturnal HD was associated with improved serum phosphate and hypertension control. No improvement was seen in cognitive performance, depression scores, nutrition, anemia management, or hospitalization rates. The FHN Nocturnal Trial patient enrollment goal was 250 patients in the original study design, but this goal was reduced to 125 due to enrollment difficulties, and only 87 patients were randomized. This makes drawing firm conclusions from the trial problematic.[49]

Other non-randomized studies have consistently reported improvements in blood pressure control, when assessed, but variable changes in left ventricular hypertrophy, anemia, bone mineral metabolism, and quality-of-life measures.[50] Longer and more frequent dialysis sessions allow ultrafiltration to occur at a lower rate, which has been associated with less intradialytic hypotension and consequently less myocardial stunning and inflammation.[51] Pauly et al.[52] compared outcomes in a cohort of 177 NHD patients with 531 renal transplant recipients over 5 years and found survival rates were comparable between the 2 groups; however, in the most recent retrospective cohort study of intensive home HD patients and kidney transplant recipients, kidney transplantation was associated with superior treatment and patient survival.[53] Small cohort studies have demonstrated improvement in sleep apnea syndrome, sleep patterns, and restless leg syndrome with short daily HD and NHD.[54,55]

There are a few small cohort studies describing the potential for improved fertility and successful pregnancy outcomes using frequent NHD.[56-58] Hladunewich et al.[59] compared cohorts of female patients undergoing home daily NHD and CHD patients in Toronto, Canada, and the United States, respectively, over a 13-year period and found a dose-response relationship between the intensity of dialysis and pregnancy outcomes, including live birth rate, gestational age, and birth weight. If home NHD is not an option for a pregnant patient, an intensive, in-center NHD-like regimen (ie, 35 to 45 hours per week on dialysis) should be offered.[60]

Patients Who May Benefit from this Prescription

Daily home NHD is ideal for patients who are employed or have daytime commitments. Dialyzing during sleep allows patients to receive maximum renal replacement therapy with minimal burden, helps prevent patient and care partner burnout, and provides free time during waking hours for work or leisure activities. Patients with multiple medical problems—including those who have failed PD or transplant, or are on a transplant waiting list and are > 60 years of age—benefit from increased time and frequency of HD sessions, which maximizes stability during their treatment; this increases their quality of life and decreases comorbid events while they are on dialysis. Patients who are pregnant or planning to become pregnant should have their dialysis

Table 5. Traditional Nocturnal Home HD Prescription Using Standard Dialysate Flow Machines

Frequency	4-6 sessions per week
Session Duration	6-8 hours
Blood Flow Rate	250-350 mL/min
Dialysate Flow Rate	200-300 mL/min
Membrane	1.4-2.1 m^2 high flux
Dialysate Sodium	138 mmol/L
Dialysate Potassium	3 mmol/L
Dialysate Total Calcium	1.5-1.75 mmol/L (3.0-3.5 mEq/L)
Dialysate Bicarbonate	28-35 mmol/L
Anticoagulation	• Standard heparin bolus (50 U/kg) with heparin pump, providing 500-1500 U/hr. Heparin should be stopped 1 hour before end of treatment if the patient has an AVF or AVG, and at the end of treatment if the patient has a CVC • Low-molecular-weight heparin is also effective, but is used less commonly due to cost. Dose is typically administered as a bolus; it may be fixed or weight-based, depending on the patient and local policies
Assessment of Adequacy	• Provide a standardized weekly Kt/V ≥ 4.0 • Control phosphorus without the use of binders • Control blood pressure without the use of antihypertensive medication • Provide ≥ 24 hours of RRT per week
Special Considerations	• The majority of patients will dialyze 4-5 times per week, which is a minimal increase in supply cost compared with typical alternate-day home HD • Most patients who dialyze using NHD an average of 5 days per week can maintain their phosphate levels in adequate range by increasing phosphate intake. Only 20-30% of patients will need to add additional phosphate to their dialysate. Addition of phosphate to the acid component of the dialysate in the form of Fleet® 5-40 mL may be required if serum phosphate predialysis is < 1 mmol/L and post-dialysis is lower than the recommended normal reference range, and when phosphate binders have been ceased and dietary phosphate intake has been encouraged • A standard renal replacement vitamin and vitamin C 500 U daily provides adequate water-soluble vitamin replacement • Requires reliable monitoring for blood leak. Blood leak sensor and alarm system are recommended. There appears to be no advantage in remote monitoring • Because the dialysate flow is 200-300 mL/min, there is no need for additional acid or bicarbonate jugs to provide adequate dialysate for a 6- to 8-hour treatment • Starting with a calcium bath of 1.5 mmol/L with the ability to increase to 1.75 mmol/L is standard of care and critical in the management of traditional NHD

HD = hemodialysis;
AVF = arteriovenous fistula;
AVG = arteriovenous graft;
CVC = central venous catheter;
NHD = nocturnal hemodialysis;
RRT = renal replacement therapy.

hours per week increased, and this can be conveniently offered by a home NHD prescription. Daily home NHD also suits patients who value maximized dietary freedom while maintaining optimized blood chemistry. A standard renal replacement multivitamin and vitamin C 500 U daily provides adequate water-soluble vitamin replacement.

The majority of NHD patients will dialyze 5 times per week, which generates a moderate increase in cost and the need for increased storage space in the home compared with alternate-day home HD. Patients with cannulation phobias or vascular access that is difficult to cannulate or those prone to complications may be less suited to NHD regimens (see "The Care and Keeping of Vascular Access in Home Hemodialysis Patients" module).

Low-Flow Dialysate Short Daily Home HD

Low-Flow Dialysate HD Machine

Specifically designed low-flow dialysate HD machines are typically used only in the United States. Dialysate volume for the low-flow dialysate HD machine is 15 to 60 L per short daily treatment, or 90 to 360 L per week.[61] In comparison, the typical dialysate volume for traditional CHD machines is 90 to 200 L per treatment (270 to 600 L per week).

While uncommon in most areas of the world, in the United States more than 85% of the > 6000 patients on home HD use a low-flow dialysate machine to perform short daily home HD.[2,62] This machine was approved by the US Food and Drug Administration (FDA) and Health Canada in July 2003[63] for HD, hemofiltration, and/or ultrafiltration for treatment of renal failure or fluid overload in the in-center dialysis and acute-care settings, and was evaluated[64] and approved for home HD by the FDA in June 2005.

Short daily home HD prescriptions using a low-flow dialysate HD machine (Table 6) are not based on time per treatment, but rather on a flow fraction of 30% to 35% (a ratio of blood flow rate to dialysate flow rate of 3 to 1) to maximize urea saturation of dialysate used, shorten dialysis time per treatment, meet the minimal adequacy KDOQI standards, and decrease the amount of sterile fluid used per treatment.[64,65]

A web-based HD dose calculator is available to help physicians prescribe low-flow dialysate HD and to better meet prescription goals and needs of their patients (see https://dosingcalculator.nxstage.com/Account/Login.aspx). This calculator allows the physician to suggest a weekly standardized Kt/V goal, blood flow rate, weekly ultrafiltration rate, maximum ultrafiltration rate per hour, minimal hours per week, and frequency of treatments per week. Once the physician completes the required fields, the calculator will provide varied prescriptions that meet the physician's specified goals. This approach moves away from flow fraction–based prescribing and providing minimally adequate dialysis, and toward frequency and time per week of HD for more optimal dialysis.

It should be noted that clearances with low-flow dialysate systems are reduced in efficiency compared with other currently available HD systems. Thus, most patients will require an increased intensity HD prescription to maintain optimal health. Great care is needed to ensure adequate dialysis is maintained as residual renal function wanes and patients gradually modify their HD schedules at home.

Outcome Data

There are no randomized, controlled studies supporting the use of low-flow dialysate short daily HD for the management of ESRD; however, there are several observational studies that support the efficacy and safety of this prescription.

Table 6. Low-flow dialysate short daily home HD prescription

Frequency	5-6 sessions per week
Session Duration	2.5-4 hours
Blood Flow Rate	300-400 mL/min
Dialysate Flow Rate	83-300 mL/min (20-60 L of dialysate per treatment)
Membrane	1.8 m² high flux
Dialysate Sodium	138 mmol/L
Dialysate Potassium	2.0 mmol/L
Dialysate Total Calcium	1.5 mmol/L (3.0 mEq/L)
Dialysate Bicarbonate	40-45 mmol/L
Anticoagulation	Standard heparin bolus (50 U/kg)
Assessment of Adequacy	• Provide a standardized weekly Kt/V ≥ 2.1 (meeting specified KDOQI guidelines) • Control blood pressure without the use of antihypertensive medications • Liberalize dietary intake • Provide > 12 hours of RRT weekly Note: In the United States the Center for Medicaid and Medicare Services regulates meeting specified KDOQI guideline requirements and minimizing the cost of supplies. A more optimal prescription would include five treatments per week, use of > 30 L of dialysate per treatment, and > 15 hours RRT per week
Special Considerations	• This machine has built-in moisture detectors in the pan under the machine to detect any type of leak related to the machine and artificial kidney • It is important to note that because this machine uses a lower dialysate flow rate, the clearance of small molecules is reduced compared with traditional machines • Frequency of treatment, simple set up and take down procedures, and portability make the low-flow machine unique for short daily dialysis • Low-flow machine only provides a calcium bath of 1.5 mmol/L

HD = hemodialysis; KDOQI = Kidney Disease Outcomes Quality Initiative; RRT = renal replacement therapy.
Note: This machine is typically used only in the United States.

In a study of 5 patients, the rate of removal of solutes (β_2 microglobulin, phosphorus, potassium, and urea nitrogen) from the serum per dialysis session was demonstrated to be lower with low-flow dialysate short daily HD than with thrice-weekly HD using higher dialysate flow rates.[61] While the solute removal rates were lower per session using lower flow rates, the increased frequency of sessions with short daily HD (17.5 hours per week) compared with CHD resulted in an overall increase in solute removal.[61]

Clinical outcomes, including improvements in prevalence and severity of symptoms of restless leg syndrome and sleep disturbances, have been reported with low-flow, short daily HD.[55] An observational study by Finkelstein et al.[66] enrolled 291 participants and used the SF-36 health survey to evaluate health-related quality of life (HRQOL) in home HD patients. Results indicated long-term improvements from baseline in HRQOL over the course of 12 months, including physical and mental components, when patients were initiated on low-flow daily home HD.[66] A prospective, open-label study comparing the safety of in-center and home HD using this low-flow dialysate HD machine was conducted by Kraus et al.[64] They reported lower rates of adverse events during home HD compared with in-center HD ($P = .007$). Despite a lower rate of adverse events, only a modest improvement in survival has been observed with low-flow, short daily HD compared with in-center CHD, with the cumulative incidence of death of 19.2% and 21.7%, respectively.[67]

The FHN Daily Trial was a randomized, controlled study that compared outcomes in patients managed with 6 or 3 HD sessions weekly using traditional in-center machines with higher dialysate flow rates.[45] Findings revealed a reduction in left ventricular mass and improvement in quality-of-life indicators with more frequent dialysis. While this trial included a frequent HD prescription with a similar number of dialysis hours per week to that used in a low-flow, short daily HD prescription, the improved outcomes achieved with the higher dialysate flow rate cannot be extrapolated to a low-flow dialysate system without performing a similar study using a low-flow machine.

Previous studies have elicited concern associated with low-flow dialysate HD machines and why there appears to be significant technique failure at 1 year. The FREEDOM study, which reported improvements in HRQOL with short daily HD, also reported a high study discontinuation rate.[66] A total of 291 participants completed the SF-36 health survey, of which 154 completed the 12-month follow up (47% discontinuation rate). The majority (54%) of patients who withdrew from the study did so within the first 4 months. Participants withdrew from the study for the following reasons: modality change or return to in-center dialysis (63 patients), kidney transplantation (14 patients), death (13 patients), off short daily HD for > 6 weeks (12 patients), transfer out of a participating dialysis center (7 patients), non-compliance (3 patients), recovery of kidney function (2 patients), and other reasons (23 patients). Considering only those patients who changed modalities, died, or were off short daily HD for > 6 weeks, the rate of discontinuation over a 1-year period for this low-flow dialysate machine was 30%. Additional studies are required to explain why technique failure rates appear to be higher for this prescription than for home NHD.[66]

Patients Who May Benefit from this Prescription

Patients who may benefit from low-flow short daily HD regimens are the same as those who benefit from traditional short daily regimens (refer to discussion in "Traditional Short Daily Home HD Using Standard Dialysate Flow Machines" section).

In addition, the low-flow dialysate HD machine used in the United States is particularly suited to patients who wish to use short daily HD regimens because the machine has been designed to minimize time spent setting up, cleaning, and maintaining the system. The machine allows patients to dialyze at home with limited quantity and/or poor quality water supply, and is also useful for those who are unable to significantly modify their residence (eg, temporary accommodation or apartment dwelling). Dialysate can be easily prepared from drinking-quality tap water using the disposable water purification system and built-in water quality testing, which requires no regular maintenance by the patient or routine water testing by the supervising dialysis unit. Alternatively, dialysate is available in premade sterile bags (for more information, see "Infrastructure, Water, and Machines in the Home" module).

Patients who need or wish to travel and have experienced difficulties organizing in-center HD at their desired destinations may particularly benefit from this machine, which is relatively compact and portable. Patients who intend to travel with this machine should seek information regarding associated costs, baggage restrictions, and requirements for local medical supervision at the destination (see "Psychosocial Aspects in Home Hemodialysis" and "Infrastructure, Water, and Machines in the Home" modules).

Low-Flow Dialysate Nocturnal Home HD

Outcome Data

Low-flow dialysate machines are typically used only in the United States and for short daily home HD. As such, there are no randomized studies evaluating low-flow dialysate NHD, but its use is supported by published observational studies. Pierratos et al.[68] presented the Toronto 3-year experience with nocturnal dialysis in 1998. It is important to note that this dialysis prescription for the first 3 years was a low surface area (0.7 m^2, Fresenius F40) dialyzer, blood flow rate of 250 to 300 mL/min, and a dialysis flow rate of 100 mL/min.[68] This would be considered low-flow dialysate HD, which would suggest that nocturnal dialysis could be performed utilizing the low-flow dialysate HD machine presently used in the United States.

An example prescription is presented in Table 7.

Lockridge et al.[69] presented data on 15 patients over a 3-year period who were trained on the low-flow dialysate HD machine to perform NHD. The HD machine was reprogrammed to convert it from a flow fraction–to a time-based machine using the following settings:

- Flow fraction: 100% (setting 1)
- Dialysate flow rate: Liter dialysate per treatment ÷ hours per session (setting 2)
- Dialysate volume: Liter dialysate per treatment ÷ hours per session (setting 5)
- Access pod: "Off" (setting 53)
- Cartridge: 171-B
- Heparin pump: External

Low-flow NHD was performed successfully in this diverse group of patients with a mean treatment time of 6.8 (6.0 to 7.0) hours per treatment, 4.8 (4.0 to 5.0) treatments per week, and 56 L of dialysate per treatment. After patients had been on the NHD therapy for 3 months or longer, the mean Kt/V for this dialysis prescription was 3.8 (3.10 to 4.56), and few patients required antihypertensive medications (1 of 15 patients) or phosphate binders (4 of 15 patients).[69] Reprogramming a low-flow dialysate system with the addition of an external heparin pump allowed for the convenience of NHD with optimized dialysate adequacy.

Patients Who May Benefit from this Prescription

Patients who may benefit from low-flow NHD regimens are the same as those who benefit from traditional NHD. Please (refer to discussion in "Traditional Nocturnal Home HD Using Standard Dialysate Flow Machines" section).

Table 7. Low-flow dialysate home NHD

Frequency	4-6 sessions per week
Session Duration	6-8 hours
Blood Flow Rate	300-350 mL/min
Dialysate Flow Rate	62.5-166.6 L/min (30-60 L of dialysate/treatment)
Membrane	1.8 m^2 high flux
Dialysate Sodium	138 mmol/L
Dialysate Potassium	2.0 mmol/L
Dialysate Total Calcium	1.5 mmol/L (3.0 mEq/L)
Dialysate Lactate	Lactate baths 40-45 mmol/L
Anticoagulation	• Standard heparin bolus (50 U/kg) with heparin pump, providing 500-1500 U/hr. Heparin should be stopped 1 hour before end of treatment if the patient has an AVF or AVG, and at the end of treatment if the patient has a CVC • Low molecular weight heparin is also effective, but is used less commonly due to cost. Dose is typically administered as a bolus; it may be fixed or weight-based, depending on the patient and local policies
Assessment of Adequacy	• Provide a standardized weekly Kt/V ≥ 3.0-4.5 (optimal RRT) • Control of phosphorus without the use of binders • Control blood pressure without the use of antihypertensive medications • Provide ≥ 24 hours of RRT per week
Special Considerations	• Most low-flow dialysate nocturnal patients dialyzing 5 days per week can maintain their phosphate levels in an adequate range. This low-flow dialysate machine does not offer the ability to add phosphorus to the dialyses bath • A standard renal replacement vitamin and vitamin C 500 U daily provides adequate water soluble vitamin replacement • This machine has built-in moisture detectors in the pan under the machine to detect any type of leak related to the machine and artificial kidney. Because this machine uses a lower dialysate flow rate, the clearance of small molecules is reduced compared with traditional machines. Large-molecule clearance that is time-based is the same rate as that achieved with traditional machines • The only low-flow dialysate machine available at present can only provide a calcium bath of 1.5 mmol/L, which could be problematic if there is calcium depletion associated with ultrafiltration

NHD = nocturnal hemodialysis; AVG = arteriovenous graft; AVF = arteriovenous fistula; CVC = central venous catheter; RRT = renal replacement therapy.

Note: This machine is typically used only in the United States.

Summary

There are numerous prescriptions available for ESRD patients who wish to perform HD in the home, and no single prescription can provide optimum dialysis for all patients. Comparisons of commonly used prescriptions from around the world can be found in Tables 8 and 9. Providers must weigh clinical goals against patient preferences and overall patient and care partner burden to ensure successful home HD therapy.

Table 8. Home HD Modality Prescriptions

Modality	Sessions per Week	Session Duration, hours	QB mL/min	QD mL/min	Base, mmol/L	K^+, mmol/L	Ca^{2+}, mmol/L	PO_4 added
Traditional (standard hours)	3-3.5	3-5	300-400	500-800	HCO_3, 32-36	2	1.25	none
Alternate-Night Nocturnal	3.5	6-8	250-350	300-500	HCO_3, 28-35	2	1.25	rare
Traditional Short Daily	5-6	2.5-3.5	350-400	350-600	HCO_3, 32-36	2	1.25	none
Traditional Nocturnal	4-6	6-8	250-350	300	HCO_3, 28-35	3	1.5-1.75	20-30% of time
Low-flow Dialysate Short Daily	5-6	2.5-4	300-400	90-300	Lactate, 40-45	2	1.5	none
Low-flow Dialysate Nocturnal	4-6	6-8	300-350	83-166	Lactate, 40-45	2	1.75	none

QD = dialysis fluid flow rate; QB = blood flow rate; K^+ = potassium; Ca^{2+} = calcium; PO_4 = phosphate; HCO_3 = bicarbonate.

Table 9. Comparative Efficacy Across Prescriptions Relative to Renal Transplant

Renal Replacement Therapy	Regimen Intensity: Sessions per Week	Regimen Intensity: Session Duration, hours	Efficacy Relative to Transplant (5 = Transplant, 0 = No Treatment): Controls Volume	Controls PO_4	Minimum Adequacy[a]	Optimal Adequacy[b]
Transplant	–	–	5	5	4	5
CAPD and CCPD Without Residual Renal Function	–	–	1	1	4	0
Traditional HD (Standard Hours)	3	3-5	2	1	4	1
	3.5	3-5	3	2	4	2
Traditional Short Daily HD	5-6	2.5-3.5	5	3	4	3
Traditional Nocturnal HD	3.5	6-8	4	4	4	4
	5-6	6-8	5	5	4	5
Low-flow Dialysate Short Daily HD	5-6	2.5-4.0	5	2	4	3
Low-flow Dialysate Nocturnal HD	5-6	6-8	5	4	4	4

Note: Outcomes data available to make direct comparisons between dialysis regimens and renal transplant are limited. Relative efficacy values are largely opinion-based and provided only as estimates.

[a]Minimal adequacy is the minimally adequate dialysis dose defined in the KDOQI Clinical Practice Guidelines and Recommendations 2006 Update on Hemodialysis Adequacy.[4]

[b]Optimal adequacy is the dialysis dose provided by longer and more frequent dialysis sessions.

HD = hemodialysis; PO_4 = phosphate; CAPD = continuous ambulatory peritoneal dialysis; CCPD = continuous cycling peritoneal dialysis.

References

1. US Renal Data System. USRDS 2013 Annual Data Report: Atlas of End-Stage Renal Disease in the United States. Vol 2 – Atlas ESRD. International Comparisons. National Institutes of Health, National Institute of Diabetes and Digestive and Kidney Diseases. Bethesda, MD. 2013: 333-344. Available at: www.usrds.org/2013/pdf/v2_ch12_13.pdf. Accessed June 2, 2014.
2. Lockridge RS, Pipkin M. Short and long nightly hemodialysis in the United States. Hemodial Int. 2008;12(Suppl 1):S48-S50.
3. Twardowski Z. We should strive for optimal hemodialysis: A criticism of the hemodialysis adequacy concept. Hemodial Int. 2003;7:5-16.
4. National Kidney Foundation Kidney Diseases Outcomes Quality Initiative. 2006 Update. Hemodialysis Adequacy. 2006. Available at: http://www.kidney.org/sites/default/files/docs/12-50-0210_jag_dcp_guidelines-hd_oct06_sectiona_ofc.pdf. Accessed October 10, 2014.
5. Tentori F, Zhang J, Li Y, et al. Longer dialysis session length is associated with better intermediate outcomes and survival among patients on in-center three times per week hemodialysis: Results from the Dialysis Outcomes and Practice Patterns Study (DOPPS). Nephrol Dial Transplant. 2012;27:4180-4188.
6. Nesrallah GE, Lindsay RM, Cuerden MS, et al. Intensive hemodialysis associates with improved survival compared with conventional hemodialysis. J Am Soc Nephrol. 2012;23:696-705.
7. Johansen KL, Zhang R, Huang Y, et al. Survival and hospitalization among patients using nocturnal and short daily compared to conventional hemodialysis: A USRDS study. Kidney Int. 2009;76:984-990.
8. Lacson E Jr, Xu J, Suri S, et al. Survival with three-times weekly in-center nocturnal versus conventional hemodialysis. J Am Soc Nephrol. 2012,23:687-695.
9. Pauly RP, Klarenbach SW, Pomenda, P. Comparative survival literature in intensive hemodialysis: Limitations and future directions. Semin Dial. 2011;24:629-633.
10. Kjellstrand CM, Buoncristiani U, Ting G, et al. Short daily hemodialysis: Survival in 415 patients treated for 1006 patients-years. Nephrol Dial Transplant. 2008;23:3283-3289.
11. Jadoul M, Thumma J, Fuller DS, et al. Modifiable practices associated with sudden death among hemodialysis patients in the Dialysis Outcomes and Practice Patterns Study. Clin J Am Soc Nephrol. 2012;7:765-774.
12. Flythe JE, Curhan GC, Brunelli SM. Disentangling the ultrafiltration rate-mortality association: The respective roles of session length and weight gain. Clin J Am Soc Nephrol. 2013;8:1151-1161.
13. Flythe JE, Kimmel SE, Brunelli SM. Rapid fluid removal during dialysis is associated with cardiovascular morbidity and mortality. Kidney Int. 2011;79:250-257.
14. Hecking M, Karaboyas A, Antlanger M, et al. Significance of interdialytic weight gain versus chronic volume overload: Consensus opinion. Am J Nephrol. 2013;38:78-90.
15. Foley RN, Gilbertson DT, Murray T, Collins AJ. Long interdialytic interval and mortality among patients receiving hemodialysis. N Engl J Med. 2012;365:1099-1107.
16. Zhang H, Schaubel DE, Kalbfleisch JD, et al. Dialysis outcomes and analysis of practice patterns suggests the dialysis schedule affects day-of-week mortality. Kidney Int. 2012;81:1108-1115
17. The Australia and New Zealand Dialysis and Transplant Registry (ANZDATA). The 33rd Annual Report. Chapter 5: Haemodialysis. 2012. Available at: http://www.anzdata.org.au/v1/report_2010.html. Accessed June 2, 2014.
18. Laurent G, Charra B. The results of an 8 h thrice weekly haemodialysis schedule. Nephrol Dial Transplant. 1998;13(Suppl 6):S124-S131.

References (cont'd)

19. Schipper K, Abma TA. Coping, family and mastery: Top priorities for social science research by patients with chronic kidney disease. Nephrol Dial Transplant. 2011;26:3189-3195.

20. Van Biesen W, van der Veer SN, Murphey M, Loblova O, Davies S. Patients' perceptions of information and education for renal replacement therapy: An independent survey by the European Kidney Patients' Federation on Information and Support on Renal Replacement Therapy. PLoS One. 2014;9:e103914.

21. Gotch FA, Sargent JA, Keen ML. Whither goest Kt/V? Kidney Int. 2000;58(Suppl 76):S3-S18.

22. Lowrie EG, Laid NM, Parker TF, Sargent JA. Effect of the hemodialysis prescription of patient morbidity: Report from the National Cooperative Dialysis Study. N Engl J Med. 1981;305:1176-1181.

23. Gotch FA, Sargent JA. A mechanistic analysis of the National Cooperative Dialysis Study (NCDS). Kidney Int. 1985;28:526-534.

24. Keshaviah P. Urea kinetic and middle molecule approaches to assessing the adequacy of hemodialysis and CAPD. Kidney Int. 1993;43(Suppl 40):28–38.

25. Eknoyan G, Beck GJ, Cheung AK, et al. Effect of dialysis dose and membrane flux in maintenance hemodialysis. N Engl J Med. 2002;347:2010-2019.

26. Suri R, Depner TA, Blake PG, Heidenheim AP, Lindsay RM. Adequacy of quotidian hemodialysis. Am J Kidney Dis. 2003;42(Suppl 1):42-48.

27. Szabo E, Moody H, Hamilton T, Ang C, Kovithavongs C, Kjellstrand C. Choice of treatment improves quality of life. A study on patients undergoing dialysis. Arch Intern Med. 1997;157:1352-1356.

28. Ortiz A, Covic A, Fliser D, Fouque D, Goldsmith D, Kanbay M, et al. Epidemiology, contributors to, and clinical trials of mortality risk in chronic kidney failure. Lancet. 2014;383:1831-1843.

29. Yeun JY, Ornt DB, Depner TA. Hemodialysis. In: Taal MW, Chertow GM, Marsden PA, Skorecki K, Yu AL, Brenner BM, eds. Brenner and Rector's: The Kidney. 9th ed. Philadelphia, PA: Elsevier/Saunders. 2012;2294-2346.

30. Meyer TW, Hostetter TH. The pathophysiology of uremia. In: Taal MW, Chertow GM, Marsden PA, Skorecki K, Yu AL, Brenner BM, eds. Brenner and Rector's: The Kidney. 9th ed. Philadelphia, PA: Elsevier/Saunders. 2012;2000-2020.

31. Woods JD, Port FK, Stannard D, Blagg CR, Held PJ. Comparison of mortality with home hemodialysis and center hemodialysis: A national study. Kidney Int. 1996;49:1464-1470.

32. Saner E, Nitsch D, Descoeudres C, Frey FJ, Uehlinger DE. Outcome of home hemodialysis patients: A case-cohort study. Nephrol Dial Transplant. 2005;20:604-610.

33. Charra B, Calemard E, Ruffet M. et al. Survival as an index of adequacy of dialysis. Kidney Int. 1992;41:1286-1291.

34. Ok E, Duman S, Asci G, et al. Comparison of 4- and 8-h dialysis sessions in thrice-weekly in-centre nocturnal haemodialysis. Nephrol Dial Transplant. 2011;26:1287-1296.

35. The Australia and New Zealand Dialysis and Transplant Registry (ANZDATA) 35th Annual Report, 2012. Available at: http://www.anzdata.org.au/v1/report_2012.html. Accessed June 2, 2014.

36. Jun M, Jardine MJ, Gray N, et al. Outcomes of extended-hours hemodialysis performed prominently at home. Am J Kidney Dis. 2013;61:247-253.

37. van Eps CL, Jeffries L, Haluska B, et al. Cardiac and vascular structure and function parameters do not improve with alternate nightly home hemodialysis: An interventional cohort study. BMC Nephrol. 2011;12:51.

References (cont'd)

38. van Eps CL, Jeffries JK, Anderson JA, et al. Mineral metabolism, bone histomorphometry and vascular calcification in alternate night nocturnal haemodialysis. Nephrology (Carlton). 2007;12:224-233.

39. van Eps CL, Jeffries JK, Johnson DW, et al. Quality of life and alternate nightly nocturnal home hemodialysis. Hemodial Int. 2010;14:29-38.

40. van Eps C, Hawley C, Jeffries J, et al. Changes in serum prolactin, sex hormones and thyroid function with alternate nightly nocturnal home haemodialysis. Nephrology (Carlton). 2012;17:42-47.

41. van Eps CL, Jones M, Ng T, et al. The impact of extended-hours home hemodialysis and buttonhole cannulation technique on hospitalization rates for septic events related to dialysis access. Hemodial Int. 2010;14:451-463.

42. Suri RS, Nesrallah GE, Mainra R, et al. Daily hemodialysis: A systematic review. Clin J Am Soc Nephrol. 2006;1:33-42.

43. Culleton B, Asola M. The impact of short daily and nocturnal hemodialysis on quality of life, cardiovascular risk and survival. J Nephrol. 2011;24:405-15.

44. Diaz-Buxo JA, White SA, Himmele R. Frequent hemodialysis: A critical review. Semin Dial. 2013;26:578-589.

45. The FHN Trial Group, Chertow GM, Levin NW, et al. In-center hemodialysis six times per week versus three times per week. N Engl J Med. 2010;363:2287-2300.

46. Daugirdas JT, Chertow GM, Larive B, et al. Effects of frequent hemodialysis on measures of CKD mineral and bone disorder. J Am Soc Nephrol. 2012;23:727-738.

47. Daugirdas JT, Greene T, Rocco MV, et al. Effect of frequent hemodialysis on residual kidney function. Kidney Int. 2013;83:949-958.

48. Culleton BF, Walsh M, Klarenbach SW, et al. Effect of frequent nocturnal hemodialysis vs conventional hemodialysis on left ventricular mass and quality of life: A randomized controlled trial. JAMA. 2007;298:1291-1299.

49. Rocco MV, Lockridge RS Jr, Beck GJ, et al. The effects of frequent nocturnal home hemodialysis: The Frequent Hemodialysis Network Nocturnal Trial. Kidney Int. 2011;80:1080-1091.

50. Walsh M, Culleton B, Tonelli M, Manns B. A systematic review of the effect of nocturnal hemodialysis on blood pressure, left ventricular hypertrophy, anemia, mineral metabolism, and health-related quality of life. Kidney Int. 2005;67:1500-1508.

51. Jefferies HJ, Virk B, Schiller B, Moran J, McIntyre CW. Frequent hemodialysis schedules are associated with reduced levels of dialysis-induced cardiac injury (myocardial stunning). Clin J Am Soc Nehrol. 2011;6:1326-1332.

52. Pauly RP, Gill JS, Rose CL, et al. Survival among nocturnal home hemodialysis patients compared to kidney transplant recipients. Nephrol Dial Transplant. 2009;24:2915-2919.

53. Tennankore KK, Kim SJ, Baer HG, Chan CT. Survival and hospitalization for intensive home hemodialysis compared with kidney transplantation. J Am Soc Nephrol. 2014;25:2113-2120.

54. Hanley PJ, Pierratos A. Improvement of sleep apnea in patients with chronic renal failure who undergo nocturnal hemodialysis. N Engl J Med. 2001;344:102-107.

55. Jaber BL, Schiller B, Burkart, JM, et al. Impact of short daily hemodialysis on restless legs symptoms and sleep disturbances. Clin J Am Soc Nephrol. 2011;6:1049-1056.

56. Gangji AS, Windrim R, Gandhi S, Silverman JA, Chan CT. Successful pregnancy with nocturnal hemodialysis. Am J Kidney Dis. 2004;44:912-916.

57. Barua M, Hladunewich M, Keunen J, et al. Successful pregnancies on nocturnal home hemodialysis. Clin J Am Nephrol. 2008;3:392-396.

References (cont'd)

58. Craig KL, Podymow T, Pauly R. Intensifying renal replacement therapy during pregnancy: The role for nocturnal home hemodialysis. Int Urol Nephrol. 2010;42:137-139.

59. Hladunewich MA, Hou S, Odutayo A, et al. Intensive hemodialysis associates with improved pregnancy outcomes: A Canadian and United States cohort comparison. J Am Soc Nephrol. 2014;25:1103-1109.

60. Thompson S, Marnoch CA, Habib S, Robinson H, Pauly RP. A successful term pregnancy using in-center intensive quotidian hemodialysis. Hemodial Int. 2011;15(Suppl 1):S59-S63.

61. Kohn OF, Coe FL, Ing TS. Solute kinetics with short-daily home hemodialysis using slow dialysate flow rate. Hemodial Int. 2010;14:39-46.

62. Centers for Medicare and Medicaid Services. End Stage Renal Disease Network Organization Program 2011 Summary Annual Report. Baltimore, MD: CMS; 2012. Available at: www.esrdncc.org/index/cms-filesystem-action/resources/SAR2011_website_posting.pdf. Accessed June 3, 2014.

63. Clark WR, Turk JE Jr. The NxStage System One. Semin Dial. 2004;17:167-170.

64. Kraus M, Burkart J, Hegeman R, Solomon R, Coplon N, Moran J. A comparison of center-based vs. home-based daily hemodialysis for patients with end-stage renal disease. Hemodial Int. 2007;11:468-477.

65. Leypoldt JK, Kamerath CD, Gilson JF, Friederichs G. Dialyzer clearances and mass transfer-area coefficients for small solutes at low dialysate flow rates. ASAIO J. 2006;52:404-409.

66. Finkelstein FO, Schiller B, Daoui R, et al. At-home short daily hemodialysis improves the long-term health-related quality of life. Kidney Int. 2012;82:561-569.

67. Weinhandl ED, Liu J, Gilbertson DT, Arneson TJ, Collins AJ. Survival in daily home hemodialysis and matched thrice-weekly in-center hemodialysis patients. J Am Soc Nephrol. 2012;23:895-904.

68. Pierratos A, Ouwendyk M, Francoeur R, et al. Nocturnal hemodialysis: Three-year experience. J Am Soc Nephrol. 1998;9:859-868.

69. Lockridge R, Hara F, Pipkin M. Nightly home hemodialysis (NHHD): Can it be done with NxStage System I? (abstract). Hemodial Int. 2013;17:167.

10a Psychosocial Aspects in Home Hemodialysis: A Review

Paul N Bennett, RN, PhD[1, 2]

Dori Schatell, MS[3]

Kamal D Shah[4]

[1]Western Health, Deakin University, Melbourne, Victoria, Australia; [2]Medical Education Institute, Inc., Madison, Wisconsin, USA; [3]NephroPlus Dialysis Centres, Hyderabad, India

Implementing Hemodialysis in the Home
A Global Perspective

ISHD
International Society for Hemodialysis

CONTENTS

Abstract

Psychosocial aspects related to home hemodialysis (HD) play an important role in the success of home HD programs. Once patients commence HD at home, unique psychosocial issues related to patient and care partner burden can emerge. Proactive professional support, peer support, respite care, travel support, and financial support from the home HD healthcare team must be a priority for patient care. If the psychosocial aspects are not proactively addressed, patients receiving HD at home may return to in-center HD and the program may struggle as a result. This review provides a psychosocial guide for new start-up home HD programs.

Introduction

Home hemodialysis (HD) is far more than a medical treatment: it is a lifestyle. Home HD delivers the physical requirements needed for patients with end-stage renal disease (ESRD) to prolong their lives at a higher quality while they perform treatments in their homes. The impact of performing therapy at home and the ability of both patients and care partners (when present) to take an active part in productive day-to-day life activities requires psychosocial support from family, friends, peer groups, and the center to ensure success. There needs to be a clarification of dialysis roles for both patients and care partners through effective communication and education, with an understanding of the financial impact of performing home HD.[1-4] Appropriate support from a multidisciplinary team, including nephrologists, nurses, health psychologists, and social workers, must be a priority to ensure that patients and care partners receive the psychosocial care they need.[3,5] This review provides a psychosocial guide for new start-up home HD programs.

Professional Psychosocial Support

Patients who have any chronic disease, and those who use dialysis, in particular, are at a high risk of depression and anxiety. The Dialysis Outcomes and Practice Patterns Study (DOPPS), using the Center for Epidemiological Screening – Depression (CES-D) index, identified depression in 43% of 9382 standard in-center HD patients from 12 countries compared to nephrologists who suggested only 13.9%.[6] Diagnosing and treating depression is vital, as its presence has been strongly associated with mortality.[7] Depressed HD patients tend not to follow their treatment plans,[8] and depression among patients on HD predicts the decision to withdraw from therapy.[9]

Depression has been found to be significantly less prevalent in the home HD population (8%) than among in-center HD patients (42.3%).[10] Results from the Rehabilitation, Economics, and Everyday-Dialysis Outcomes Measurements (FREEDOM) study, indicated that 128 participants who completed 12 months of short daily home HD had a significant decrease in their depressive symptoms over the course of the study, from 41% to 27%.[11] Patients enrolled in the Frequent Hemodialysis Network (FHN) trial who received short daily HD in-center did not experience an improvement in depression.[12] While the nocturnal HD branch of the FHN trial did not find a significant difference in depression vs conventional home HD therapy, it is important to note that this study was underpowered, and that home HD of any sort may convey enough benefit that there is insufficient separation between home HD options.[13]

It is important to formally assess all HD patients, in-center and home, for depression upon initiating treatment and periodically thereafter, particularly if symptoms are observed or the patient has a change in life status (divorce, death in the family, loss of a job, hospitalization, etc.). However, many countries may not have the capacity to formally assess patients and thus a cheaper, more efficient screening process may be an option. In the United States, the Kidney Disease Quality of Life survey (KDQOL-36) is required for adult dialysis patients annually for use in care planning. More specific depression scales can also be used as a preliminary screener for depression such as the Mental Component Summary (MCS), the Patient Health Questionnaire -2 (PHQ-2), and the Beck inventory.[14] Because home HD has been found to improve health-related quality of life (HRQOL) –including mental functioning[15, 16] – and better HRQOL scores predict lower morbidity and mortality,[17] dialysis programs can consider home HD as an intervention for medically appropriate patients with failure to thrive or depression who are at risk for poor outcomes.

Patients undergoing home HD also experience mental health concerns that are not typically experienced by patients undergoing other dialysis modalities,[18] and these distinct problems are not always considered or recognized by the treatment team. It is important to proactively involve a psychologist or counselor at the beginning of training and at regular intervals of treatment to ensure that a patient's potential for anxiety and depression is explored. This approach may help keep the patient from withdrawing from home HD completely. Depression and other psychological assessment tools have been used to assess those patients considering home HD[10] and may be useful instruments to use in developing a successful start-up home HD program.

Peer Psychosocial Support

A feeling of isolation can be an issue for those patients who dialyze at home.[19] Group peer support or time spent with others who dialyze at home can help reduce isolation among home HD patients and care partners.[19, 20] Home HD training teams must acknowledge a patient's need for peer support, given the higher potential for isolation for these patients compared with patients undergoing in-center dialysis where on-site social networks develop naturally.[21] Several options for peer support are available, for example, local support groups, web-based groups, or "buddy" support from fellow patients.

Local support groups

Consumer networks and face-to-face peer support groups for patients on home HD and their care partners are increasingly more accessible. Such support groups can offer understanding and friendship from others facing similar life challenges, and can be led by healthcare professionals or other home HD patients. There may be challenges in motivating patients to attend a professionally run group, however, as patients may not welcome professionals as guest speakers or facilitators and would prefer socializing with dialysis patients going through challenges similar to their own. Peer-run groups that meet away from the dialysis clinics in more social settings, such as a restaurant, library, place of worship, or home, may be more acceptable to patients and thus better attended. The most engaging support groups will be those that are driven by the members of each group, with nephrology staff providing encouragement and support to sustain the activities and initiatives that arise.

Web-based support

Increasing numbers of dialysis patients are using the Internet for information and support.[22-24] Internet-based support and information is available 24 hours a day anywhere in the world in the form of social media discussion groups, message boards, email distribution lists, chat rooms, and others. It is important that healthcare professionals are aware of these options and encourage patients to share their stories and offer others virtual support. The Interned-based method of accessing a wide variety of information and support increases healthcare professional responsibility to ensure that patients are provided with appropriate, accurate, and evidence-based information.[22]

Individual support

One-on-one interaction between home HD patients, including care partners (if present), can lend emotional support, and get-togethers can be logistically easier to arrange than group gatherings. Such support can take place face to face or via telephone or the Internet. The center's home HD team can advocate this "buddy" system by encouraging current home HD patients and care partners to provide support to others. Contact information and basic demographic data (eg, age, gender, work status) can be recorded (with permission) to enable patients with similar situations and interests to be matched. A patient who has expressed interest in being a support "buddy" previously but has not immediately been serving in this role should be contacted again before his or her name is given to a patient; this ensures that the prospective support patient is still interested in participating in the buddy program. Background information about the patient who needs support should also be communicated to the potential buddy at this time. Buddies should be cautioned to divert all specific medical questions a patient may have to the care team as each patient's treatment and prescriptions are different. This buddy system can be easily set up within each dialysis program, region, or country.

Dialysis Partner or Solo?

A patient can dialyze independently or with the assistance of a care partner who may be a spouse, parent, child, sibling, friend, or neighbor. There is a range of care partner involvement, from a self-dialyzing patient with no partner[25]—a model that is encouraged or required in some countries,[26, 27] but discouraged or forbidden in others—to full care in those cases where a patient requires total assistance with all activities of daily living, including management of home HD.[3, 25] Any time a care partner is present for home HD, his or her involvement can fall anywhere along this care continuum. A partner's level of participation in care may also vary over time, as the patient becomes more confident and adept or if a health setback reduces the patient's physical or cognitive abilities. Nephrologists, nurses, social workers, and especially home HD training staff who encourage the maximal degree of patient independence for self-care may help minimize dialysis care partner burnout.[28] In particular, cannulation can be extremely stressful for dialysis care partners. It is best that patients learn to self-cannulate, if possible, to minimize care partner burnout associated with this task.[29] If a care partner becomes unable or unwilling to provide care, a patient on home HD who requires care partner assistance may be unable to continue treatment at home.

The chances for home HD success may improve if dialysis patients and partners offer social and emotional support to each other and clearly define their healthcare roles.[30] Center staff who create an expectation that self-dialysis is the norm and provide positive feedback for each step along this path goes a long way toward helping patients and dialysis care partners succeed. A study conducted by Wise et al[3] identified four dialysis partner-patient team types: "thriving", "surviving", "martyrdom", and "seeking [other options]". Home HD with thriving and surviving teams was more successful than home HD with the martyrdom and seeking partnerships team types. Observing warning signs of martyrdom and looking for other options may mean that psychosocial support may be needed to reduce the potential for home HD burnout and withdrawal.[3]

Care partners who show an interest in home HD, who are encouraging and express open communication about expectations, and who urge the patient to do as much as he or she is able to do independently are strategies that can improve the success rate of the program. It is wise to confront the issue of care partner burnout up front during training and explain how it can be addressed (eg, shifting of care tasks onto the patient, identifying backup care partners, and using respite services).[31] This way, patients will not be surprised if one day the therapy becomes untenable for the care partner.

Dialysis Care Partner Considerations

It is important that patients and their care partners are educated regarding all aspects of home HD. Ensuring that dialysis care partners learn how to access respite and relevant resources is a critical part of a home HD program that involves or requires care partners.[32] Proactive monitoring of patients by the overseeing unit and identifying potential stressors early may help eliminate care partner fatigue and assuage a partner's feelings of guilt about wanting, or needing, to take a break.[19, 33] Comprehensive resources may be of benefit to those care partners who are responsible for coping with a home HD patient's activities of daily living (i.e., feeding, bathing, toileting, etc) and performing medical tasks (suctioning, cannulating, supply monitoring and ordering, etc.). Intermittent respite care by dialysis professionals can relieve care partner burden and may make the difference between a patient's remaining in home HD or withdrawing from this modality entirely.

Care partners, regardless of level of involvement with home HD treatments, may benefit from peer support from other home dialysis partners to help them to reduce their own feelings of isolation. Just as for patients, centers should develop local face-to-face and online support options for care partners.[20] Good communication between patients on home HD and their respective dialysis care partners (if involved) is vital. The home dialysis team needs to develop strategies to identify the early signs of isolation, poor partner communication, and partner-patient friction, and provide the necessary support tools to address these problems.

The term "care partner" (not "caregiver" or "carer") has been deliberately used in this module. "Caregiver" and "carer" imply an individual who is deeply immersed in and feels responsible for the patient's day-to-day home HD treatments, including machine set-up, cannulation, monitoring, clean-up, reporting, and supply ordering. While assistance from a care partner may be a necessity for some patients, without appropriate support mechanisms, this is a recipe for burnout and is, at least anecdotally, a substantial cause of patient withdrawal from the home HD program. The "patient-does-most" model has achieved the greatest success, as long as patients are capable of learning and performing home HD safely and independently.[26]

Respite Care for Home HD

Proactive respite for patients and dialysis care partners may make the difference between home HD success and failure. Both patients and partners should be informed about the availability of respite care during and after training, and ensure that they know how to access these services when it is wanted or needed (ie, due to a sudden illness or travel of a care partner). Respite programs may offer a nurse or other paid respite care provider who could visit the home on a temporary basis to perform the designated care partner's dialysis tasks, allowing the designated care partner to take time off from the role.[33] This respite model is likely to be preferred by both patients and care partners, as the patient's setting and dialysis prescription will not change, and the respite care provider may be trusted by both individuals (particularly important when the patient does not self-cannulate). Program respite may also require access to a dialysis machine at a local satellite unit or other home training unit that can offer this service.[34] This in-center respite model may be much less appealing, particularly if patients who use frequent and/or extended home HD must switch to conventional, thrice-weekly treatments and also use an unknown cannulator. Respite care could be automatically planned for 1 to 4 weeks per year in the home HD program. The type of respite required will be determined by the patient and dialysis care partner to fit their own unique situation.

Trained dialysis assistance

In some countries, professionals who are trained in dialysis may come to the home and assist the patient with dialysis treatments. Government-sponsored financial support is available in some regions, but it is not common.[35] So-called staff-assisted home HD could be a convenient alternative for patients who do not have a dialysis care partner, who do not want to do dialysis-related activities by themselves, and who can afford to pay a salary or a per-treatment fee to a helper.[36] However, there is a danger that patients may rely on these assistants too heavily[37]; therefore, appropriately vigilant management of this role by the home HD team is required to prevent overreliance.

Travel and Holidays

Travel and holidays are an important part of many patients' lives and, depending on the machine used, can be a great challenge to those on home HD.[38, 39] Although there may be an increased risk of complications such as infection,[40] assisting and encouraging home HD patients to enjoy a holiday may provide them with some normality, improve their quality of life, and keep them on home HD longer.[41] Because some patients may believe that travel is not possible while they undergo dialysis, it is vital that healthcare professionals make every effort to help patients to see the possibilities.[42] Independent or organized holidays[43] can improve quality of life, self-image, and self-confidence.

Newer, smaller home HD machines specifically designed to be more mobile can enable patients to travel more independently.[44] Many international airlines now accept these smaller machines as essential medical equipment at no charge. Typically, supplies must be shipped to the patient's travel destination, and there may or may not be a fee the patient must pay, depending on distance and location. Regional travel in caravans or recreational vehicles fitted with a hemodialysis machine is possible.[44, 45] It is necessary for the home HD team to advise patients to research and identify clinics at their destinations that can support them if necessary during their trips.[43]

To travel safely can be a logistical challenge that can be mitigated with help from the home HD team. Home HD patients who want to travel may need to plan for holidays from several months to as much as a year in advance.[46] Home HD staff can assist patients with travel dialysis bookings, review the administration tasks involved during travel, revisit blood test requirements, provide medication storage information as patients travel, and deliver specific nutrition education. Those home HD patients wanting to travel who switch from frequent and nocturnal home HD treatments to thrice weekly dialysis sessions to accommodate their travel plans may need to consider the increased dietary restrictions required for this regimen. This may mean that patients should schedule a renal dietitian consult before a trip[43] as a refresher to review the importance of restricting potassium in the diet to eliminate the chance of lethal high serum potassium levels and to review the symptoms of hyperkalemia. Furthermore, if patients will be away for an extended period, they should be encouraged to undergo blood testing at a clinic at their destination.

Financial Consideration

Home HD is considered more cost-effective than hospital or community satellite hemodialysis.[47] Some costs, however, may shift from the center to the patient, and these costs are perceived by some patients as a barrier to home HD.[48] It is vital that patients who choose home HD not be financially burdened. Considering the unique financial issues to home HD care is particularly important for those centers establishing new home HD programs. Reimbursement models may not take into consideration the cost shifting associated with home HD care. Costs beyond the machine and water treatment systems include ongoing dialysis partner payments (country dependent); disability pensions; electricity and water usage; medications; dialysis consumables; dialysis chairs; dressings; and equipment for health monitoring, such as scales and blood pressure machines.[49] Assistance with these costs through reimbursement can be facilitated by the home HD team to avoid financial burden, however small it may appear, and help maintain patients on home HD.

Dialysis care partner costs may include accommodation or travel during training. In some countries, care partners may be eligible for a Carer's Pension or other financial support through local or regional government sources. In some countries, government-supported Social Security or pension systems may make annual payments to patients whose home energy costs increase due to the use of essential medical equipment for a disability or health condition, and these payments may apply to home HD therapies. In other countries, there is minimal government or insurance company support for home HD; patients may pay out of pocket.[50] Some providers have begun to offer home HD programs where patients pay a monthly equipment rental fee and do not have to purchase the equipment. In such cases, insurance companies may pay the equivalent of an in-center HD session, while the rest of the cost is borne by the patient. Such programs mainly offer staff-assisted HD. There are still cost hurdles to overcome in many countries and these need to be explored thoroughly before attempting to develop a home HD program.

Summary

Psychosocial aspects for patients and care partners in home HD are an important component to consider when starting a new home HD program. Many patients around the world who perform home HD have been able to fit dialysis into their lifestyles rather than allowing the restrictions of dialysis to dominate their lives. Although the improved lifestyle aspects associated with home HD are appealing, healthcare teams must monitor each patient and care partner to ensure the therapy does not increase their psychosocial burden. Strategies to prevent increased burden include initiating proactive professional support, peer support, respite support, travel support, and financial support, all of which contribute to a sustainable home HD program.

References

1. Culleton BF, Asola MR. The impact of short daily and nocturnal hemodialysis on quality of life, cardiovascular risk and survival. J Nephrol. 2011; 24:405-415.
2. Nearhos J, Van Eps C, Connor J. Psychological factors associated with successful outcomes in home haemodialysis. Nephrology. 2013;18:505-509.
3. Wise M, Schatell D, Klicko K, Burdan A, Showers M. Successful daily home hemodialysis patient-care partner dyads: Benefits outweigh burdens. \Hemodial Int. 2010;14:278-288.
4. Young BA, Chan C, Blagg C, et al. How to overcome barriers and establish a successful home HD program. Clin J Am Soc Nephrol. 2012;7:2023-2032.
5. Bennett P, Oppermann W. Are nurses the key to the increased uptake of frequent nocturnal home haemodialysis in Australia? Ren Soc Aust J. 2006;2:22-29.
6. Lopes AA, Albert JM, Young EW, et al. Screening for depression in hemodialysis patients: Associations with diagnosis, treatment, and outcomes in the DOPPS. Kidney Int. 2004;66:2047-2053.
7. Farrokhi F, Abedi N, Beyene J, Kurdyak P, Jassal SV. Association between depression and mortality in patients receiving long-term dialysis: A systematic review and meta-analysis. Am J Kidney Dis. 2014;63:623-635.
8. Rosenthal Asher D, Ver Halen N, Cukor D. Depression and nonadherence predict mortality in hemodialysis treated end-stage renal disease patients. Hemodialysis Int. 2012;16:387-393.
9. McDade-Montez EA, Christensen AJ, Cvengros JA, Lawton WJ. The role of depression symptoms in dialysis withdrawal. Health Psychol. 2006;25:198-204.
10. Griva K, Davenport A, Harrison M, Newman S. An evaluation of illness, treatment perceptions, and depression in hospital- vs. home-based dialysis modalities. J Psychosom Res. 2010;69:363-370.
11. Jaber BL, Lee Y, Collins AJ, et al. Effect of daily hemodialysis on depressive symptoms and postdialysis recovery time: Interim report from the FREEDOM (Following Rehabilitation, Economics and Everyday-Dialysis Outcome Measurements) study. Am J Kidney Dis. 2010;56:531-539.
12. Unruh ML, Larive B, Chertow GM, et al. Effects of 6-times-weekly versus 3-times-weekly hemodialysis on depressive symptoms and self-reported mental health: Frequent Hemodialysis Network (FHN) trials. Am J Kidney Dis. 2013;61:748-758.
13. Rocco MV, Lockridge RS Jr, Beck GJ, et al. The effects of frequent nocturnal home hemodialysis: the Frequent Hemodialysis Network Nocturnal Trial. Kidney Int. 2011;80:1080-1091.
14. DeOreo PB. Hemodialysis patient-assessed functional health status predicts continued survival, hospitalization, and dialysis-attendance compliance. Am J Kidney Dis. 1997;30:204-212.
15. Heidenheim AP, Muirhead N, Moist L, Lindsay RM. Patient quality of life on quotidian hemodialysis. Am J Kidney Dis. 2003;42(1 Suppl):36-41.
16. Ting GO, Kjellstrand C, Freitas T, Carrie BJ, Zarghamee S. Long-term study of high-comorbidity ESRD patients converted from conventional to short daily hemodialysis. Am J Kidney Dis. 2003;42:1020-1035.
17. Lowrie EG, Curtin RB, LePain N, Schatell D. Medical Outcomes Study Short Form-36: A consistent and powerful predictor of morbidity and mortality in dialysis patients. Am J Kidney Dis. 2003;41:1286-1292.
18. Richmond JM, Lindsay RM, Burton HJ, Conley J, Wai L. Psychological and physiological factors predicting the outcome on home hemodialysis. Clin Nephrol. 1982;17:109-113.
19. Tong A, Palmer S, Manns B, et al. The beliefs and expectations of patients and caregivers about home haemodialysis: An interview study. BMJ Open. 2013;3:1-14.
20. Wong J, Eakin J, Migram P, Cafazzo JA, Halifax NV, Chan CT.

References (cont'd)

Patients' experiences with learning a complex medical device for the self-administration of nocturnal home hemodialysis. Nephrol Nurs J. 2009;36:27-32.

21. Bennett PN. Satellite dialysis nursing: technology, caring and power. J Adv Nurs. 2011;67:149-157.
22. Buettner K, Fadem SZ. The Internet as a tool for the renal community. Adv Chronic Kidney Dis. 2008;15:73-82.
23. Schatell D, Wise M, Klicko K, Becker BN. In-center hemodialysis patients' use of the Internet in the United States: A national survey. Am J Kidney Dis. 2006;48:285-291.
24. Seto E, Cafazzo JA, Rizo C, Bonert M, Fong E, Chan CT. Internet use by end-stage renal disease patients. Hemodial Int. 2007;11:328-332.
25. Guza J. "Solo" hemodialysis. Nephrol Nurse. 1982;4:26-28.
26. Agar JWM. Home hemodialysis in Australia and New Zealand: Practical problems and solutions. Hemodial Int. 2008;12:S26-S32.
27. Malmström R, Muroma-Karttunen R, Kilpiä M, Honkanen E. Experiences on home hemodialysis without an assistant. Hemodial Int. 2003;7:73-104.
28. Lowry MR, Atcherson E. Spouse-assistants' adjustment to home hemodialysis. J Chronic Dis. 1984;37:293-300.
29. Moran J, Kraus M. Starting a Home Hemodialysis Program. Semin Dial. 2007;20:35-39.
30. Courts NF. Psychosocial adjustment of patients on home hemodialysis and their dialysis partners. Clin Nurs Res. 2000;9:177-190.
31. Belasco AG, Sesso R. Burden and quality of life of caregivers for hemodialysis patients. Am J Kidney Dis. 2002;39:805-812.
32. Mollaoğlu M, Kayataş M, Yürügen B. Effects on caregiver burden of education related to home care in patients undergoing hemodialysis. Hemodial Int. 2013;17:413-420.
33. Peterson KJ. Psychosocial adjustment of the family caregiver: home hemodialysis as an example. Soc Work Health Care. 1985;10:15-32.
34. Kerr PG, Agar JWM, Hawley CM. Alternate night nocturnal hemodialysis: The Australian experience. Semin Dial. 2011;24:664-667.
35. McGregor D, Buttimore A, Robson R, Little P, Morton J, Lynn K. Thirty years of universal home dialysis in Christchurch. N Z Med J. 2000;113:27-29.
36. Lindsay R, Leitch R. Home hemodialysis. In: Hörl W, Koch K, Lindsay R, Ronco C, Winchester J, eds. Replacement of Renal Function by Dialysis. Dordrecht, the Netherlands, Springer. 2004;1553-1566.
37. Blagg C. Quality of care in home dialysis. In: Henderson L, Thuma R, eds. Quality Assurance in Dialysis. Dordrecht, the Netherlands, Springer. 1994;63-83.
38. Bennett PN, Bonner A, Andrew J, Nandkumar J, Au C. Using images to communicate the hidden struggles of life on dialysis. J Commun Healthc. 2013;6:12-21.
39. Morton RL, Tong A, Webster AC, Snelling P, Howard K. Characteristics of dialysis important to patients and family caregivers: a mixed methods approach. Nephrol Dial Transplant. 2011;26:4038-4046.
40. Corbett RW, Prout V, Haynes D, Edwards C, Frankel AH. Problems associated with hemodialysis and travel. J Travel Med. 2014:21:255-259.
41. Thodis ED, Oreopoulos DG. Home dialysis first: a new paradigm for new ESRD patients. J Nephrol. 2011;24:398-404.
42. Agar JW, Mahadevan K, Knight R, Antonis ML, Somerville CA. 'Flexible' or 'lifestyle' dialysis: Is this the way forward? Nephrology. 2005;10:525-529.
43. Black K. Travel and dialysis: How can nurses help? Educational supplement. Ren Soc Aust J. 2009;5:152-154.
44. Doss-McQuitty S. Alternative dialysis therapies–why all the interest? Nephrol Nurse J.. 2013;40:17-20.

References (cont'd)

45. Schatell D. Five practical steps you can take to promote successful home dialysis. Dial Transplant. 2010;39:326-327.

46. Kotton CN, Hibberd PL, the AST Infectious Disease Community of Practice. Travel medicine and transplant tourism in solid organ transplantation. Am J Transplant. 2013;13(Suppl 4):337-347.

47. Walker R, Marshall M, Morton RL, McFarlane P, Howard K. The cost-effectiveness of contemporary home haemodialysis modalities compared to facility haemodialysis: A systematic review of full economic evaluations. Nephrology. 2014;19:459-470.

48. Pipkin M, Eggers PW, Larive B, et al. Recruitment and training for home hemodialysis: experience and lessons from the Nocturnal Dialysis Trial. Clin J Am Soc Nephrol. 2010;5:1614-1620.

49. McFarlane P, Komenda P. Economic Considerations in Frequent Home Hemodialysis. Semin Dial. 2011;24:678-683.

50. Komenda P, Sood MM. The economics of home dialysis: acting for the individual while planning responsibly for the population. Adv Chronic Kidney Dis. 2009;16:198-204.

10b Psychosocial Guide for Healthcare Professionals

Paul N Bennett, RN, PhD[1]

Dori Schatell, MS[2]

Kamal D Shah[3]

[1]Western Health, Deakin University, Melbourne, Victoria, Australia; [2]Medical Education Institute, Inc., Madison, Wisconsin, USA; [3]NephroPlus Dialysis Centres, Hyderabad, India

Implementing Hemodialysis in the Home
A Global Perspective

ISHD
International Society for Hemodialysis

CONTENTS

Introduction

Home hemodialysis (HD) is far more than a medical treatment: it is a *lifestyle*. For patients and dialysis care partners* (when present) to succeed, we must pay attention to such psychosocial aspects of care as the impact of therapy on day-to-day life, including offering support for patients and care partners, gaining social support from peers, defining partner roles, opening lines of communication, addressing depression, taking advantage of opportunities to travel, and considering the financial impact of home HD. Psychosocial factors are significant in a home HD program,[1] and psychosocial support from nephrologists, nurses, health psychologists, and social workers should thus be a priority for patient care.

Care Partner

A care partner is someone who assists a patient with home HD treatment, often a family member or friend, but not all home HD patients require a care partner. Please note the deliberate use of the term "care partner"—not "caregiver." While in the United States there is a regrettable tendency to turn a care partner into a de facto dialysis technician who undertakes machine set-up, cannulation, monitoring, clean-up, reporting, and even supply ordering, this model is not the case in most of the rest of the world, nor is it ideal. Rather, it is best for each patient to take on as many of the responsibilities for dialysis treatment as she or he is capable of learning and performing safely and independently, with the partner present for emotional support. (The amount of self-care a patient can do is likely to change over time.) The term "caregiver" implies an individual who is deeply immersed in the patient's day-to-day home HD treatments, which is a recipe for burnout and, at least anecdotally, a substantial cause of home HD dropout.

Psychosocial Support

Isolation can be an issue for those who dialyze at home and their care partners. Group peer support or time spent with individual "buddies" can help reduce isolation among home HD patients and partners. It is wise for home training teams to acknowledge the need for peer support, given the numbers of patients who may stay in-center because they have no other social outlet. Several options for peer support are described below.

Local Support Groups

Your country may have consumer networks and face-to-face peer support groups for people on dialysis, and perhaps even specifically for home HD. Such groups can offer understanding and friendship to others who are faced with similar life challenges. If there is a local group near your clinic, provide the contact information to patients and encourage them to attend.

If your area does not have these types of support groups, interested home HD patients and/or dialysis care partners may wish to start one of their own. Clinics often report challenges getting patients to attend clinic- or professional-run groups. Peer-run groups that meet outside of the dialysis clinic in a social setting such as a restaurant, library, place of worship, or home may be more acceptable to patients, and thus better attended. Patient groups may—or may not—welcome professionals as guest speakers or facilitators. Each group may differ, and the choice of speakers needs to belong to the members. Patients and dialysis care partners may benefit from having separate groups so members of each group can speak freely without worrying about upsetting a loved one.

Web-based Support

For Internet-savvy patients, online support is available 24 hours a day anywhere in the world, in the form of social media discussion groups, message boards, email listservs, chat rooms, and others. For example, a Facebook discussion group that includes patients undergoing home HD can be found here, and other groups are available online in Google+, Yahoo, etc. Because each person's treatment and prescriptions are different, caution patients not to follow medical advice of any kind discussed in these groups without first checking with their own care teams.

Buddy Support

One-on-one "buddy" support can help patients and/or dialysis partners, and can be logistically easier to arrange than group support. Such support can be face-to-face or via telephone or the Internet. Talk to patients and dialysis partners and see if they would like to provide support to others. If so, keep their contact information and basic demographics (age, gender, work status, cause of kidney disease, etc), so you can attempt to match like individuals. It may be wise to recontact a potential buddy before giving out his or her name to a patient, to protect the buddy's privacy and ensure that he or she is still available and interested in participating. It is important to provide participating buddies with some general nonmedical background information about the patient who needs support. Caution buddies to divert all medical questions to the care team, as each person's treatment and prescriptions are different.

Useful Resources*

For those who want to start a peer support group.

- The Community Toolbox. Creating and Facilitating Peer Support Groups
- Manuals and Workbooks for Starting and Running Support Groups

*For hyperlinks see Web version of Manual on ISHD.org

Practice Tip

An example of a buddy support system can be found at http://homedialyzorsunited.org/hdu-buddies/. This system could be set up in your own program, region, or country.

Dialysis Partner or Solo?

The patient is always involved in home HD as the recipient of treatment. However, there is a continuum of care partner involvement, from 0% (self-dialyzing patient with no partner; a model that is encouraged or required in some countries, but discouraged or forbidden in others) to 100% (severely disabled patient who requires total care for all activities of daily living as well as home HD). Dialysis care partners are most often spouses or significant others. However, some are parents, children, siblings, friends, or neighbors. Any time a partner is present for home HD, his or her involvement can fall anywhere along the 0% to 100% continuum, and the level of care partner participation in care may vary over time, either as a patient becomes more confident and adept, or if a health setback reduces his or her physical or cognitive abilities.

Nephrologists, nurses, social workers, and especially home HD training staff who *encourage the maximal degree of patient independence for self-care* may help minimize dialysis partner burnout. In particular, cannulation can be extremely stressful for dialysis partners and is best undertaken by the patients themselves, if possible (See "The Care and Keeping of Vascular Access for Home Hemodialysis Patients" module). If a partner becomes unable or unwilling to provide care, a patient on home HD who requires partner assistance is unlikely to be able to continue at home.

The chances for home HD success may improve if dialysis care partners (when present) offer social and emotional support to the able patient, while taking on as few of the instrumental tasks as possible.[2] Creating an expectation that self-dialysis is the norm and providing positive feedback for each step along this path can go a long way toward helping patients and dialysis care partners succeed. A study conducted by Wise et al identified 4 dialysis partner/patient team types, 2 of which in the study appeared, at least in the short run, to be far more successful than the others.[2]

1. *Thriving* – Both the patient and dialysis partner flourish with the new challenge they face together. They work as a team and use the HD time as couple time to strengthen their relationship.
2. *Surviving* – Home HD does not make a patient and the dialysis partner stronger, but they successfully adjust to the challenges and succeed.
3. *Martyrdom* – A patient expects support from a dialysis partner who provides it resentfully. Research suggests that burdening a partner is associated with home HD failure.
4. *Seeking Other Options* – A patient may insist that his or her home treatment is burdening the dialysis partner—even though the care partner may not agree. The patient plans to switch to in-center care.

Dialysis Partner Considerations

Ensuring that dialysis partners learn how to access relevant resources is a critical part of a home HD program that involves or requires partners. Dialysis partners who are moderately or highly involved in day-to-day home HD treatments need to feel that their questions will be answered by a very patient home dialysis staff at any time of the day or night. Dialysis partners may need to take time off to refresh themselves and renew their energy by socializing with friends or family or pursuing a hobby, even if only for a few hours at a time. (And they need to hear from dialysis staff that time away will not only help the patient, but also themselves, and that partners should not feel guilty about wanting a break.) Partners also need to know that they or the patient can get short- or longer-term respite care when and if it is needed.

Generic care partner resources may be of benefit to those partners whose role in home HD and other activities of daily living and medical tasks is all encompassing (ie, feeding, bathing, toileting, suctioning, etc). Given the high degree of dialysis care partner burnout, support for both patients and care partners is vital to ensure home HD program success.

All care partners, regardless of level of involvement with home HD treatments, may benefit from peer support from other home HD partners. Tell them about local face-to-face and online support options that may help them to reduce their own isolation. Good communication between patients on home HD and dialysis partners is vital. Encouraging patients and dialysis partners to work as a team can bring them closer together (Table 1).

Practice Tip

Observing couples who show an interest in home HD, encouraging open communication about expectations, and urging the patient to do as much as he or she is able are strategies that may help improve the success rate of your program. It is wise to confront the issue of care partner burnout up front during training, and explain how it can be addressed (ie, through shifting of care tasks onto the patient, identifying backup care partners, and using respite services). This way, patients will not be surprised if one day the therapy becomes untenable for the partner.

Useful Resources*

- Caregiving Basics: Tips for Caregivers
- Caregiver.com
- Caring for Caregivers
- Family Caregiver Support Network
- US Administration on Aging – What states are required to do to help caregivers
- Carers UK
- Carers Support UK

*For hyperlinks please see Web version of Manual on ISHD.org

Table 1. Communication Strategies for Trainers to Share with Patients and Care Partners
Make eye contact–look at your partner
Tell your partner that you appreciate things he or she does
Use forms of touch that you are both comfortable with (eg, a pat on the back or hug)
Celebrate milestones (ie, each year on dialysis as 1 year more of life together)
Negotiate home dialysis task changes if your situation changes
Talk about your goals and dreams, and steps you'll take to reach them

Respite Care for Home HD

Respite care is the provision of temporary or part-time care by healthcare professionals and provides relief to the patient and their care partner from having to perform HD at home. Proactive respite care for patients and dialysis partners may make the difference between home HD success and failure, although there are no studies in adults that examine this premise. Encourage both partners to exercise, get out socially, support others, engage in hobbies, and be active in a community. Life should NOT be about dialysis! Alert both patients and partners to the availability of respite care during training and afterward, and ensure that they know how to access the service when it is wanted or needed (ie, due to a sudden illness or travel of a care partner).

Respite programs may offer a nurse or other paid care assistance who could visit the home on a temporary basis to take on the chosen care partner's dialysis tasks, providing the partner with time off from the role. This respite model is likely to be preferred by both patients and care partners, as the patient's setting and dialysis prescription will not change, and the respite care provider may be trusted by both individuals (particularly important when the patient does not self-cannulate).

Program respite may also require access to a dialysis machine at a local satellite unit or other home training unit that can offer this service. This respite model may be much less appealing, particularly if patients who use frequent and/or extended home HD must switch to conventional, thrice weekly treatments and also use an unknown individual as the cannulator.

Plan to include 1 to 4 weeks per year of respite care in your renal program. The type of respite required will be determined by the patient and dialysis partner and their own unique situation.

Trained Dialysis Assistance

In some countries, professionals who are trained in dialysis may come to the home and assist with dialysis treatments. So-called "staff-assisted" home HD could be a convenient alternative for patients who do not have a dialysis partner, do not want to do everything by themselves, and can afford to pay a monthly salary or a per-treatment fee to a helper. The salary or fee would vary depending on the tasks a helper would need to do.

Depression

In a small study of nocturnal home HD (N = 67) participants and care partners, depression criteria were met by 47% of patients and 25% of care partners.[3] Other research has found that depression will not subside without treatment,[4] and can substantially reduce the ability of an individual to follow the treatment plan. The Kidney Disease Quality of Life survey (KDQOL-36; required to be performed at least annually in the United States) can be used as an initial assessment tool for determining depression, with a mental functioning score of 42 or less suggesting that additional screening is needed. The Center for Epidemiologic Studies Depression Scale Revised (CESD-R)
is a valid, reliable, 20-question tool to assess for clinical depression that is easily scored by hand. You can access the CES-D in English here.

Proactively involving a psychologist at the beginning of training and at regular intervals of treatment can ensure that the potential for anxiety and depression for both patients and care partners are explored, and may help keep patients from withdrawing from home HD unnecessarily (Table 2).

Table 2. Informal Questions to Detect Anxiety and Depression
Are you often struggling to get out of bed and do daily activities?
Do you cry often?
Do you feel angry easily for no reason?
Have you stopped paying attention to how you look?
Are you eating for comfort or refusing to eat at all?
Are you thinking of harming yourself?

Travel and Holidays/ Vacations

Travel and holidays/vacations are an important part of many peoples' lives. Assisting and encouraging home HD patients to enjoy a holiday/vacation may provide them with some normality, improve their quality of life, and keep them on home HD longer. Because some patients may believe that travel is not possible while they are undergoing dialysis, it is vital that health professionals make every effort to help patients to see the possibilities. Patients on home HD can indeed travel, but may require staff assistance, depending on the machine. Machines that are more portable allow the patient to bring the machine along in a carrier in a car, plane, ship, or train. Many international airlines now accept the machines as essential medical equipment at no charge, and some allow 2-days' worth of dialysate to accompany the machine as long as the dialysate is in the original packaging. Supplies must be shipped to the travel destination, for which there may or may not be a fee the patient must pay, depending on distance and location. A hotel may charge a package receiving fee; it is worth asking if this fee can be waived due to the lifesaving nature of the delivery. Advise patients who bring their own machines along for travel to identify a clinic at their destination that can support them if necessary during the trip. Dialysis travel checklists and information can be found at:

- http://www.davita.com/services/travel-support/travel-tips-and-articles/travel-checklist-for-people-on-dialysis/s/5734
- http://www.nwkidney.org/dialysis/traveling/checklist.html
- http://www.kidney.org.au/ForPatients/DialysisandTravel/tabid/608/Default.aspx

For those patients with a non-portable machine, planning for holidays/vacations may be required from several months to as much as a year in advance. Clinic staff must assist with travel dialysis bookings and the administration that is involved (blood tests, treatment information).

Travel can change dialysis logistics. The food at another location may be different, as may the treatment schedules, so patients will need to be flexible regarding their own self-care. Further, blood pressure may change with travel, so dose adjustment of antihypertensive medications may be necessary. Special medication storage may be required for drugs such as erythropoietin and insulin that must be kept within a certain temperature range.

Financial and Cost Considerations

Real and perceived costs may determine the success of maintaining people on home HD. People who choose home HD should not be financially burdened by it. If in-center HD incurs minimal or no cost to the patient, home HD must provide a comparable cost structure, or cost will be a disincentive. Sharing the cost implications with interested patients may dispel myths and make home HD more appealing. In some countries, patients wrongly believe that they must buy a home HD machine, and many do not know that their government-funded healthcare helps pay for most dialysis, dialysis partners, utility costs, and equipment (see "Funding and Planning: What You Need to Know for Starting or Expanding a Home Hemodialysis Program" module).

Practice Tip

Patients who switch from nocturnal and home HD treatments to standard ones during travel risk lethal hyperkalemia if they do not adapt their diets. A visit with a renal dietitian or at least a revisiting of the need to restrict potassium (and reexamining which foods and beverages contain it) and discussing the symptoms of hyperkalemia before a trip can help avert high serum potassium. Blood tests are encouraged at the destination clinic if patients will be away for an extended period.

Costs for dialysis care partners may include accommodation or travel during training. In some countries (not the United States), care partners may be eligible for a Carer's Pension or other financial support through local or regional government sources. Examples of funding support in Australia can be found here.

Healthcare financing systems vary by country, and in some cases within regions of the same country. For home HD, costs beyond the machine and water treatment include ongoing dialysis partner payments (country-dependent), disability pensions, electricity and water usage, medications, dialysis consumables, dialysis chairs, medications, dressings, and equipment for health monitoring, such as scales and blood pressure machines.

In some countries, the social security/pension system may make annual payments to people whose home energy costs increase due to the use of essential medical equipment for a disability or health condition, and these payments may apply to home HD therapies.

In other countries, such as India, there is currently minimal government or insurance company support for home HD; patients must pay out of pocket. Some providers have started to offer home HD programs where patients pay a monthly equipment rental fee and do not have to buy the equipment. In such cases, insurance companies may pay the equivalent of an in-center HD session, while the rest of the cost is borne by the patient. Such programs mainly offer staff-assisted HD.

Infrastructure Support

In countries that have infrastructure support in place for home HD, it may be hard to imagine its absence. However, in some parts of the world where home HD is relatively new, there may not be adequate infrastructure in place to fully support home HD (eg, telephone backup for home patients and technicians to make electrical and water updates for a home HD machine). It is important to acknowledge that patients who lack such support may feel even more anxious and isolated than they already would at the prospect of having to dialyze at home. Providing answers to questions like, "What do I do if I have a problem?" is vital to allow these patients to succeed at home. In these cases, online peer support may make the difference between success and failure (see "Patient Safety in Home Hemodialysis" module).

Summary

In this module, we have provided you with information regarding the psychosocial aspects related to home hemodialysis. Although there are many other important facets to consider, many people around the world who perform home HD have been able to fit dialysis into their lifestyles rather than allowing the restrictions of dialysis to dominate their lives. We wish you all the best with the development of your program and encourage you to consider the information we have provided above.

References

1. Nearhos J, Van Eps C, Connor J. Psychological factors associated with successful outcomes in home haemodialysis. Nephrology (Carlton). 2013;18:505-509.
2. Wise M, Schatell D, Klicko K, Burdan A, Showers M. Successful daily home hemodialysis patient-care partner dyads: benefits outweigh burdens. Hemodial Int. 2010;14:278-288.
3. Rioux JP, Narayanan R, Chan CT. Caregiver burden among nocturnal home hemodialysis patients. Hemodial Int. 2012;16:214-219.
4. Soykan A, Boztas H, Kutlay S, et al. Depression and its 6-month course in untreated hemodialysis patients: a preliminary prospective follow-up study in Turkey. Int J Behav Med. 2004;11:243-246.

10c Psychosocial Guide for Patients, Families, and Dialysis Partners

Kamal D Shah[1]

Dori Schatell, MS[2]

Paul N Bennett, RN, PhD[3]

[1]Director and Cofounder, Nephroplus, Hyderabad, India, [2]Executive Director, Medical Education Institute, Inc, Catonsville, Maryland, United States; [3]Associate Professor, Western Health, Deakin University, Melbourne, Victoria, Australia

Implementing Hemodialysis in the Home
A Global Perspective

ISHD
International Society for Hemodialysis

CONTENTS

This module was predominantly authored by Kamal D Shah, a dialysis patient since July 1997. Kamal lives in India and has been on home hemodialysis (HD) since May 2006. He does nocturnal HD 7 hours each night, 6 nights per week, assisted by a trained dialysis technician. Kamal works full-time, blogs, swims every day, and travels regularly— things, he says, have been made possible only due to his home HD! A video describing his experience can be found on www.ishd.org in module 10 of the on-line manual.

Introduction

Home hemodialysis (HD) is far more than a medical treatment: it is a lifestyle. To ensure success, you, your care partner (if you have one), and your family must think through home HD therapy and the impact it will have not only on your daily life, but on the lives of your support team as well. In this module, we answer some common questions asked by home HD patients:

- "How will my lifestyle be affected by home HD?"
- "Will home HD be a burden for my care partner?"
- "I'm concerned about dealing with the machine. Will it be hard for me to adjust to home HD?"
- "What will my home HD training consist of?"
- "How much will home HD cost?"
- "How do I manage supplies at home?"
- "What kind of support can I find as I go through my home HD treatment?"

No doubt, other questions will arise as you start home HD. Never hesitate to ask your doctor, nurse, or dialysis care team for help about any questions you may have.

How will my lifestyle be affected by home HD?

Home HD is convenient. Gone are the days of fitting your life into the clinic's schedule. At home, you can dialyze when you want. Occasionally, you may choose not to dialyze on a given day. If, for example, you stay late at work and need to start dialysis an hour later, no problem! You are free to fit your home HD treatment around your busy life.

Better social life. When you are home, you can choose when to dialyze—during the day or overnight. The prescription can be tailored to what you prefer. Some people choose to dialyze for 2.5 to 4 hours each day, and can choose which hours. When you do your home HD treatment every day, there is less time for toxins and fluid to build up in your body. This means you can have a little more fluid and a more normal diet.[1]

Some people choose to dialyze longer—7 to 9 hours each night while sleeping. If you choose this method, your days and evenings are free to spend time with your family and friends. Doing home HD longer at night also lets you remove most limits on your fluids and diet, so you will have more options when you plan social events with friends and family.

Few limits on travel. Home HD can allow you the flexibility to travel more. Some machines are smaller than the standard ones you might see in a clinic. These are reasonably portable. They can be carried with you in a car, plane, boat, or train. Most airlines now take the machines as essential medical equipment, at no extra charge. (Airlines will also accept about 2-days' worth of dialysate fluid. Just make sure the fluid is in its original box and clearly labeled.)

Less time wasted. If you dialyze each night while you sleep, you will not waste any of your waking hours during the day. You can work full-time, complete tasks, socialize, and just be more productive overall.[2]

Fewer complications. The more you dialyze—during the day or at night—the less fluid you need to remove at 1 time. People who do home HD say that they don't have the "washed-out" or "energy-drained" feeling they had when performing standard in-center HD. With nocturnal home HD, blood pressure drops are rare and your heart is less strained.[3,4] Nocturnal home HD uses blood flow rates that are much lower than those used in-center, so you feel more like yourself during and after the session.

Most people who do daily or nocturnal home HD say that they feel much better and healthier.[5] They have more energy, better appetites, fewer hospital stays, and more active sex lives. In general, they are living fuller, productive lives.

Will home HD be a burden for my care partner?

A care partner is someone who helps a person with home HD treatment, often a family member or friend. Not everyone needs a care partner, and home HD does not have to be a burden for a care partner if you have one. Some countries, such as the United States, require training with a care partner for most people who do home HD. Others, such as Australia and New Zealand, will NOT train a partner! They expect you to do your treatments yourself. Because the number of people who perform home HD in these countries is larger than the number of people who perform home HD in the United States, it's apparent you don't have to put a big burden on a partner, even if you do have one. The key is to learn to do your own treatments and do as much as you can yourself.

Most importantly, you should always cannulate yourself (ie, put in your own needles), if at all possible. Asking a partner to do this scary task may be one reason why assisting with home HD does not always work out for the partner. If you put in your own needles, you always have your own best cannulator with you. Self-cannulation not only helps a fistula or graft last much longer, but it frees you up to travel.

Do you have other disabilities and need total care? If so, it may be less of a burden for a partner to learn to do your home HD than to help you get to and from a clinic 3 times per week for standard treatments. Be sure to let your care partner know often how much you appreciate his or her help.

I'm concerned about dealing with the machine. Will it be hard for me to adjust to home HD?

You won't need to make many changes to fit home HD into your life. Home HD machines have been designed to give you the freedom you want without sacrificing safety. Some machines may require some minor updates to your home's plumbing and wiring. If you rent your home, many landlords will allow the changes, but some will not.

Choose your home treatment room. Living area or bedroom, the choice is yours. Some who do daily home HD prefer to sit in an easy chair in their living room. If you do nocturnal home HD, you can sleep in the room you chose as your treatment room. In fact, couples can even sleep in the same bed. Whichever option you use, you will need to keep your treatment room clean and safe. More information, including a checklist of home infrastructure requirements, can be found in the "Infrastructure, Water, and Machines in the Home" module.

Pets. If you have pets, watch them closely if you want to have them in your treatment room during home HD. Many people have said that they do their home HD with their pets sitting on their laps, but this may not work with all pets. Some pets may be startled by the machine's alarms and sounds. Other pets may play with or bite the hoses or blood tubing, which can result in damage or cause an infection for you. If you dialyze at night while you sleep, it is best to keep pets out of the room.

Infection. Dialysis at home or in the clinic always comes with a risk of infection, which can require treatment in the hospital. You can help prevent infection by regularly washing your hands, using a sterile technique to insert needles, and keeping your home HD room clean. Your clinic training program will teach you how to avoid infections and make sure you feel safe at home.

There is no infection risk for families living with patients who do home HD. When you use the sterile techniques your clinic will teach you, there is no chance a family member will get an infection simply by being with you as you dialyze.

What will my home HD training consist of?

Training will be performed by a training nurse or other dialysis staff at your clinic. You will be trained to use the machine you have chosen and the prescription your doctor wrote for you. The time required for training will be based on your machine. Training for small portable machines that have been designed for easy use may take 2 to 4 weeks. Training for larger, more complex machines may take 5 to 8 weeks. During this time, you will learn how to place the needles, set up and run the machine, fill out treatment forms, and track your supplies. You won't take the machine home and begin home HD until both you and your trainer are confident that you can succeed. Your trainer may come to your home to support you during your first treatment to ensure your peace of mind. In most countries, your clinic will give you 24/7 phone support in case you have questions. Be sure to ask your trainer how your clinic will support you at home.

It's normal to worry about things that can go wrong during home HD. Your trainer will teach you how to have a comfortable, safe, and successful treatment. Here are some key facts to keep in mind while you are training:

Home HD is much gentler than in-center HD. Home HD is less stressful on your body than in-center HD. Much less fluid is removed at a time. This means you have a much lower risk of blood pressure drops and cramping. These are common problems in-center, but are very rare with home HD.

Putting in your own needles hurts less than having someone else do it for you. People who do home HD say that they focus so intently on placing their needles correctly, they feel much less pain than they do when a care partner or nurse does it. Also, when you are able to place your own needles, your access can last much longer.[6] For more information, see "The Care and Keeping of Vascular Access for Home Hemodialysis Patients" module.

Good taping and alarms keep you safe. If you dialyze at night, you will learn how to tape the needles securely and safely so they won't come out as you sleep. If you use an alarm (like a bed wetting alarm) you will have even greater peace of mind. With an alarm under your access arm and one under the dialyzer, you can sleep without fear that you will bleed and not know it.

Fewer clinic visits. You will still need to meet with your nephrologist, but less often than if you were getting your treatments at a clinic. During the visit with your doctor, you will review your prescription, medicines, and blood test results. It is helpful to set up a fixed schedule for your visit. For example, you may want to set up your visits on the first Monday of each month. That way, you can plan around the visit. You can draw your blood samples, deliver or send them to your lab, and have the results in time for your visit.

How much will home HD cost?

In countries with national healthcare systems, you may not have to pay for dialysis no matter which type you choose. In some countries, like the United States, you may pay the same amount out of pocket for home HD as you would for in-center HD (you do not have to buy the machine). In other countries, you will have to pay for home HD yourself. If you live in a country that does not cover home HD, you will need to buy the machine and the water treatment equipment. Or, you may be able to pay a monthly rental fee to a clinic that will set up the machine and water treatment system and maintain the equipment for you. You and your dialysis care team will need to find out what your insurance or national healthcare service will cover. Here are some costs you may have:

Cost of the machine. In most cases, you will have a choice of home HD machines. You and your dialysis staff will discuss the costs of each brand of machine, compare ease of use, and look at maintenance costs.

Costs for water treatment. You and your dialysis staff will look at the volume of water your machines will need and calculate how this will affect your water bill.

Cost of supplies. You will need supplies for home HD. Your center may provide these. Ask your dialysis staff for an estimate of the monthly costs for supplies (see the "Supplies" section for more details).

Cost of maintenance. Normally, your center will provide the fittings and arrange for an electrician to do the wiring, a plumber to do plumbing fittings and install piping, a biomedical waste disposal service to handle waste products that are generated by dialysis, and a technician to clean your water tank and pipes and maintain your machine. Ask your dialysis staff how this is set up and whether you will have any costs.

How do I manage supplies at home?

Some clinics will keep track of the supplies you need and send you more before you run out. Others will require you to order what you need when you need it. Either way, keep track of supplies you are using and budget enough time to get more supplies before you run out. A good rule to follow is to keep 2 to 3 weeks of supplies on hand at any one time.

You will need a fair amount of space to store all of the supplies. You may need to empty a closet in or near your dialysis room, add open shelves or closed cabinets to the room for storage, or store supplies in a dry garage or basement (be sure they won't get too hot or cold). If you do not have space, talk to your dialysis staff. The center may be able to send you supplies for a week or 2 at a time, instead of 1 delivery per month. You will need to keep a close watch on your stock levels to make sure you don't run out.

Practice Tip

To make sure you never run out of any supplies, keep an "emergency" set-up kit for 1 full home HD session in a small bag in a safe, secure place. This way, if you notice just before a treatment that you have run out of an item, you can use your kit. Make sure you review the kit periodically to make sure you replace things that are about to expire.

What kind of support can I find as I go through my home HD treatment?

Peer support. Group support can help you to feel less alone. Your country may have consumer networks and face-to-face peer support groups. Such groups can help you meet others who have similar life challenges. If your area does not have support groups, you may wish to start one of your own. You might form a group of other home HD patients that meets outside your clinic in a social setting (eg, restaurant, library, place of worship, or your home). Your care partner, if you have one, might want to form a group for other care partners. You may want to ask professionals to be guest speakers or facilitators. One-on-one "buddy" support can also be helpful, and may be easier to arrange than group support. Such one-on-one support can also be done via telephone or the Internet. Talk to your dialysis staff to see if they know of any buddy support programs or might be willing to start one. An example of a buddy support system can be found here. This system could be set up in your own program, region, or country.

Web-based support. If you have Internet access, you can find online support in the form of Facebook groups, message boards, email listservs, chat rooms, and others. For example, a Facebook group for home dialysis can be found here. You could also search Google (http://www.google.com) for "dialysis support". Remember to check with your care team before you follow any medical advice discussed on any sites.

Useful Resources*

If you want to start a peer support group, we recommend the following websites:

- The Community Toolbox. Creating and Facilitating Peer Support Groups
- Manuals and Workbooks for Starting and Running Support Groups

*For hyperlinks see Web version of Manual on ISHD.org.

Summary

We have given you some general information about the impact of home HD on your lifestyle. We haven't touched on every issue, but we hope that this module will act as a springboard to stimulate other questions you may have. ***Never hesitate to contact your dialysis staff with any questions you may have about your home care.*** Many people around the world who do home HD have reported great success. They have been able to fit dialysis into their lifestyles rather than letting dialysis limitations dominate their lives. We wish you every success as you think about doing treatment with home HD.

References

1. Schorr M, Manns BJ, Culleton B, et al. The effect of nocturnal and conventional hemodialysis on markers of nutritional status: results from a randomized trial. J Renal Nutr. 2011;21:271-276.
2. Faratro R, Chan CT. Nocturnal hemodialysis improves productivity of end-stage renal failure patients. Hemodial Int. 2003;7:73-04.
3. Culleton BF, Walsh M, Klarenbach SW, et al. Effect of frequent nocturnal hemodialysis vs conventional hemodialysis on left ventricular mass and quality of life: a randomized controlled trial. JAMA. 2007;298:1291-1299.
4. Chan CT, Floras JS, Miller JA, Richardson RMA, Pierratos A. Regression of left ventricular hypertrophy after conversion to nocturnal hemodialysis. Kidney Int. 2002;61:2235-2239.
5. Pierratos A. Nocturnal home haemodialysis: an update on a 5-year experience. Nephrol Dial Transplant. 1999;14:2835-2840.
6. Mott S, Moore H. Using "tandem hand" technique to facilitate self-cannulation in hemodialysis. Nephrol Nurse J. 2009;36:313-316.

Index

T

U

V

Made in the USA
Las Vegas, NV
07 November 2025

33959554R00174